Beliefs and Illness
A Model for Healing

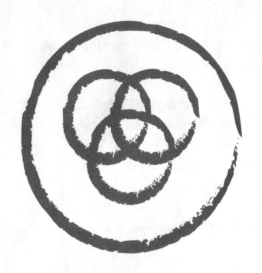

Other Books by the Authors:

Wright, L.M., & Leahey, M. (2009). *Nurses and families: A guide to family assessment and intervention* (5th ed.). Philadelphia: F.A. Davis. (previous editions: 1st ed. 1984; 2nd ed. 1994; 3rd ed. 2000; 4th ed., 2005)

Wright, L.M. (2005). *Spirituality, suffering, and illness: Ideas for healing.* Philadelphia: F.A. Davis.

Wright, L.M., Watson, W.L., & Bell, J.M. (1996). *Beliefs: The heart of healing in families and illness.* New York: Basic Books.

Feetham, S.L., Meister, S.B., Bell, J.M., & Gilliss, C.L. (Eds.). (1993). *The nursing of families: Theory/research/education/practice.* Newbury Park, CA: Sage. (selected papers from the Second International Family Nursing Conference.)

Bell, J.M., Watson, W.L., & Wright, L.M. (Eds.). (1990). *The cutting edge of family nursing.* Calgary, Alberta, Canada: Family Nursing Unit Publications. (selected papers from the First International Family Nursing Conference.)

Leahey, M., & Wright, L.M. (Eds.). (1987). *Families & life-threatening illness.* Springhouse, PA: Springhouse.

Leahey, M., & Wright, L.M. (Eds.). (1987). *Families & psychosocial problems.* Springhouse, PA: Springhouse.

Wright, L.M., & Leahey, M. (Eds.). (1987). *Families & chronic illness.* Springhouse, PA: Springhouse.

Beliefs and Illness
A Model for Healing

by

Lorraine M. Wright, RN, PhD
Janice M. Bell, RN, PhD

www.lorrainewright.com
www.janicembell.com
www.illnessbeliefsmodel.com

Due to the sensitive nature of some of the clinical narratives and
exemplars within Beliefs and Illness, some names may have been
changed to protect the identities of those involved.

Wright, Lorraine M.,
Beliefs and illness : a model for healing / Lorraine M. Wright,
Janice M. Bell.

Includes bibliographical references and index.
ISBN 978-1-897530-09-2

1. Sick--Psychology. 2. Sick--Family relationships.
3. Family psychotherapy. I. Bell, Janice M., II. Title.

R726.5.W75 2009   616.89'156   C2009-901985-X

Published by 4th Floor Press, Inc.
www.4thfloorpress.com
1st Printing 2009
Printed in Canada

Cover design by Aaron De Simone
Author photographs © Chipperfield Photography

To Dr. Chintana Wacharasin, dear friend and colleague, who brought forth and introduced me to her beliefs about families, illness, and living life (all contextualized within her Buddhist beliefs) in a way that caught my attention and admiration.

Lorraine M. Wright

To my mother, Violet Luchak Melenchuk, who showed by example how to live fully an unexpected life alongside illness with creativity, courage, and compassion for others, and whose enormous influence for good continues to live on in my life and in the life of my family in countless ways.

Janice M. Bell

TABLE OF CONTENTS

ILLNESS BELIEFS MODEL
A MAP FOR HEALING

PART I
BELIEFS: THE HEART OF THE MATTER

PART II
THE ILLNESS BELIEFS MODEL

PART III
ADDITIONAL RESOURCES RELATED TO THE ILLNESS BELIEFS MODEL

ILLNESS BELIEFS MODEL
A MAP FOR HEALING

We believe:

Beliefs are the heart of healing. Constraining beliefs increase illness suffering and facilitating beliefs decrease illness suffering.

Illness suffering can be physical, emotional, relational, and/or spiritual. Likewise, healing in individuals and families can be physical, emotional, relational, spiritual, and/or all four.

Softening suffering is the heart, the center, and the essence of caring in our relationships with individuals and families in health care. One of the most useful ways to soften suffering is to invite more facilitating beliefs.

Illness is a family affair. Everyone in a family experiences the illness; no one family member "has" cancer, depression, chronic pain, or renal failure. From the onset of symptoms, through diagnosis and treatment, other family members are impacted by and reciprocally influence the illness.

Serious illness invites a wake-up call about life, which usually leads one into the spiritual domain as the meaning of life is queried or reviewed.

There is a distinction between disease and illness and between medical narratives and illness narratives. We believe illness narratives include stories of sickness and suffering as well as stories of survival and strength that need to be told.

Cellular and "soulular" changes occur through conversations. Our network of conversations and our relationships can contribute to illness or wellness.

A clinician's worldview can open or close opportunities for family members to diminish their illness suffering. We believe a worldview that facilitates healing is one that acknowledges another person as a legitimate other, even though one may not embrace or agree with the other's beliefs. This also implies that the clinician is willing to challenge his or her own beliefs.

One key to therapeutic change is a respectful, curious, and compassionate relationship between a clinician and family members that facilitates discussion of even the most difficult topics and invites the consideration of alternative or modified beliefs.

Therapeutic change is enabled when the core constraining belief—the belief at the heart of illness suffering—is distinguished and challenged.

Changes in beliefs involve changes in the bio-psychosocial-spiritual structures of both family members and clinicians. The direction and pace of change cannot be predicted.

Therapeutic change involves invitations to reflection by family members and the clinician.

Distinguishing therapeutic change sustains and maintains change by strengthening facilitating beliefs.

The privilege of participating in therapeutic conversations about individuals/families' illness experiences provides opportunities for learning and possibilities for changing the biology of the clinician.

The more a clinician is able to embrace a reality of objectivity-in-parentheses, the more he or she becomes a particular kind of person who brings forth healing conversations in a context of compassion and love.

"It is hard to let old beliefs go. They are familiar. We are comfortable with them and have spent years building systems and developing habits that depend on them. Like a man who has worn eyeglasses so long that he forgets he has them on, we forget that the world looks to us the way it does because we have become used to seeing it that way through a particular set of lenses."
—Kenichi Ohmae

PART I

BELIEFS: THE HEART OF THE MATTER

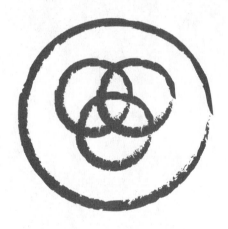

CHAPTER ONE
From Illness Suffering to a Clinical Practice Model for Healing

"The world breaks everyone and afterward
many are strong at the broken places."
—Ernest Hemingway, *A Farewell to Arms*

When Linda and George, a married couple in their early fifties, first arrived at our outpatient clinic, the Family Nursing Unit, University of Calgary, there was obviously something broken between them. Remnants of their last argument, one of the first in their six-year marriage, intermingled with uncomfortable tension and strain—as though one wrong word could send them reeling. Yet, under all that, glimpses of the humor and strong bond between them could still be seen.

At 53, Linda was facing multiple chronic illnesses: diabetes, high blood pressure, fibromyalgia, obesity, depression, and PTSD (Post-Traumatic Stress Disorder) from early childhood trauma. Her most troubling and limiting illness symptoms at the time were pain and fatigue. She could no longer work outside the home and had begun seeing herself as a burden to her husband, on almost every level.

George, a 50-year-old patient care attendant at a local nursing home, was coping as well as he could, but the stress and strain on his marriage was taking its toll. The couple denied any explicit perception of their experience as "suffering" and saw it only as a part of life. They had labeled Linda's health issues "The Monster," making it a third party in their home. The Monster was swiftly taking over their lives and negatively influencing their marriage, which had always been a primary source of comfort and support.

During a series of seven sessions, George revealed to the clinician, Dr. Janice Bell, that the couple was "used to discussing most everything. She shut me out, so everything seemed to go to the side. There was no communication."

Prior to their work with our clinical team, Linda had fallen into a pattern of keeping her feelings from George, in order to protect him, or so she thought.

"It seemed all we had to talk about anymore was my health, and we started to snip and snap at each other," Linda wrote in a letter to the clinical team after finishing at the Family Nursing Unit.

"I was in a constant state of worry and anxiety," George chimed in. "The tension was so thick. It was making me increasingly unhappy, and so was Linda. I wanted so much to be able to ease her pain, make her feel better, and [make her] interested in what we used to enjoy together. So much of our focus was Linda's health we were unable to find our joy in each other."

Within the first few sessions, the couple showed remarkable ability and resourcefulness to take up the clinical team's suggestions. They even created their own experiment called the NIFT Day—No Illness-or Fatigue-Talk Day (2006). This break in their routine of dealing with Linda's illness symptoms was just what they needed—dedicated time to simply enjoy each other's company again. The day could be spent at an outing, if Linda was strong enough, or on their couch cuddled up with a bowl of popcorn. The activity didn't matter, just that for a dedicated period of time, they had only each other: no chronic illness, no talk of pain and medications, just moments of levity and connection.

This intervention focused on challenging the family's belief that they were powerless to exert any influence over Linda's illness symptoms. We believed NIFT Day would encourage them to begin experimenting with a belief that they had more influence over the illness than they imagined; that they could influence illness symptoms and reclaim their relationship from "The Monster" of illness.

George and Linda's story of how illness impacted their couple-relationship, and how they joined together to influence the illness, underscores the reality that illness, disability, and death are universal human experiences. The question for individuals and families is not "Will I or my loved ones be spared these experiences?" but rather "When, which illness, how serious will it be, and for how long?" (Rolland, 2003). As families respond to the emotional and practical demands of illness and deal with major changes within the family unit, their needs are often overlooked and unattended by the health care system, with unfortunate immediate and long-term consequences. Clinical practice models are needed that address illness suffering and attend to healing, not just with individual family members, but also at the level of the family unit.

In these pages, we'll explain our clinical practice model, the *Illness Beliefs Model*, for addressing the suffering of families as they experience the challenges of serious illness. The focus is uniquely on *illness beliefs* and the connection between beliefs, suffering, and healing. Rich in clinical exemplars, *Beliefs and Illness: A Model for Healing* takes the reader inside the therapeutic conversation between the health care provider and family members to show the model in action. We'll first describe the systemic, relational nature of the model and then highlight the research and clinical practice that has shaped the model's development.

Illness Suffering is a Relational Phenomenon

Nurses and other health care providers are altering and/or modifying their usual patterns of clinical practice as they shift from caring for only the "individual patient" to seeing the "family as the patient" and increasingly including families in health care (Schober & Affara, 2001; Wright & Leahey, 1990, 2009). To realize that illness is a family affair, and thus focus on the family as the unit of care, requires a conceptual shift, even a paradigm shift, by health care providers. They must now consider a number of factors: the interaction and reciprocity between illness suffering and family functioning, the interaction between themselves and the families in their care, and the larger systems within which families and health care providers exist. A vogue term for this increasing ability of the health care provider to think systemically, recursively, and interactionally is relational practice (Doane & Varcoe, 2005; Robinson, 1996; Silverstein, Bass, Tuttle, Knudson-Martin, & Huenergardt, 2006; Tapp, 2000; Wright & Leahey, 2009). Involving families in a systemic, relational way in health care is called many different names within the literature, depending on the context of the practice and the health care provider: family-focused practice, family centered practice, family health and healing, family nursing, Family Systems Nursing, systemic health care, family medicine, family psychology, medical family therapy, medical social work, etc.

Beliefs and Illness: A Model for Healing is written for clinicians from a variety of disciplines: nursing, medicine, social work, psychology, rehabilitation studies, occupational health, medical family therapy, and others. Because illness suffering is a relational phenomenon (Marshall, 2007), health care providers in all of these disciplines require advanced practice knowledge and skills to assess and intervene at the level of illness suffering within and across multiple systems levels in order to "soften" illness suffering in individuals and families (Wright, 2005, 2007, 2008). We are grateful to Marga Thome, University of Iceland (personal communication, June 6, 2006) for offering us the meaningful phrase "softening suffering" to describe lessening the intensity of suffering. This is now our preferred description rather than "diminishing", "reducing", or "alleviating" suffering, which suggest suffering can be measured, and of course this painful human phenomena cannot be calculated (Wright, 2005).

This book was written primarily for health care providers who work with ill individuals and families, but those who are experiencing illness suffering may also benefit from an understanding about how beliefs can increase illness suffering or invite healing.

How the Illness Beliefs Model Was Developed
Our Clinical Experience and Context

For twenty-five years, our clinical practice has been a central anchor to both our teaching and research that led to the development and refinement of the *Illness Beliefs Model*, as well as to the many practice examples included in *Beliefs and Illness: A Model for Healing*. The clinical practice occurred at the Family Nursing Unit, University of Calgary (1982-2007), a unique outpatient clinic for families suffering with serious illness. Dr.

Lorraine Wright established the clinic in 1982 for the purpose of education, clinical scholarship, and research (Bell, 2002, 2008; Flowers, St. John, & Bell, 2008; Gottlieb, 2007; Wright, Watson, & Bell, 1990; Wright, Watson, & Duhamel, 1985). Faculty and graduate students worked together as a clinical team to collaborate and consult with families to soften emotional, relational, physical, and/or spiritual suffering. Direct involvement in clinical practice enabled us to examine the practice, offer descriptions of the practice, and continuously learn from families. This resulted in the discovery, organization, analysis, synthesis, and transmission of knowledge about caring practices with families experiencing illness (Bell, 2003; Diers, 1995).

The medium of offering healing to families experiencing illness is the *therapeutic conversation.* An extensive database of videotaped therapeutic conversations between nurse clinicians, clinical teams, and families served as the unit of data collection and analysis across our program of research at the Family Nursing Unit (Bell, 2008; Bell & Wright, 2007).

Research about Therapeutic Change

As a clinical team, we were grounded in the everyday complexities and uniqueness of each family we served. While we benefited from the extensive research literature that offered a description of family responses to illness, we were intimately involved in *doing* intervention and consequently became intrigued with questions about the intervention process itself. This kind of research is complicated and comprehensive to design and implement because it is a) discovery oriented, b) attempting to account for a relational process that involves both the clinician and family members, and c) focusing data collection and analysis on more than one individual. The research that underpins the *Illness Beliefs Model* sought to describe, explore, and evaluate our clinical practice to gain an understanding of *what* was working in the moment. What were we as nurses actually doing and saying that was helpful to families in their experience of illness suffering?

The complexity of accounting for what is happening *inside* the intervention was overwhelming. Rather than trying to simplify the phenomena, we rose to the challenge of its complexity and utilized hermeneutic inquiry (Benner, 1994; Chesla, 1995; Gadamer 1960/1989,

1976; Moules, 2002a; Packer & Addison, 1989) to account for what was happening *inside* the therapeutic conversation. We routinely asked families for permission to videotape each therapeutic conversation for clinical learning and research purposes. Over the past twenty-five years we developed a rich data set of videotaped therapeutic conversations, and extensive clinical documentation about each therapeutic conversation, with families who were experiencing serious illness.

The purpose of family nursing intervention is to effect change that will soften suffering and promote family healing; therefore, a beginning step in our program of research was to focus on *significant change events*. In our clinical work with families at the Family Nursing Unit, we have experienced many incredible changes within families that have invited healing and a return to a peaceful and satisfying health status. To understand these changes, we embarked on a funded research project that helped us learn about what accounted for this therapeutic change. Specifically, our research project was entitled "Exploring the process of therapeutic change in Family Systems Nursing practice: An analysis of five exemplary cases." The investigators were Drs. Janice Bell, Lorraine Wright, and Wendy Watson Nelson. Other research team members included Lori Limacher and Dianne Tapp (research assistants), and our consultant Dr. Catherine (Kit) Chesla from the Department of Family Health Nursing, University of California, San Francisco. Our research question was: "How does therapeutic change occur?" Our research team reviewed all the families we had worked with from 1988-1992 and chose five exemplary cases. The family sessions with these selected families were conducted by two expert family clinicians/nurse educators (Drs. Lorraine Wright and Wendy Watson Nelson). In each case, the families showed dramatic cognitive, affective, or behavioral change during the Family Systems Nursing therapeutic conversations, which ranged from two to five sessions. The families also reported improvement in the presenting problem when they were interviewed six months after the completion of the clinical sessions for our Family Nursing Unit outcome study.

Direct observation of the previously videotaped clinical sessions constituted our data set. We first viewed the videotapes to get an understanding of the whole of the clinical work with the family. Next, each member of the research team selected segments of the therapeutic conversations she considered salient to the process of therapeutic change (Gale, Chenail, Watson, Wright, & Bell, 1996). Each therapeutic conversation was examined to see how the nurse clinician responded to the family and how the family responded to the nurse. The members of the research team then convened to discuss their choice of change segments to see if consensus among team members could be reached. The change segments were then transcribed and interpretive analysis was done on the text of the change segments. Questions were asked of the data such as: What is happening here from the nurse's perspective and from the family's perspective? Is this move or intervention unique or is it similar to another? Has it happened before? Do we have a usual name for this move? What else could we call it?

This process uncovered the personal, contextual, and cognitive processes that form the clinician's formulation of any given case and the overall model of intervention. The study helped us uncover new understandings about our clinical practice approach and gave us a language with which to describe the therapeutic process. Our approach for intervention was described in our 1996 publication *Beliefs: The Heart of Healing in Families and Illness* (Wright, Watson, & Bell, 1996) with translation in Japanese and Swedish.

Research Findings: A Book, and A Model without a Name

The impact of this research project on our practice was substantial. The project illuminated, clarified, and offered new descriptions of our clinical practice that shaped and changed our subsequent clinical work with families at the Family Nursing Unit. Despite the publication of the *Beliefs* book in 1996, we did not give the clinical practice model an actual name, which, in hindsight, was probably a mistake or oversight on our part.

Part of our hesitancy came from humility and perhaps some fear. The discipline of Nursing during this era loved the language of "nursing models," and we frankly did not feel worthy to be included in the list of distinguished contributors. Part of our hesitancy also came from disagreement among our clinical research team. We simply could not agree about the name of the approach and were not sure whether having "therapy" in the name might limit its appeal to some health care providers.

We also wondered if we really wanted to use a staid and somewhat pompous word like "model" to name the clinical practice approach. Over the next few years, we, along with our graduate students, referred to our clinical approach using several names. For a few years it was called "Systemic Belief Therapy" (SBT). Our colleague, Dr. Wendy Watson Nelson, accepted an academic position at Brigham Young University in 1992 and taught scores of family therapy students this clinical approach calling it "SBT" in presentations, publications, and dissertations. Our own graduate nursing students at the University of Calgary affectionately dubbed the approach the "Wright, Watson, Bell" clinical approach and used the acronym "WWB" in their written case studies and conceptual framework papers for several years. By the late 1990s, frustrated with the multiplicity of names, we decided to end the confusion. We daringly named the clinical practice the *Illness Beliefs Model* and were encouraged by a reassuring note from then doctoral student, Dr. Nancy Moules (who later became a Family Nursing Unit faculty colleague). She reminded us that the term "model" was a synonym for "something set before one for guidance or imitation" (Merriam-Webster's Collegiate Dictionary).

The Conversation about the Illness Beliefs Model Continues

Out of many domains of family functioning, the *Illness Beliefs Model* pulls to the foreground an emphasis on beliefs, recognizing that family members as well as health care professionals have beliefs that are both facilitating and constraining in the ways they influence lives, relationships, behavior, illness suffering, and healing (see Chapters 2-6). Beliefs that are constraining can be explored, challenged, and altered (see Chapters 7-9); those that are facilitating can be acknowledged, strengthened, and amplified (see Chapter 10). The *Illness Beliefs Model* is based upon the principle that it is not necessarily the clinical problem or illness but rather *beliefs* about the clinical problem or illness that serve as the greatest source of individual and family suffering; furthermore, beliefs also lie at the heart of individual and family healing.

Within the *Illness Beliefs Model*, the language of "moves" is utilized in addition to interventions for the purpose of underscoring the process and flow that are co-evolved between the clinician and family members. The model is comprised of four macromoves:

- Creating a Context for Changing Beliefs
- Distinguishing Illness Beliefs
- Challenging Constraining Beliefs
- Strengthening Facilitating Beliefs

These macromoves are operationalized through micromoves (or interventions), which are the specific clinical practices that guide therapeutic conversations with families. In view of the diversity of beliefs about the etiology, diagnosis, and prognosis of illness as well as beliefs about the role of family members and health care providers in illness care, beliefs hold significant possibilities for both family suffering and family healing.

In subsequent research and published case studies, the *Illness Beliefs Model* has been described with families experiencing chronic illness (Bell, Moules, Simonson, & Fraser, 2004; Robinson, 1994, 1998; Robinson & Wright, 1995; Wright, 1997); loss and grief (Levac et al., 1998; Moules, 1998; Moules, Thirsk, & Bell, 2006); cardiac illness (Bohn, Wright, & Moules, 2003; Tapp, 1997, 2001, 2004); cancer (Duhamel & Dupuis, 2004); mental illness (Marshall & Harper-Jaques, 2008; Watson & Lee, 1993); violence (Robinson, Wright, & Watson, 1994); and palliative care (Duhamel & Dupuis, 2003). The usefulness of particular interventions within the *Illness Beliefs Model* have been studied from the perspectives of the families who received the interventions and the nurses who offered these skilled practices, including therapeutic letters (Bell, Moules, & Wright, 2009; Moules, 2000, 2002b, 2003, 2009a, 2009b); commendations (Houger Limacher & Wright, 2003, 2006; Houger Limacher, 2003, 2008); spiritual conversations about illness suffering (McLeod, 2003; McLeod & Wright, 2001, 2008); and the "One Question Question" (Duhamel, Dupuis, & Wright, in press). The Family Nursing Unit collection of archived publications is available for public access on DSpace at the University of Calgary Library: *https://dspace.ucalgary.ca/handle/1880/44060*. (For a list of publications by Dr. Lorraine M. Wright and/or Dr. Janice M. Bell and other faculty and graduates associated with the Family Nursing Unit, please see Part III, Resource One.)

Through numerous professional workshops and graduate courses, Family Nursing Externships, and conference presentations, the *Illness*

Beliefs Model has been taught to thousands of graduate students, academics, and health care providers in Australia, Brazil, Canada, Chile, Finland, Japan, Hong Kong, Iceland, Italy, Israel, Germany, New Zealand, Portugal, Poland, Singapore, Scotland, Spain, Sweden, Switzerland, Thailand, Viet Nam, and the United States. Part III, Resource Two, provides a listing of the international application, implementation, and dissemination of the *Illness Beliefs Model* in publications related to research and clinical practice authored by our colleagues and/or their students.

Conclusion

Understanding illness suffering through a systemic, relational lens is the first step to expanding healing opportunities and inviting innovative approaches to health care with not only individuals but families and larger systems as well. *The Illness Beliefs Model* is a clinical practice model for health care providers who care for families experiencing serious illness. Developed from clinical scholarship and a modest program of research at the Family Nursing Unit, University of Calgary, the *Illness Beliefs Model* uncovers and expands the therapeutic possibilities for helping and healing families who are suffering in their experience of serious illness. This clinical practice model has been introduced to numerous international health care providers over the past twenty-five years. *Beliefs and Illness: A Model for Healing* offers an expanded view of the 1996 publication of *Beliefs* with further embellishment of the model and inclusion of recent research and clinical practice examples.

In the chapters that follow, we will elaborate on the central focus of illness beliefs (Part I: Chapters 2-6) and then describe in detail how health care providers can use the *Illness Beliefs Model* to soften illness suffering in individuals and families and promote individual and family healing (Part II: Chapters 7-10). We have invited our Family Nursing Unit colleague, Dr. Nancy Moules, to offer the final chapter in Part II that features her astute clinical application of the *Illness Beliefs Model* to a special population: families who are grieving (Part II: Chapter 11). Finally, Part III of this book offers additional resources related to the *Illness Beliefs Model*.

References

Bell, J.M. (2002). 20th Anniversary of the Family Nursing Unit [Editorial] *Journal of Family Nursing, 8*(3), 175-177.

Bell, J.M. (2003). Clinical scholarship in family nursing [Editorial] *Journal of Family Nursing, 9*(2), 127-129.

Bell. J.M. (2008). The Family Nursing Unit, University of Calgary: Reflections on 25 years of clinical scholarship (1982-2007) and closure announcement [Editorial]. *Journal of Family Nursing, 14*(3), 275-288.

Bell, J.M., Moules, N.J., Simonson, K., & Fraser, J. (2004). Marriage and illness: Therapeutic conversations with couples who are suffering. *Vision 2004: What is the future of marriage?* (pp. 47-52). Minneapolis, MN: National Council on Family Relations.

Bell, J.M., Moules, N.J., & Wright, L.M. (2009). Therapeutic letters and the Family Nursing Unit: A legacy of advanced nursing practice. *Journal of Family Nursing, 15*(1), 6-30.

Bell, J.M., & Wright, L.M. (2007). La recherché sur la pratique des soins infirmiers a la famille [Research on family interventions]. In F. Duhamel (Ed.), *La sante et la famille: Une approche systemique en soins infirmiers* [Families and health: A systemic approach in nursing care] (2nd ed.). Montreal, Quebec, Canada: Gaetan Morin editeur, Cheneliere Education. (An English version of this book chapter is available from DSpace at the University of Calgary Library: https://dspace.ucalgary.ca/handle/1880/44060.)

Benner, P. (1994). The tradition and skill of interpretive phenomenology in studying health, illness, and caring practices. In *Interpretive phenomenology: Embodiment, caring, and ethics in health and illness* (pp. 99-127). Thousand Oaks, CA: Sage.

Bohn, U., Wright, L.M., & Moules, N.J. (2003). A family systems nursing interview following a myocardial infarction: The power of commendations. *Journal of Family Nursing*, 9(2), 151-165.

Chesla, C. A. (1995). Hermeneutic phenomenology, an approach to understanding families. *Journal of Family Nursing, 1*(1), 63-78.

Diers, D. (1995). Clinical scholarship. *Journal of Professional Nursing, 11*, 24-30.

Doane, G.H., & Varcoe, C. (2005). *Family nursing as relational inquiry.* Philadelphia: Lippincott, Williams, & Wilkins.

Duhamel, F., & Dupuis, F. (2003). Families in palliative care: Exploring family and health-care professionals' beliefs. *International Journal of Palliative Nursing, 9*(3), 113-119.

Duhamel, F., & Dupuis, F. (2004). Guaranteed returns: Investing in conversations with families of cancer patients. *Clinical Journal of Oncology Nursing, 8*(1), 68-71.

Duhamel, F., Dupuis, F., Wright, L.M. (in press). Families' and nurses' responses to the "One Question Question": Reflections for clinical practice, education, and research in family nursing. *Journal of Family Nursing.*

Flowers, K., St. John, W., & Bell, J.M. (2008). The role of the clinical laboratory in teaching and learning family nursing skills. *Journal of Family Nursing, 14*(2), 242-267.

Gadamer, H.G. (1960/1989). *Truth and method* (2nd rev. ed.) (J. Weinsheimer & D.G. Marshall, Trans.). New York: Continuum.

Gadamer, H.G. (1976). *Philosophical hermeneutics* (D.E. Linge, Ed. & Trans.). Berkeley, CA: University of California Press.

Gale, J., Chenail, R.J., Watson, W.L., Wright, L.M., & Bell, J.M. (1996). Research and practice: A reflexive and recursive relationship. Three narratives and five voices. *Marriage and Family Review, 24*(3/4), 275 295. [Special issue: Methods and Methodologies of Qualitative Family Research.]

Gottlieb, L. (2007). A tribute to the Calgary Family Nursing Unit: Lessons that go beyond family nursing [Editorial]. *Canadian Journal of Nursing Research, 39*(3), 7-11.

Houger Limacher, L. (2003). *Commendations: The healing potential of one family systems nursing intervention.* Unpublished doctoral thesis, University of Calgary, Alberta, Canada.

Houger Limacher, L. (2008). Locating relationships at the heart of commending practices. *Journal of Systemic Therapies, 27*(4), 90-105.

Houger Limacher, L., & Wright, L.M. (2003). Commendations: Listening to the silent side of a family intervention. *Journal of Family Nursing, 9*(2), 130-135.

Houger Limacher, L., & Wright, L.M. (2006). Exploring the therapeutic family intervention of commendations: Insights from research. *Journal of Family Nursing, 12,* 307-331.

Levac, A.M.C., McLean, S., Wright, L.M., Bell, J.M., "Ann" & "Fred". (1998). A "Reader's Theater" intervention to managing grief: Posttherapy reflections by a family and clinical team. *Journal of Marital and Family Therapy, 24*(1), 81-93.

Marshall, A.J. (2007). *Relational suffering: A concept analysis*. Unpublished manuscript, University of Calgary, Alberta, Canada.

Marshall, A.J., & Harper-Jaques, S. (2008). Depression and family relationships: Ideas for healing. *Journal of Family Nursing, 14*(1), 56-73.

McLeod, D.L. (2003). *Opening space for the spiritual: Therapeutic conversations with families living with serious illness*. Unpublished doctoral thesis. University of Calgary, Alberta, Canada.

McLeod, D., & Wright, L.M. (2001). Conversations of spirituality: Spirituality in family systems nursing–making the case with four clinical vignettes. *Journal of Family Nursing, 7*(4), 391-415.

McLeod, D.L., & Wright, L.M. (2008). Living the as-yet unanswered: Spiritual care practices in Family Systems Nursing. *Journal of Family Nursing, 14*(1), 118-141.

Merriam-Webster's Collegiate Dictionary. Retrieved January 14, 2009, from http://www2.merriam-webster.com/cgi-bin/mwdictsn?va=models

Moules, N.J. (1998). Legitimizing grief: Challenging beliefs that constrain. *Journal of Family Nursing, 4*(2), 138-162.

Moules, N.J. (2000). *Nursing on paper: The art and mystery of therapeutic letters in clinical work with families experiencing illness*. Unpublished doctoral thesis, University of Calgary, Alberta, Canada.

Moules, N.J. (2002a). Hermeneutic inquiry: Paying heed to history and Hermes. *International Journal of Qualitative Methods, 1*(3), Article 1. Retrieved September 2002, from http://www.ualberta.ca/~ijqm/

Moules, N.J. (2002b). Nursing on paper: Therapeutic letters in nursing practice. *Nursing Inquiry, 9*(2), 104-113.

Moules, N.J. (2003). Therapy on paper: Therapeutic letters and the tone of relationship. *Journal of Systemic Therapies*, 22(1), 33-49.

Moules, N.J. (2009a). The past and future of therapeutic letters: Family suffering and healing words. *Journal of Family Nursing, 15*(1), 102-111.

Moules, N.J. (2009b). Therapeutic letters in nursing: Examining the character and influence of the written word in clinical work with families experiencing illness. *Journal of Family Nursing, 15*(1), 31-49.

Moules, N.J., Thirsk, L.M., & Bell, J.M. (2006). A Christmas without memories: Beliefs about grief and mothering—A clinical case analysis. *Journal of Family Nursing, 12*(4), 426-441.

NIFT Letter. (2006). A letter written by George and Linda Jensen. Available from: www.janicembell.com.

Packer, M.J., & Addison, R.B. (Eds.). (1989). *Entering the circle: Hermeneutic investigation in psychology.* Albany, NY: State University of New York Press.

Rolland, J. S. (2003). Mastering family challenges in serious illness and disability. In F. Walsh (Ed.), *Normal family processes* (3rd ed., pp. 460-489). New York: Guilford.

Robinson, C.A. (1994). *Women, families, chronic illness and nursing interventions: From burden to balance.* Unpublished doctoral dissertation, University of Calgary, Alberta, Canada.

Robinson, C.A. (1996). Health care relationships revisited. *Journal of Family Nursing, 2*(2), 152-173.

Robinson, C.A. (1998). Women, families, chronic illness, and nursing interventions: From burden to balance. *Journal of Family Nursing, 4*(3), 271-290.

Robinson, C.A., & Wright, L.M. (1995). Family nursing interventions: What families say makes a difference. *Journal of Family Nursing, 1*(3), 327-345.

Robinson, C.A., Wright, L.M., & Watson, W.L. (1994). A nontraditional approach to family violence. *Archives of Psychiatric Nursing, 8*(1), 30-37.

Schober, M., & Affara, F. (2001). *The family nurse: Frameworks for practice.* Geneva, Switzerland: International Council of Nurses.

Silverstein, R., Bass, L.B., Tuttle, A., & Knudson-Martin, C., & Huenergardt, D. (2006). What does it mean to be relational? A framework for assessment and practice. *Family Process, 45*(4), 391-405.

Tapp, D.M. (1997). *Exploring therapeutic conversations between nurses and families experiencing ischemic heart disease.* Unpublished doctoral dissertation, University of Calgary, Alberta, Canada.

Tapp, D.M. (2000). The ethics of relational stance in family nursing: Resisting the view of "nurse as expert". *Journal of Family Nursing, 6*(1), 69-91.

Tapp, D.M. (2001). Conserving the vitality of suffering: Addressing family constraints to illness conversations. *Nursing Inquiry, 8*(4), 254-263.

Tapp, D.M. (2004). Dilemmas of family support during cardiac recovery: Nagging as a gesture of support. *Western Journal of Nursing Research, 26,* 561-580.

Watson, W.L., & Lee, D. (1993). Is there life after suicide?: The systemic belief approach for "survivors" of suicide. *Archives of Psychiatric Nursing, 7*(1), 37-43.

Wright, L. M. (1997). Multiple sclerosis, beliefs, and families: Professional and personal stories of suffering and strength. In S. H. McDaniel, J. Hepworth, & W. J. Doherty (Eds.), *The shared experience of illness: Stories of patients, families, and their therapists* (pp. 263-273). New York: Basic Books.

Wright, L.M. (2005). *Spirituality, suffering, and illness: Ideas for healing.* Philadelphia: F.A. Davis.

Wright, L.M. (Producer). (2007). *Spirituality, suffering, and illness: Conversations for healing.* [DVD]. (available from: www.lorrainewright.com)

Wright, L.M. (2008). Softening suffering through spiritual care practices: One possibility for healing families. *Journal of Family Nursing, 14*(4), 394-411

Wright, L.M., & Leahey, M. (1990). Trends in the nursing of families. *Journal of Advanced Nursing, 15,* 148-154.

Wright, L.M., & Leahey, M. (2009). *Nurses and families. A guide to assessment and intervention* (5th ed.). Philadelphia: F.A. Davis.

Wright, L.M., Watson, W.L., & Bell, J.M. (1990). The Family Nursing Unit: A unique integration of research, education and clinical practice. In J.M. Bell, W.L. Watson & L.M. Wright (Eds.), *The cutting edge of family nursing* (pp. 95-109). Calgary, Alberta, Canada: Family Nursing Unit Publications.

Wright, L.M., Watson, W.L., & Bell, J.M. (1996). *Beliefs: The heart of healing in families and illness.* New York: Basic Books.

Wright, L.M., Watson, W.L., & Duhamel, F. (1985). The Family Nursing Unit: Clinical preparation at the Masters' level. *The Canadian Nurse, 81,* 26-29.

CHAPTER TWO
Understanding Beliefs

"The outer condition of a person's life will always be found to reflect their inner beliefs."
—James Allen

What exactly are beliefs? How do we come to believe what we do? Our beliefs are the lenses through which we view the world, guiding the choices we make, the behaviors we choose, and feelings with which we respond. Our beliefs are the blueprint from which we construct our lives and intertwine them with the lives of others. Beliefs distinguish who we inherently are and how we present ourselves in our relationships and to the world.

But what influences our beliefs? What causes or invites us to believe what we do? How do beliefs arise? Ultimately, what one believes is determined by one's present bio-psychosocial-spiritual makeup. Each person has his or her own unique makeup or "structure" based on their genetic history and history of interactions with others and the environment (Maturana & Varela, 1992).

Surprisingly, it is not only our genes but our beliefs that control our cells, bodies, minds, and thus our lives (Lipton, 2005). Through our interactions with others and our environment we are continually acquiring, evolving, refining, solidifying, confirming, and challenging our beliefs.

Our beliefs are shaped and substantially shifted through our interactions with others and oneself in concert with the conditions in which one is living. The answer to the question "Do beliefs reside in cognition, in affect, or in behavior?" is a resounding yes: Beliefs reside in all three.

How can we learn and find out about our own and others' beliefs? In daily life, the best medium for hearing our own and others' beliefs is the stories we tell ourselves and others about our lives and relationships. Our beliefs are embedded in the stories we exchange with one another in our conversations as we move about daily life.

Beliefs distinguish one person from another, yet they also join us together. Through our living and being together, we influence each other's beliefs, for better or worse. We develop our identities within our families, friendships, professions, and communities through the belief systems that we share and do not share with others. But most amazing is that we often live our lives only slightly aware, and sometimes not at all, of our beliefs and the effect they have on our own lives and the lives of others.

The irony and challenge of life is that to survive and progress in the world, one needs both a commitment to strong beliefs and the ability to question those beliefs when they are no longer useful (Cecchin, Lane, & Ray, 1994). New ways of viewing ourselves, our relationships, and our experiences such as illness can be both enlightening and frightening.

Illness experiences occur in an interpersonal, relational context affecting beliefs, behavior, and emotion. The beliefs derived from these experiences form the text, or illness narratives, of our lives. A family who believes that a physician misdiagnosed an illness or did not appropriately treat the early symptoms of a serious illness will likely experience anger and regret, and perhaps even show suspicion and mistrust in their future encounters with health care providers. A mother who believes that her schizophrenic son's suicide was an act of love and thoughtful consideration grieves differently and recounts a different story from a mother who believes that her son's suicide was an act of rage and purposive cruelty.

What is equally fascinating is how we cling to some beliefs as if they are "truths" even when there is strong evidence to the contrary. As humans, we tend to accept only information that confirms our existing views and to ignore information, ideas, or opinions that contradict our established beliefs. This behavior is particularly evident in the area of health and illness beliefs and practices.

Tavris and Aronson (2007) in their fascinating book about the effects of cognitive dissonance report that tribes in Sudan routinely extract most of the permanent front teeth of their children, producing major facial deformities and speech impediments. They began this practice as a healing intervention during a tetanus (lockjaw) epidemic so that their children could drink liquids through the gap in their teeth and thus survive the illness. The tetanus epidemic is now long past and the beliefs about cure, which were once life-saving, are no longer useful and might even be considered abusive to an outside observer.

Similar beliefs invade our practices as health care providers all the time. Nurses working on maternity wards often believe that more babies are born when the moon is full, while health care providers working in mental health believe that patients become more disturbed and upset under that same moon. However, neither of these beliefs is supported by research evidence. Yet the belief is handed down from one generation of health care providers to the next. It begs the question, "What data do we choose to believe?"

From these examples, it appears that even research evidence does not convince most people to relinquish the beliefs they embrace. To fully understand why people believe what and the way they do, perhaps we must first look at some core definitions of the word and its many different connotations.

What is a Belief?

"Man prefers to believe what he prefers to be true."
—Francis Bacon

Many words have been used synonymously with the word *belief*— words like attitude, explanation, construct, premise, assumption, preference, values, anticipation, meaning, prejudice, and cognitive representation. We prefer the term *belief*. We think it better captures family members' and health care providers' efforts to make sense of illness and loss, and find it is used more commonly in conversational language than other synonyms.

The sentence stem "I believe" can be a useful statement of belief about the etiology of an illness: *I believe my rash is an allergic reaction*; of a belief in a health care provider: *I believe my doctor will find a treatment for my pain*; of a prediction of future events: *I believe my cancer will be cured*; or of a belief about the role of a family member when illness arises: *A good daughter cancels her vacation to care for her ill parent.*

In addition to the wide range of meanings for the word, there are two other important aspects to understanding beliefs. First, the word *belief* contains the idea of a persisting set of premises about what is taken to be true; second, there exists a set of assertions with an emotional basis about what "should" be true. For example, a person can express the belief, "I'm very healthy." This statement contains the premise that this statement is "true" and also the implication that this is a desirable state. If this belief were challenged by the discovery of a malignant tumor during an annual physical checkup, however, the person may very likely become anxious or even angry when a core belief about their identity as a healthy person has now been challenged.

Constraining and Facilitating Beliefs

Some of our beliefs are more useful than others. Some allow more solutions to challenges and problems that arise in our lives and relationships, and some are more acceptable in particular cultures or contexts than in others. The usefulness or non-usefulness of a belief, however, is dependent on the judgment of an observer and the context in which the belief arises.

We have chosen to distinguish useful from non-useful beliefs through the dichotomy of *facilitating beliefs* versus *constraining beliefs*. We do not find it useful to think about beliefs as *erroneous beliefs, false beliefs,* or *correct beliefs,* but rather whether beliefs are useful or non-useful within the particulars of one's relationships, life challenges, and coping strategies. A facilitating belief for one person might be constraining for another in a different circumstance or experience.

By constraining beliefs, we refer to beliefs that decrease possibilities for discovering solutions or resolution to challenges and/or problems and often enhance suffering; facilitating beliefs, on the other hand, increase solution possibilities, decrease suffering, and invite healing. The distinction about whether a belief is facilitating or constraining is often a clinical judgment, made by a health care provider at one point in time and subject to change based on further evidence. When illness enters a person's life, our core beliefs are brought to the fore. Therefore, in order to understand people's experience with an illness, loss, or disability, we need to understand and explore their core beliefs.

Beliefs, Stories, and Illness

It is now well accepted among health care providers and supported with research documentation that illness has a significant impact on individual and family functioning and, reciprocally, that family functioning can influence the physical health of its members (Campbell, 2003; Gilliss & Knafl, 1999; Knafl & Gilliss, 2002; Matire, Lustig, Schulz, Miller, & Helgeson, 2004; Ruddy & McDaniel, 2008; Weihs, Fisher, & Baird, 2002). At no time are family and individual beliefs more affirmed, challenged, or threatened than when illness emerges. An emerging body of literature supports that how individuals and families suffer, cope, manage, and treat an illness arises more from their beliefs about the illness than the illness itself (Haller, Sanci, Sawyer, & Patton, 2008; Hekler et al., 2008; Horne & Weinman, 1999; Kinderman, Setzu, Lobban, & Salmon, 2006; King, Baxter, Rosenbaum, Zwaigenbaum, & Bates, 2009; Lau-Walker, Cowie, & Roughton, 2009). These beliefs may be influenced by the stage in the life cycle of the individual, the family, and the illness (Rolland, 1994).

Beliefs, stories, and illness are intricately intertwined. For example, if clinicians challenge constraining beliefs that enhance suffering, new stories are drawn forth that may influence the illness experience. If a clinician assists persons and their families in reconstructing stories (revising or constructing new ones), old constraining beliefs are refuted and frequently suffering is softened. The preferred emphasis may be on reconstructing stories or on altering constraining beliefs; each approach has merit and influences the other. While Moules (2006) cautions clinicians that the word "story" might mean something different to clients, the approach to dealing with beliefs and stories is not an either/or one; it is a synergistic both/and approach.

When families present with emotional, relational, physical, and/or spiritual suffering, the most pressing concern of health care providers is assisting them with healing through the therapeutic process. We routinely ask ourselves, "Have we helped this family?" and if so, "How have we helped them?" According to our clinical and research experience, focusing on the beliefs of family members and of clinicians from a systemic perspective offers great promise for assisting families to soften emotional, relational, spiritual, and physical suffering. In the process, our lives and relationships as clinicians are also profoundly affected.

The Intersecting of Three Kinds of Beliefs

Any potential healing conversation involves at least three sets of beliefs: those of the ill patient, those of other family members, and those of the health care providers. Indeed, understanding the beliefs of the health care providers involved with a family is key to being able to help that family. Imagine all the health care providers involved with a family meeting in one room displaying placards stating their beliefs about fundamental issues: Families have problems because . . .; illness arises when…; the role of the clinician is to . . . ; change occurs when… Imagine how different the process of that team meeting would be. Would it not be easier to understand the divergent ideas that the health care providers would offer about discharge, medication, and time of the next session? Might it not be interesting to have the family read the placards? What impact would such clinician transparency have on the healing of family members? Would their selection of a health care provider to assist them in their process of healing and change be altered?

It is becoming well recognized that health care providers can have a positive or negative impact on families' beliefs and thus can enhance or soften their suffering. One clinical example is the experience of a couple that presented at the Family Nursing Unit with marital conflict eight months following the husband's second myocardial infarction. As the story of this couple's recovery experience unfolded, the constraining influence of the hospital nurses' beliefs on the wife's behavior throughout her husband's recovery became evident. The iatrogenically constraining beliefs of the nurses constrained the wife from voicing her concerns to her husband because she believed she could increase his stress and make him ill (Wright, Bell, Watson, & Tapp, 1995). As health care providers, we believe that change and healing occurs at the intersection of patient, family members' and health care providers' beliefs. We are also mindful that all of these beliefs are reciprocally influenced by the beliefs of larger systems, including the culture and society within which people are nested.

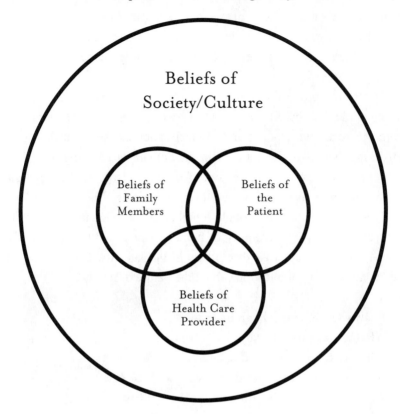

Figure 1: Illness Beliefs Model—Intersection of Beliefs

Reflections and Review about the Notion of Beliefs

There are many lenses that can be worn to explain, describe, and define the lens of "belief." We have looked through several lenses, tried them on for a time, and liked the fit and view of some more than others. Some of those lenses come from sociology, philosophy, anthropology, psychology, spirituality-religion, family therapy, and biology. By examining beliefs through a variety of lenses, we acknowledge a wide assortment of explanations about beliefs, believing, and belief systems.

Extensive reading is available in all of these domains with differing explanations of beliefs and belief systems. Overall, the literature concerning beliefs is characterized by diverse opinions and interpretations that are based on personal reflection and empirical evidence; however, the literature is also characterized by many similarities, and the differences often involve subtle shades of meaning. Despite the existence of these various lenses, there are few instruments for examining individual and family illness beliefs in research and clinical practice (see Part III, Resource Three).

In both our professional and personal lives, we unavoidably embrace particular lenses based on our bio-psychosocial-spiritual structures. From our extensive reading and clinical experiences, we have come to realize that beliefs occur not only in the domain of meaning, but also in the domain of emotion and behavior. We have also come to appreciate that beliefs influence even our cellular functioning. Many of the lenses overlap. They are cleverly brought together in the following poem, which captures the dizzying circularity of beliefs, reality, and truth. One of the greatest movements across disciplines in the late twentieth century has been the reopening of questions about the nature of reality.

> Reality is what we take to be true.
> What we take to be true is what we believe.
> What we believe is based upon our perceptions.
> What we perceive depends on what we look for.
> What we look for depends on what we think.
> What we think determines what we take to be true.
> What we take to be true is our reality. (Zukav, 1979, p. 328)

However, the explanation of beliefs that is a fit for us and that we have found most useful is a biological explanation. Biology is a concern for how living takes place (Maturana, 1998). We wonder if our attraction to a biological explanation of beliefs is related to the biological foundation of one of our "home" disciplines, nursing.

To understand our own and others' beliefs, we must understand the contexts in which we all live: the interactional, social, and cultural contexts. Beliefs arise out of distinctions that evolve through our history of interactions (ontogeny) with those we encounter in our lives as well as out of our own structure or genetic makeup (phylogeny) all within the contexts of our lives.

The definition of belief that we most favor is as follows:

A belief is the "truth" of a particular reality that influences bio-psychosocial-spiritual structure and functioning.

In our conversations, we speak and listen to one another from these domains of "truths"—explanations, values, and obligations based on our beliefs—that have arisen from the social, interactional, religious, and cultural domains in which we live.

The Lens of Biology

The Biology of Cognition, as described by the Chilean biologists, Humberto Maturana and Francesco Varela (1992) in "The Tree of Knowledge", is a worldview that has influenced our thinking about reality, beliefs, and clinical practice with families. Beliefs, or systems of meanings, arise through our history of interactions across time in a variety of contexts. Individuals can experience changes in their bio-psychosocial-spiritual structures through these interactions and vice versa. Cousins (1989) and Lipton (2005) simply but profoundly offer the notion that "beliefs become biology." Certain beliefs may conserve or maintain an illness and/or suffering; others may exacerbate symptoms; while others may alleviate or soften suffering.

Our beliefs help us to explain the various worlds in which we live. Maturana and Varela, both neurobiologists, offered the idea that there are two possible avenues for explaining our world or our reality: *objectivity* and *objectivity-in-parentheses*.

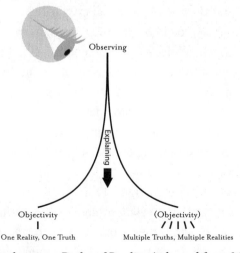

Figure 2. Two Explanatory Paths of Reality (adapted from Maturana, 1998)

The view of objectivity assumes that there is one ultimate domain of reference for explaining the world. Within this domain, entities are assumed to exist independent of the observer. Such entities are as numerous and broad as imagination might allow and may be explicitly or implicitly identified as truth, mind, knowledge, and so on. Within this avenue of explanation, we come to believe we have access to one objective reality that is true and correct. Interventions offered in this explanation of the world are believed by the health care provider to be correct and effective; therefore, patients and families experience "instructive interaction" in their conversations with health care providers. As a result, patients and families are told, instructed, and directed as to what to do, with little or no consideration as to whether the intervention is a fit for the patient and family.

To increase possibilities for healing, clinicians need to help themselves and their clients drift toward objectivity-in-parentheses. This explanation of our world offers the idea that there are many realities and thus many perspectives and beliefs about our world. Interventions in this domain will be offered collaboratively to the family to ascertain if the intervention is a fit or useful for the family. The clinician will be neither invested in the outcome of the intervention nor be judgmental, blaming, or withdraw from the family if they do not utilize the intervention(s) or do not find it useful. If the intervention is useful for the family, suffering will be softened and healing will begin. If the intervention is not useful, the clinician and family will once again collaborate and the clinician will offer other ideas and recommendations (interventions) that might be more useful.

When objectivity is placed in parentheses, there is a recognition that objects brought forth are not independent of the living system that brings them forth. The only truths that exist are those brought forth by observers, including health care providers and family members. One's view is not a distortion of some presumably correct interpretation. Instead of one objective universe waiting to be discovered or correctly described, Maturana has proposed a "multiverse," where many observer "verses" coexist, each valid in its own right. From this stance we emphasize a collaborative and consultative relationship between health care providers and the families with whom they work. Our approach of drawing forth family members' constraining beliefs and co-evolving facilitating beliefs is based on a respect for the present bio-psychosocial-spiritual structures of family members and a belief in multiverse. Whether a health care provider operates within the domain of *objectivity* or *objectivity-in-parentheses* profoundly influences his or her worldview, which in turn, influences what kind of relationship she or he prefers to have with others.

Of course it is difficult, and sometimes not even desirable, to only operate within one explanatory domain. As Maturana and Varela (1992) suggest, we must be able to walk the "razor's edge" and operate in both explanatory domains depending on the clinical context. For example, if someone expresses suicidal ideation, then we as health care providers will find ourselves in the explanatory domain of objectivity, i.e., we *will* behave as if we have the true and correct reality that life is worth living and will impose that belief upon the patient by whatever means are available to us. This could be through medication or even constant observation to prevent the patient from having time alone. However, if the person embraces life once again, then we will once again drift towards objectivity-in-parentheses in our therapeutic conversations with the patient and have the facilitating belief that there are many ways that this person might embrace and live their life.

Reality does not reside "out there" to be absorbed; rather, persons exist in many domains of the realities that we bring forth to explain our experiences. The ability to bring forth personal meaning and to respond and interact with the world and with each other, but always with reference to a set of internal coherences, can be seen as the essential quality of living.

In a phone interview, Maturana (1988b) embellished this notion as follows: "When an argument ensues between two persons, therefore, both make statements on the basis of their particular premises or beliefs. Each rational argument is constituted through the operation of preferences a priori; therefore, we have to look at each person's premises or beliefs." Maturana suggested that this is not a rational but an emotional domain; disagreements about politics, religion, or medication are examples. These differences can be resolved only in the domain of objectivity-in-parentheses, not in the domain of objectivity.

In the same telephone conversation, Maturana (1988b) discussed and drew the distinction between two paths that can cloud our understanding and prevent a stance of objectivity-in-parentheses. He offered the idea that there are two temptations into which one can fall that obscure understanding: objectivism and solipsism. Objectivism is the idea that one can make claims about a reality that is valid independent of oneself. All one's cognitive statements then become demands to others for obedience.

In the other path that can screen understanding—solipsism—everything is an idea in the mind of an observer because the observer is the only source of validation. To avoid this trap, one must realize that understanding is a reflection of an observer who is a participant in what is being observed. This understanding can be obtained through comprehension of how we are involved in language and how we are involved through our language in what we know. If one adopts a particular view of reality, it follows that one inadvertently encompasses a particular view of persons, their functioning, relationships, and illness.

The idea that humans bring different perspectives to their understanding of events is not new, but Maturana's perspective on observation is much more radical: It is based on biology and physiology, not philosophy (Wright & Levac, 1992). This biological lens has had a tremendous influence on our clinical work. There are many aspects of the *Illness Beliefs Model* that we now understand and explain according to Maturana and Varela's theoretical framework, the Biology of Cognition (1992).

Core Beliefs: The Heart of the Matter
"As a man thinketh in his heart, so is he."
—Proverbs 23:7

There are numerous beliefs operating and emerging within every person every day, about every situation, and every person encountered. But not all beliefs matter in daily life; not all beliefs invite an emotional or physiological response. But the beliefs that do matter are our *core* beliefs. We all possess core beliefs, which are very personal and usually invisible. Core beliefs are fundamental to how we approach the world; they are the basic concepts by which we live. Our core beliefs form our identity. Our core beliefs are generally about our beliefs of the nature of reality, and thus we live as if certain absolutes were true.

Core beliefs are the beliefs that are at the heart of the matter and therefore hold the most power in our lives. These beliefs are accompanied by intense affective and physiological responses. Core beliefs powerfully and profoundly influence the family system and its functioning. Core beliefs are the beliefs that matter and are most relevant to how family members cope and/or suffer with illness. They involve certitude about the issue at hand and are central to our individual lives and relationships.

Core beliefs differ from perceptions and thoughts. A perception varies more easily and is based on observation. For example, the perception "My father is very ill" is based on the observations of a daughter that her father's skin is pale and breathing is slow. She may think, "My father needs help." This is the offering of an opinion or idea. Core beliefs are based on believing the truth of some statement and are *laden* with affective and physiological responses. In this example, a core belief may be, "Responsible daughters care for their ill parents." Rules for behaving follow. The daughter may ask for time off from work to care for her ill father.

Core beliefs can be good or bad for one's health; they can be constraining or facilitating. On the positive side, a belief that one is loved and cared for is more likely to motivate individuals to take care of their health. However, we want to emphasize that it is not simply thinking positive thoughts or beliefs that leads to physical cures. We need more than just positive thinking to take control of our bodies and our lives. We need to also tackle the debilitating, limiting, and constraining beliefs that are embedded in our minds, hearts, and even cells. Unfortunately, some of our constraining or self-sabotaging beliefs were downloaded into our subconscious minds when we were children (Lipton, 2005).

From this discussion, it can be seen that beliefs arise out of the life one is living. Therefore, it is not surprising that family members and clinicians often have different beliefs about illness. To effectively assist individuals and families who are suffering, we must first listen with curiosity and then understand with sensitivity the core illness beliefs of those with whom we are privileged to work.

Social versus Therapeutic Conversations

The art of conversation has long held implications of social status and success. However, there is an important distinction between social and therapeutic conversations. Our beliefs are embedded in all our conversations whether they are social or therapeutic in nature. Social and therapeutic conversations involve both internal and external conversations, but the similarity ends there.

Social conversations are those that occur as we move about in our daily life and interact with those we encounter. Therapeutic conversations are purposeful and time-limited, as are the relationships. Persons and clinicians engaged in therapeutic conversations come together for a particular purpose, generally because the clinician, a family member, or both, have identified some emotional, spiritual, or physical suffering that needs to be alleviated, reduced, or softened. Although the clinician's job is to invite the client-family to an alternative, facilitating belief of what is needed to get past a problem or cope with an illness, the client-family's job is to invite the clinician to an appreciation of the illness experience. Between the two, a therapeutic conversation co-evolves.

Both client-family and clinician bring their expert knowledge to the therapeutic conversation. The clinician brings his or her expert knowledge of ideas to soften suffering and manage an illness; the client-family brings their expert knowledge of the illness experience and how the illness has affected their lives and relationships, such as the impact on their marriage, their family, or their ability to work. As the expertise of both the family and the clinician is acknowledged, appreciated, and expressed, both clinician and family change or challenge their beliefs together through their conversations.

Therapeutic conversations are the medium for change; that is, the medium for challenging constraining beliefs and ultimately bringing forth facilitating beliefs and changing hearts, minds, cells, and souls.

Rules and Norms of Conversations

The rules and norms of both social and therapeutic conversations are influenced by context, gender, beliefs, and previous history of interactions; however, the rules and norms for a therapeutic conversation are not the same as those for a social conversation. Interrupting is one example of a difference in rules. In social conversations, there are implicit rules of not interrupting while another is speaking. To do otherwise is considered impolite or controlling. In a therapeutic conversation, however, an implicit rule exists that permits interrupting; for example, in situations where family members are not being given an opportunity to offer their ideas and opinions—when their voices are not being acknowledged.

Another predominant difference between social and therapeutic conversations is the rule, or norm, about asking questions. In social conversations with family and friends, it is expected that there will be a mutual exchange of asking questions, telling stories, and taking an interest in one another. When reciprocal questioning is absent in social conversations, one may believe that the other person does not care or is not interested. In therapeutic conversations, however, there is no expectation that clients and family members will ask questions or take an interest in the clinician. We have a strong belief that the focus of a therapeutic conversation is to be on softening the suffering of individuals and families.

The persistence with which questions are asked may also be different in social versus therapeutic conversations. Because we know the world through our explanations, clinicians may continue to ask questions concerning problems or solutions if the explanations from families are not clear to them. Clinicians must be free, or at least believe they are free, to ask any and all questions about a family member's experience with illness. If clinicians are constrained to ask only certain questions, it is because of their own constraining beliefs about problems, change, their "role," and so on.

In both social and therapeutic conversations, the art of listening and being fully present is paramount. Both of these activities of listening and being fully present in the moment require great discipline of mind and spirit. However, when these behaviors of relational listening are fully practiced, they are an immense gift we give to another. The need to communicate what it is like to live in our individual, separate worlds of experience is a powerful need in human relationships. Consequently, nothing can be more frustrating or painful than the sense that those with whom we are close are not really interested in our lives or seem to be distracted or "somewhere" else. This kind of relationship does not validate our experience of living and thus can diminish self-worth and/or enhance suffering. All our conversations matter because no conversation is ever trivial. Each conversation in which we participate influences changes in our bio-psychosocial-spiritual structures and ultimately our beliefs.

Human beings exist in language. It is not possible to refer to ourselves or to anything else without language. But language does not take place in the brain. Languaging is a social phenomenon rather than a phenomenon of the nervous system (Maturana, 1998). Every reflection takes place in language, which is our unique way of being human. Every human act takes place in language, and therefore all of our social acts have ethical implications (Maturana & Varela, 1992).

Languaging interaction is as powerful as physical interaction. A loving conversation can be experienced as a caress; an angry conversation as a hit. Such interactions trigger structural changes of many different types, including changes in blood pressure and respiration. We do not believe the childhood saying "sticks and stones will break my bones but words will never hurt me." Words can and do influence our bio-psychosocial-spiritual structures.

The braiding of languaging plus emotioning equals conversation (Maturana, 1998). Emotioning is interconnected with the notion of languaging. In our conversations, we may observe a range of emotions from anger to joy. Emotions arise from structural changes caused by the mutual perturbations between individuals that have occurred through their languaging. Recursively, emotions may give rise to structural changes that may trigger an "illness" response or an interactional dilemma.

It is important to emphasize and clarify that emotions do not require language. As humans, we experience emotions but we language feelings. There is a difference between emotions and feelings. For example, if a person says, "I feel angry about my diagnosis," this is an expression of feelings about how that person is experiencing emotion, but it is not the emotion itself. Our description in language of our emotions constitutes our feelings. These strong emotions are triggered by our beliefs and vice versa. Our relationships with patients and families always occur within conversation. Our conversations are dramatically influenced by our beliefs and our beliefs invite particular behaviors.

Conversations that Invite Reflections

There are numerous types of conversations and each has the potential to hurt or heal. People usually participate in many different conversations, simultaneously or successively. Drawing forth facilitating beliefs in therapeutic conversations is one way to help create new, healthier, and healing conversations. Clinicians distinguish themselves from other conversationalists by the way they enter and create novel conversations with individuals and families. Curiosity is an important characteristic of therapeutic conversations (Cecchin, 1987). The other important characteristic is to invite family members to a reflection which will challenge constraining beliefs or strengthen facilitating beliefs. As family members contemplate their behaviors and subsequently their beliefs about themselves, their relationships, and their illnesses, they are able to open space for new patterns of relating. By inviting family members to distinguish their distinctions—to think about their thinking—the clinician is inviting family members to participate in the process of self-reflection. The process of self-reflection is foundational to the co-evolution of new, more facilitating beliefs.

Different kinds of conversations give rise to different emotions based on one's view of reality (see the earlier description of objectivity and objectivity-in-parentheses in this chapter.) Some conversations are simply obscured by actions and emotionally inert, whereas others are emotionally saturated. Conversations can range from emotionally violent to emotionally loving.

Conversations that can be distinguished as emotionally violent are generated by the belief that one has access to a true, right, or correct reality. We have found Maturana's (1998) definition of emotional violence to be a useful one in our clinical practice: holding an idea or opinion to be true, such that another person's opinion is not only untrue but must change. The first part of his definition is characteristic of any good argument: people try to convince others of the correctness of their point of view. But the conversation becomes violent when one person insists that another person's opinion must change and be in accordance with the first person's. This behavior of emotional violence, if over a number of years in an intimate relationship, may lead to emotional suffering, physical violence, physical illness, or all three. Whatever the manifestation, the bio-psychosocial-spiritual structure is changed.

The belief that we are right and others are wrong and must change generates conversations of accusations, recriminations, and negative characterizations (Mendez, Coddou, & Maturana, 1988). On the other hand, loving interactions or conversations are based on a belief that there are many views and realities and, therefore, many ideas and opinions:

"multi verses." There are many equally legitimate views, but all are not equally desirable or pleasant to live in (Maturana & Varela, 1992).

Conversations where there exists a belief that there are many realities compels each of us to be a particular kind of person; a person who is open to others' ideas and beliefs; does not blame or judge others' choices or decisions; and is even open to having their own ideas and beliefs challenged or altered. Of course becoming this kind of person is not an easy path for living one's life. It requires giving up the need to be right in exchange for respect for others' ideas; of letting go and forgiving the actions of others; and of being able to give our love away, rather than demand the receiving of love according to our "right" ideas of how persons should behave towards us. This preferred way of being enables and enhances the possibility for healthy, peaceful, healing relationships.

We call conversations that draw forth love "conversations of affirmation and affection" and "conversations of growth and change." We have embraced Maturana and Varela's (1992) definition of *love:* "the acceptance of the other person beside us in our daily living" (p. 246). Furthermore, love is the domain of those actions that constitute another as a legitimate other in coexistence with one's self (Maturana, 1998). Consequently, even the admonition "love your enemies," as in the Judeo/Christian Bible, can be an acknowledgment that your enemy is a legitimate other. If we believe that our enemies are mistaken and must change, however, we are operating in the domain of objectivity-without-parentheses.

Clinicians are socially empowered to bring forth either health or pathology in our therapeutic conversations. Clinicians are most interested, therefore, in altering, modifying, softening or stopping conversations of negative characterizations and conversations of accusations and recriminations, which are types of conversations that we believe bring forth pathology. Our primary goal as clinicians is to bring forth conversations that invite new or renewed beliefs about problems, persons, and relationships: conversations of affirmation and affection and conversations of growth and change.

We propose that the most powerful way to change the nature or character of a conversation is to change one's beliefs. Beliefs can be altered or modified by inviting individuals and families to a reflection; i.e., the clinician operates from a worldview of objectivity-in-parentheses and invites family members into that world. Here is where the passion and the commitment of the clinician should appear, not as a passion or commitment to change others, but as the passion for bringing forth a type of conversation that allows family members to put objectivity into parentheses.

One of the tasks of health care providers, therefore, is to help families reflect on their thoughts and actions and move into living with their illness experiences primarily in objectivity-in-parentheses. By putting objectivity into parentheses, the validation, worth, and ability to love others comes naturally, as we become more accustomed to bringing forth that kind of person. We recognize that we generate and validate all reality through living together in language, deriving consensus, and drawing distinctions.

Conversations that Hurt or Heal

These types of conversations may include conversations of characterizations, conversations of accusations and recriminations, conversations of command and obedience, conversations inviting change and healing, and conversations of affirmation and affection. These types of conversations are briefly described in the following sections, with accompanying examples. They are not inclusive of, but only introductory to, the full range of conversations that we have found useful in our clinical practice.

Conversations of Characterizations

The reciprocal assigning of positive or negative characteristics of the person involved in a conversation is typical of conversations of characterizations (Maturana, 1988a). The following is an example of a conversation including a positive characterization:

"I appreciate you visiting my ill husband. You are such a thoughtful person."

"Well, thank you for the nice compliment."

By criticizing, one is attacking and usually blaming another's personality or character rather than a specific behavior. The following is an example of this type of conversation:

"Where have you been? I thought you were someone I could count on to be on time."

"But this is one of the few times I've been late."

"No, you're self-centered and disrespectful of people's time."

Conversations of Accusations and Recriminations

Complaints of unfulfilled expectations occur within conversations of accusations and recriminations (Maturana, 1988a). These types of conversations give rise to emotional contradiction because they make claim to knowledge of an objective reality and thus there exists a mutual negation. With these conversations, opinions and descriptions take place in a domain of rejection and frustration. These conversations may lead to emotional, spiritual, and physical suffering, deny the existence of others, and interfere with structural coupling between members, leading to possible disintegration of a relationship. The following is one example:

"I had so much hope that you were going to finally stop drinking."

"Well, you know that I've been trying. If you had more confidence in me, I'd be farther along now."

"Oh, so it's all my fault, is it? Well, you're the one with the problem."

"That's right, my problem is you."

Conversations of Command and Obedience

Conversations of command and obedience occur against an emotional background of mutual negation and self-negation in which some of the participants obey (Maturana, 1988a). This behavior results in the negating of self by the one who obeys and, simultaneously and ironically, negates the one who commands. The negation of the "commander" also occurs because he negates those who obey by accepting their negation as legitimate. For example, in a nursing home, a health care professional may command an elderly person to get out of bed, negating the elderly person (and herself):

"Mr. Valquez, get out of bed. You've been sleeping too long," the nurse says forcefully.

"Not yet," Mr. Valquez replies weakly. "I'm tired."

"You're tired because you sleep all the time and don't move around enough, now get up."

"Okay," he resigns. "You're the nurse."

Conversations Inviting Change and Healing

Conversations inviting change and healing work through disagreements, differences, and conflict. Co-evolving conversations that facilitate the resolving of disagreements, hurts, and suffering involve letting go of certainty or the need to be right, validating the other person's experience, listening with one's heart and drawing forth the other's heart, giving up being defensive, letting the other know one understands or is trying to, and staying calm. These behaviors, and hopefully reflections, lead to the possibility of healing. An example follows:

"I know we haven't been getting along well these last few weeks," the wife says to her husband. "What do you think is wrong?"

"Well, I can only speak for myself," he responds, taking her hand gently. "But I've been really stressed with our son being ill and you don't seem to want to talk about it."

"I do want to talk about it. It's just that I don't want to make you worry more. I don't know how to stop you from worrying."

"I don't need you to stop me worrying; I just need to be able to say that I'm worried," he says.

"Okay, let's sit down right now. I'd like to learn what you're worried about ....and then I've got a couple of things to say, too."

"Great, thanks for bringing this up. It's been a really hard time."

Conversations of Affirmation and Affection

Conversations of affirmation and affection consist of reciprocal confirmations of another's worth and value as a human being and particularly that they are loved. This type of conversation opens space for the existence of another. These conversations assist in emotional healing by triggering structural and biological changes as beliefs about oneself are changed.

Detailed examples of this type of conversation are offered in Chapter 9. We believe that clinicians need to make an effort toward drawing forth and co-evolving conversations of affirmation and affection, because these are conversations that promote healing. These are conversations where participants are operating within objectivity-in-parentheses and thus open to multiple views and multiple realities of how to live in the world.

One example of this kind of conversation is with a couple who had recently lost a son in a car accident:

"I want to tell you that our son had sixteen precious years with the best mother in the world," the husband says to his wife. "He could not have been loved more by you."

His wife responded, "I so appreciate you telling me that. I've often wondered if there was more I could have done to be a better mother. And he could not have had a better father."

In summary, we become our conversations and we generate the conversations that we become (Mendez et al., 1988). We indeed become a particular kind of person through the conversations that we engage in. Therapeutic conversations constitute deliberate and purposeful actions on the part of the clinician based on his or her beliefs. It is hoped that these actions will trigger biological changes in family members such that they will no longer participate in negative characterizations, accusations, and recriminations. Eliminating these kinds of conversations can soften emotional, relational, physical, and/or spiritual suffering and offer hope for family healing.

The privilege of working with families invites clinicians to consider that our participation in therapeutic conversations also influences emotional and structural changes in ourselves as we witness the healing in others. Our own beliefs are, hopefully, challenged as we open space to the individuals/ families with whom we have the privilege of knowing. But how do we co-evolve and draw forth conversations that invite change and healing? Through research about our clinical practice (Wright, Watson, & Bell, 1996), we have uncovered interactions in our therapeutic conversations with families that have triggered dramatic changes. These macromoves and micromoves (interventions) are described in Chapters 7 through 10.

Conclusion

This chapter has offered a discussion of our preferred explanation of beliefs using the lens of biology. This lens has dramatically influenced our clinical practice over the years. In both our personal and professional lives, we unavoidably embrace particular beliefs that guide us in living. We currently define a belief as the "truth" of a particular reality that influences a person's bio-psychosocial-spiritual structure and functioning. Core beliefs are the "beliefs that matter" within our relationships and within significant events in our lives, such as illness, loss, and disability. Our beliefs and our believing inevitably influence the way we interact and behave and ultimately what kind of clinician and how kind a clinician we are.

We also offered various types of conversations that are brought forth depending on whether one operates within the explanation of reality as *objectivity* or *objectivity-in-parentheses*. Understanding the difference between the two is essential to facilitating the conversations families need to have to begin healing when faced with serious illness, loss, or disability.

References

Campbell, T.L. (2003). The effectiveness of family interventions for physical disorders. *Journal of Marital and Family Therapy, 29*(2), 263-281.

Cecchin, G. (1987). Hypothesizing, circularity, and neutrality revisited: An invitation to curiosity. *Family Process, 25*(4), 405-413.

Cecchin, G., Lane, G., & Ray, W.A. (1994). Influence, effect and emerging systems. *Journal of Systemic Therapies, 13*(4), 13-21.

Cousins, N. (1989). Beliefs become biology [Videotape]. Victoria, British Columbia, Canada: University of Victoria.

Gilliss, C.L., & Knafl, K.A. (1999). Nursing care of families in non-normative transitions. The state of science and practice. In A.S. Hinshaw, S.L. Feetham, & J.L. Shaver (Eds.), *Handbook of clinical nursing research* (pp. 231-249). Thousand Oaks, CA: SAGE.

Beliefs and Illness: A Model for Healing

Beliefs and Illness: A Model for Healing

Haller, D.M., Sanci, L.A., Sawyer, S.M., & Patton, G. (2008). Do young people's illness beliefs affect health care? A systematic review. *Journal of Adolescent Health, 42*(5), 436-449.

Hekler, E., Lambert, J., Leventhal, E., Leventhal, H., Jahn, E., & Contrada, R. (2008). Commonsense illness beliefs, adherence behaviors, and hypertension control among African Americans. *Journal of Behavioral Medicine, 31*(5), 391-400.

Horne, R., & Weinman, J. (1999). Patients' beliefs about prescribed medicines and their role in adherence to treatment in chronic physical illness. *Journal of Psychosomatic Research, 47*(6), 555-567.

Knafl, K.A., & Gilliss, C.L. (2002). Families and chronic illness: A synthesis of current research. *Journal of Family Nursing, 8*(3), 178-198.

Kinderman, P., Setzu, E., Lobban, F., & Salmon, P. (2006). Illness beliefs in schizophrenia. *Social Science & Medicine, 63*(7), 1900-1911.

King, G., Baxter, D., Rosenbaum, P., Zwaigenbaum, L., & Bates, A. (2009). Beliefs systems of families of children with autism spectrum disorders or Down syndrome. *Focus on Autism and Other Developmental Disabilities, 24*(1), 50-64.

Lau-Walker, M.O., Cowie, M.R., & Roughton, M. (2009). Coronary heart disease patients' perception of their symptoms and sense of control are associated with their quality of life three years following hospital discharge. *Journal of Clinical Nursing, 18*(1), 63-71.

Lipton, B. (2005). *The biology of belief: Unleashing the power of consciousness, matter, and miracles.* Santa Rosa, CA: Elite Books.

Matire, L.M., Lustig, A.P., Schulz, R., Miller, G.E., & Helgeson, V.S. (2004). Is it beneficial to involve a family member? A meta-analysis of psychosocial interventions for chronic illness. *Health Psychology, 23*(6), 599-611.

Maturana, H.R. (1988a). Reality: The search for objectivity or the quest for a compelling argument. *Irish Journal of Psychology, 9*(1), 25-83.

Maturana, H.R. (1988b). *Telephone conversation: The Calgary/Chile coupling* [Phone conversation with Dr. Lorraine Wright and graduate students]. (Transcript available from www.lorrainewright.com)

Chapter 2: Understanding Beliefs

Maturana, H.R. (1998). *Biology of cognition and biology of love.*
[Videotapes of a workshop presented at the Faculty of Nursing, University of
Calgary in 1998]. (Available from www.janicembell.com)

Maturana, H.R., & Varela, F.J. (1992). *The tree of knowledge: The biological
roots of human understanding* (rev. ed.). Boston: Shambhala.

Mendez, C.L., Coddou, F., & Maturana, H.R. (1988). The bringing forth of
pathology. *Irish Journal of Psychology, 9*(1), 144-172.

Moules, N.J. (2006).A cautionary tale about stories [Guest Editorial]. *Journal of
Family Nursing, 12*(3), 231-233.

Rolland, J.S. (1994). *Families, illness, and disability: An integrative treatment
model.* New York: Basic Books.

Ruddy, N.B., & McDaniel, S.H. (2008), Couples therapy and medical illness:
Working with couples facing illness. In A.S. Gurman (Ed.), *Clinical handbook
of couple therapy* (4th ed., pp. 618-640). New York: Guilford.

Tavris, C., & Aronson, E. (2007). *Mistakes were made (but not by me). Why we
justify foolish beliefs, bad decisions, and hurtful acts.* Orlando, FL: Harcourt.

Weihs, K., Fisher, L., & Baird, M. (2002). Families, health, and behavior: A section
of the Commissioned Report by the Committee on Health and Behavior:
Research, Practice, and Policy, Division of Neuroscience and Behavioral
Health and Division of Health Promotion and Disease Prevention, Institute
of Medicine, National Academy of Sciences. *Families, Systems, & Health,
20*(1), 7-46.

Wright, L.M., Bell, J.M., Watson, W.L., & Tapp, D. (1995). The influence of the
beliefs of nurses: A clinical example of a post-myocardial-infarction couple.
Journal of Family Nursing, 1(3), 238-256.

Wright, L.M., & Levac, A.M. (1992). The non-existence of non-compliant
families: The influence of Humberto Maturana. *Journal of Advanced Nursing,
17*, 913-917.

Wright, L.M., Watson, W.L., & Bell, J.M. (1996). *Beliefs: The heart of
healing in families and illness.* New York: Basic Books.

Zukav, G. (1979). *The dancing Wu Li masters: An overview of the new
physics.* New York: Morrow.

43

CHAPTER THREE
Beliefs about Families

"Families are about love overcoming emotional torture."
—Matt Groening

Everyone has beliefs about families because most, if not all, of us have grown up in a family context. For instance, your beliefs about how a "good mother" should respond when her child becomes ill have likely been shaped by many life experiences, including the behaviors you saw modeled in your family of origin. Health care providers bring their strong personal and professional beliefs about families to the clinical domain. Beliefs about what is "normal" behavior in families or how a "good" family should function in the presence of illness shape how health care providers view, assess, and most importantly, care for, facilitate healing, and intervene with families. For example, a health care provider who believes addiction is a consequence of irresponsibility, early childhood trauma, or personal weakness will likely respond differently to a family experiencing addiction than to a family experiencing the effects of a congenital heart defect, an illness which he or she believes is not related to trauma, behavior, or responsibility.

Our beliefs as health care providers determine whether we view families as "dysfunctional" or "healthy;" see them as pathological or resourceful; put them on the "Board of Directors" by involving them in their health care or foster dependency; and even determine if we are able to move from an individual focus to a systemic focus with our clinical assessments and interventions. Our beliefs of who constitutes a family and how they influence health are among the beliefs that impact clinical practice, affecting who we include in our practice and how we offer assistance to those experiencing illness suffering. *Figure 3* illustrates five core beliefs about families that influence our clinical practice using the *Illness Beliefs Model*.

Figure 3. Illness Beliefs Model: Beliefs about Families

- **A family is a group of individuals who are bound by strong emotional ties, a sense of belonging, and a passion for being involved in one another's lives**

- **Individuals experiencing illness are best understood in their relational contexts**

- **Individuals are structurally determined**

- **Problems do not reside within individuals but between persons in language and beliefs**

- **All families have strengths, often unappreciated or unrealized**

A Family is a Group of Individuals who are Bound by Strong Emotional Ties, a Sense of Belonging, and a Passion For Being Involved in One Another's Lives

In our current world of varied and diverse family structures, we need a definition of family that moves beyond the traditional boundaries of limiting family membership by blood, adoption, and marriage to account for all of those significant relationships one can't live without. To begin to understand just whom these people include, health care providers need to listen carefully to how individuals prefer to define "family". A favorite colloquial definition of family is those individuals who "give a damn" about one another. Another useful definition proposes that the "family is who they say they are" (Wright & Leahey, 2009, p. 50).

With a curiosity about these preferences, the clinician is open and willing to honor family members' ideas about which relationships are significant to them and how these relationships influence health and illness. Inviting the individual to define who constitutes "the family" provides access to important beliefs. Through the construction of a genogram, the clinician may learn that an individual believes support and affection received from a neighbor, friend, coworker, or even a family pet is as significant, if not more significant, than support received from a spouse or sibling.

Genograms and ecomaps are necessary clinical tools in the *Illness Beliefs Model* for accounting for significant relationships and have been used extensively in clinical work and research (McGoldrick, Gerson, & Petry, 2008; Rempel, Neufeld, & Kushner, 2007; Wright & Leahey, 2009). They quickly provide a way of engaging individuals and families and efficiently organizing complex information about family structure and important personal, social, and health care networks and relationships. They also offer an opportunity to inquire about previous and current family illness experiences that provide a portal to understanding beliefs about many aspects of family illness experiences, including beliefs about diagnosis, treatment, and about the role of family members when illness arises.

The term "family" is used in the *Illness Beliefs Model* to symbolize a conceptual systemic lens that accounts for the interaction, reciprocity, and relationships between multiple systems levels that range from the smallest level of the cell to the largest level of society. It does not matter how many people you have sitting in your consultation room. Whether it is one individual or a group of individuals who call themselves "family", a systemic lens is used to inquire about relationships and interaction at many systems levels. These include the illness, the ill individual, the family, the health care provider, and the larger systems within which they are nested. The clinician, using the *Illness Beliefs Model*, is adept at assessing beliefs at multiple systems levels and choosing interventions that target the systems level(s) that offers the greatest possibility for health and healing, i.e., the intervention might target individual beliefs, the relationship between two or more family members' beliefs, the relationship between the family's beliefs and the health care providers' beliefs, health care system beliefs,

47

societal beliefs, or some combination of these.

The *Illness Beliefs Model* is a unique model for advanced practice with individuals and families that uses a systemic conceptual lens to examine the intersection of beliefs at multiple systems levels. Within the discipline of nursing, we think about the *Illness Beliefs Model* as a clinical practice model for advanced practice, specifically, Family Systems Nursing (Wright & Leahey, 1990; Bell, 2009). Other health disciplines have also argued that a family systems perspective is critical for assessing and intervening in medicine (Engel, 1980), social work (Hartman & Laird, 1983), psychology (Kazak, Simms, & Rourke, 2002; McDaniel, Belar, Schroeder, Hargrove & Freeman, 2002), and family therapy (McDaniel, Hepworth, & Doherty, 1992; Weakland, 1977). Thus, the *Illness Beliefs Model* may be a useful practice model across a number of disciplines who lay claim to the importance of a systemic approach in helping individuals and families who suffer in their experience of illness.

Despite our keen interest in helping health care providers move from an individual to a family focus in health care, we believe that a collective meaning unit called "family" does not actually exist. The idea of the family unit as a system composed of individual family members and having characteristics of its own that transcend those of the individual members (i.e., the whole is greater than the sum of its parts) is a fundamental assumption of family systems theory. However, the distinction between family and individual family members is an important one to consider. Humberto Maturana (1998) persuasively argued that "family" is an idea brought forth in our minds through language to account for the special relationship that occurs over time among individuals who call themselves and think of themselves as part of a family; however, a family can be known only through its individual members.

Maturana and Varela's (1992) objectivity-in-parentheses proposes that an independent reality does not exist but is brought forth by the observer. The act of bringing forth an entity, that is, the describing and distinguishing of anything, is accomplished by each individual through language. If reality is observer-dependent, there are as many families as there are family members, because each family member has his or her distinct view of "the family." In a family of five, therefore, there are not five different views of one family; there are five different families! Even when meanings, beliefs, and experiences are consensually shared through language by several individuals within a family and evolved through interaction over time among the individual family members, there is no such thing as a "family belief," a "family construct," "family meaning," or "family health." Instead, there are many individual family member descriptions of family beliefs, family meanings, or family health, each one equally valid.

This belief has implications for family research as well as for clinical work with families. Asking each family member about their experience of "family" or their experience of illness recognizes that there will likely be different answers and different experiences among family members, and all are equally legitimate. This discarding of a search for the "truth" about a family acknowledges that reality is observer-dependent. Rather than believing that there should be consensus among the answers provided by family members and searching for who is telling the "truth," the family clinician or researcher respectfully encourages a variety of family member perspectives and becomes curious about the differing individual beliefs that may be at play within the family as well as the differing beliefs that may coexist between the family and the health care provider(s). Therefore, it may be more useful to talk about a "systemic" approach rather than a "family" approach when describing clinical work and research using the conceptual lens offered by the *Illness Beliefs Model*.

Individuals Experiencing Illness are Best Understood in Their Relational Contexts

Our health care systems in North America, from assessment through treatment and evaluation, are generally focused on the individual. Clinicians who take a relational or systemic perspective frequently find themselves swimming against the current within a health care system that is primarily oriented to the individual. Caring for the relational system is conceptually and empirically different than providing care to individuals or to family members and is guided by a belief that individuals are powerfully connected, not just emotionally but also biologically, in their relationships with others.

Research has shown that a powerful and reciprocal connection exists between family relationships and health. In an integrative review by Weihs,

Fisher, and Baird (2002), the authors offer an overview of what is known about characteristics of couple and family relationships that influence the experience and management of chronic illness over time. Protective family processes linked to chronic illness management include family closeness, caregiver coping skills, mutually supportive family relationships, clear family organization, and direct communication about the illness and its management. Risk factors in families experiencing chronic illness include intrafamilial conflict, criticism, and blame; psychological trauma related to diagnosis and treatment; external stress; lack of an extra-familiar support system; disease interrupting family member's developmental tasks; and perfectionism and rigidity (Weihs et al., 2002). Further hypothesizing about these factors led Fisher (2006) to later declare:

> Family characteristics that have been shown to have a powerful effect on illness management include poor couple conflict resolution skills, low relationship satisfaction, high interspouse conflict, high criticalness, high hostility, *and lack of congruence in disease beliefs and expectations* [italics supplied]. Interestingly, these characteristics emerge from *family and couple beliefs, emotional tone, and relationship skills* [italics supplied], a cross-section of family life in general. Furthermore, these characteristics apply across many chronic diseases, recognizing the differences in the demand characteristics of different diseases, and they are similar across different family developmental stages (Fisher & Weihs, 2000). For example, poor problem solving and conflict resolution are disruptive for disease management in families with ill children, adults, or elders. Even within a developmental stage, poor relationship satisfaction, for example, does not bode well for chronic disease management regardless of disease, for example, among families with diabetes, cardiovascular disease, asthma, or depression. How family members come together emotionally, *what they believe to be the cause and best treatment for disease* [italics supplied], and their skills in addressing disease-related problems and conflicts set the stage for collaboration among the people who live with the disease on a daily basis, regardless of the disease and the age of family members. These, then, are major areas of family and couple behavior that can be targeted for intervention across a broad range of chronic diseases. (p. 374)

These findings offer a compelling reason for health care providers to involve families in health care and possess the knowledge and skills to focus on beliefs and relationship issues.

One of the basic clinical tools used to gain a richer understanding of the interconnections between beliefs and relationships is the Circular Pattern Diagram (CPD) (Bell, 2000; Tomm, 1980; Wright & Leahey, 2009). The CPD allows the health care provider to draw out the loops of recursive links between the cognition, affect, and behavior of an individual or systems level and the cognition, affect, and behavior of another individual or systems level. Whereas Tomm (1980) and Wright and Leahey (2009), use the term "cognition", we prefer, within the *Illness Beliefs Model*, to use "beliefs" in the CPD.

We have found that intense and insatiable curiosity is needed to think relationally and systemically (Bell, 1998). As Cecchin (1987) offered, curiosity is the ability to be interested in all family members and yet not aligned with any one family member's point of view over another. Curiosity is absent when we think we have come to "know" a family or find ourselves feeling bored and restless within a therapeutic conversation. Questions that help invite curiosity within clinical team discussions include: What have we stopped being curious about with this individual/ family? And when did we stop being curious with this individual/family? What would be possible if we let ourselves get curious again?

Individuals are Structurally Determined

One of Humberto Maturana's ideas that has greatly influenced our clinical practice using the *Illness Beliefs Model* is the concept of *structural determinism* (Maturana & Varela, 1992). Each individual's bio-psychosocial-spiritual structure is unique and is a product of the individual's genetic history (phylogeny) as well as his or her history of interactions with others over time (ontogeny).

A living system is "structure determined" and any or all changes are determined by its structure. Maturana argues that change is constantly occurring in our environment and within each individual's unique bio-psychosocial-spiritual structure. Structural change occurs in living systems from moment to moment, either as a change triggered by information coming from the environment in which the structure exists or as a result of internal dynamics. It is important to note that it is the individual's structure that will determine the change that occurs. Triggers for change are numerous and constant, but it is the unique individual structure that decides which particular trigger it will select. A trigger for change, selected by the structure, is called a "perturbation", and this perturbation will result in structural change to the individual. It is the individual's structure—*not* the power or novelty of the trigger itself—that determines changes to the individual's structure.

Therefore, we cannot say a priori which health care interventions (triggers) of the *Illness Beliefs Model* will be selected by the individual's structure to promote change for *this* particular family member at *this* time and which will not. Change results when there is a "fit" between the individual structure and the health care intervention that is selected by the individual's structure as a perturbation. We cannot predict which of the clinician's ideas/interventions will fit for a particular person's structure and which will not. The initially static-sounding notion of structural determinism is heard differently when one considers it in conjunction with Maturana's concepts of "plasticity" and "structural coupling." Living systems are highly plastic, that is, able to make changes through interactions and through structurally coupling with other systems. There is hopefulness for change and desire for therapeutic competence that is generated through the integration of the concepts of structural determinism, plasticity, and structural coupling. Chapter 5 contains a further description of these concepts and their influence on beliefs about therapeutic change.

A deep respect for and intense curiosity about family members develops in clinicians who are cognizant of the notion of structural determinism. We become deeply curious about the "fit" between our ideas and the family member's structure. Application of Maturana's concept of structural determinism has led us to believe that the description of families as noncompliant, resistant, or unmotivated is not only "an epistemological error but a biological impossibility" (Wright & Levac, 1992, p. 913). This concept has revolutionized the way we think about families and, more important, the way we interact with families. The concept of "fit" allows us to be non-blaming of family members and ourselves.

One way we have applied the idea of structural determinism in our practice has been through the use of a particular question: "What stood out for you?" For example, when families come to a session, we routinely ask, "What stood out for you from the last session?" In so doing, we are acknowledging the uniqueness of each family member and that what is experienced as significant, meaningful, and perturbing at each session varies among family members. We are curious about which of all the ideas and opinions offered during a session stood out and were selected as meaningful perturbations for particular family members. We have found this to be a respectful way to work with families, because we realize that not everything we offer families will fit or be helpful.

During a clinical session, we frequently use the clinical intervention called a reflecting team (Andersen, 1987, 1991). (For more discussion about this intervention, see Chapter 9.) From behind a one-way mirror, individuals and families have the opportunity to listen to and observe the clinical team discussing their situation. Following the team's discussion, we encourage family members to reflect on the team's reflections by asking, "What stood out for you?" In this way, we honor the idea that each individual's structure is unique. It is not what the clinician says or does that effects change; rather, it is the fit between the individual's present structure and what the clinician offers that effects therapeutic change.

Problems do not Reside Within Individuals but Between Persons in Language And Beliefs

"The adult daughters continually fight about who should care for their ill mother. They are so dysfunctional!" These words of a health care provider, speaking about an aging family experiencing chronic illness, express particular limiting beliefs about families. It is not unusual, given the strong medical model influence of health professional education, to distinguish and draw forth pathology and problems and thus to become blind to family member's health, resources, and strengths. The influence of this prevailing deficit model on health care providers' beliefs about individuals and families is sometimes subtle and yet dangerously pervasive (Duncan, 2005).

Health care providers often struggle to define what is "healthy" family functioning. Providers in various health disciplines often pride themselves on being the first to identify what is "really wrong" with a family. Health care providers, under the influence of the medical model often believe that it is necessary to find the cause of a problem before a cure can be suggested. This belief generates a clinical approach that focuses on etiology—the endless search for "why"—and often invites blame and accusation of the ill individual and other family members.

Frequently, illnesses and other problems are seen to reside within individuals and this is reflected in the language that is used where person and illness are one and the same: the depressed cancer patient, the acting-out adolescent, the abusive father. Making a distinction between person and illness allows that an individual's illness does not solely define their life. "Families who experience childhood cancer" for instance, is a more useful term when describing a family's experience of illness, rather than being labelled a pediatric cancer family.

The pioneering work of Harlene Anderson and Harry Goolishian (1988) conceptualized problems as being distinguished in language rather than residing within individuals. A "problem-determined system" is not an individual or family, but a language system with boundaries marked by whoever communicates about a shared problem. We would add that the language system is linked to a belief system and that beliefs have the potential to perpetuate problems and suffering and to diminish relationship difficulties and suffering.

We assert that there is no such thing as a "dysfunctional" individual or family (Bell, 1995). To label a family as dysfunctional suggests that the clinician is, in Maturana's words, operating in the domain of "objectivity-without-parentheses" (Maturana &Varela, 1992). When one operates from a stance of objectivity-without-parentheses, one believes that reality is independent of the observer. There is one correct reality and it is mine. We need to ask whose point of view is being privileged in the labeling of behavior as dysfunctional. The objectivity-without-parentheses stance in the health care setting frequently honors the clinician's observations and judgments as the "truth" about a family. It implicitly and hierarchically values the clinician's observations over other observations and descriptions. It also limits both the clinician and those being labeled "dysfunctional" from proposing other distinctions. The term *dysfunctional* also serves to trivialize and minimize problems, offering only one label to capture a wide range of difficulties and challenges. We find the term itself to be dysfunctional, serving no useful purpose and prohibiting wider views of situations and families.

We have found it useful to think about difficulties as problems that are drawn forth in language and occur between, rather than within, persons. Stubbornness, for example, is a relational phenomenon brought forth in language between two people; it is hard to be stubborn alone. To be characterized as "stubborn" requires another person in interaction with the "stubborn" individual to feel that their point of view is not honored or their request for change is not acknowledged. Stubbornness arises as an interactional, between persons phenomenon. This "between persons" conceptualization removes the temptation to engage in linear thinking through conversations of causation (i.e., asking the individual "why" questions) or of accusation (blaming a particular individual). Different conversations unfold when a person experiencing depression is not asked why he is depressed but rather is asked what beliefs seem to fuel and perpetuate his depression, how family members respond to his depressed behavior, who is most or least supportive of his depressed behavior, whether there was ever a time he held beliefs that were more optimistic and hopeful about his illness, and if so, what was different then. A systemic description of interactions which maintain or perpetuate constraining beliefs or which bring forth facilitating beliefs that diminish suffering provides many more possibilities for intervention and healing to soften physical, relational, emotional, and/or spiritual suffering.

All Families Have Strengths, Often Unappreciated or Unrealized

While we emphasize that all families have strengths that need to be distinguished and encouraged, we also acknowledge that all families have problems and challenges. A famous quote reminds us, "The only normal people are the ones you don't know very well" (Joe Ancis). However, we prefer to abandon the lens that pathologizes families and adopt a belief that families experiencing illness suffering are resourceful, competent, and resilient.

We believe all families possess the strengths and abilities necessary to solve their own problems, but sometimes, in the face of serious illness suffering, their solution capabilities may be hidden, inaccessible, or forgotten. A strengths-oriented and resilience perspective has increasingly influenced health care providers to look for family strengths, remind families about their forgotten strengths and abilities, and magnify current strengths (Duncan, 2005; Feeley & Gottlieb, 2000; Walsh, 2002, 2006).

Our clinical team at the Family Nursing Unit worked with a family who had experienced childhood chronic illness for many years. Carole Robinson (1998) recruited the family for her study and asked the parents to reflect on what been helpful to them about the therapeutic conversations at the Family Nursing Unit. Despite encountering numerous health care professionals over many years, the mother of the ill child reported, "Nobody ever told me before that I was doing a good job." Similarly, another woman who came to the Family Nursing Unit following her husband's repeated life-threatening cardiac crises over four years, reflected on her experience of her first session at the Family Nursing Unit: "Yeah, I learned a lot about myself that day. I didn't realize I was strong like the clinical team saw me."

In our clinical experience, families generally seek help for problems once their own efforts at problem solving have been exhausted, they have reached an impasse, or their suffering has become unbearable. They seek professional help feeling inadequate, exhausted, fearful, frustrated, incompetent, or overwhelmed. Through an understanding of the family's experience with illness suffering, the clinician looks for opportunities to invite the members to a new view of their strengths or to help them regain a view of their competence that has been lost. Clinicians therefore need to be "strengths detectives" (Levac, Wright, & Leahey, 1997; Wright & Leahey, 2009). Drawing forth family strengths through commendations has become a key characteristic of our clinical practice using the *Illness Beliefs Model* (Bohn, Wright, & Moules, 2003; Houger Limacher, 2008; Houger Limacher & Wright, 2003, 2006). (For more information on commendations, see Chapter 9, Challenging Constraining Beliefs.) What characteristics allow clinicians to focus on strengths rather than pathology? Some beginning answers to this question are offered in Chapter 6, Beliefs about Clinicians.

Conclusion

The core beliefs that the clinician holds about families lay the essential groundwork for the *Illness Beliefs Model* and influence almost everything the clinician sees, says, and does. Therapeutic conversations, grounded in the clinician's facilitating beliefs about families, have the potential to change not only the biology of the family members but the biology of the clinician as well.

We, as clinicians, are privileged to work with families who act as teachers and guides about illness suffering and offer untold opportunities for reciprocal learning about illness and resilience in the face of life's challenges (Tapp, 2001). The clinician's core beliefs about illness and illness suffering, in particular, are examined next in Chapter 4, Beliefs about Illness.

References

Andersen, T. (1987). The reflecting team: Dialogue and meta-dialogue in clinical work. *Family Process, 26*(4), 415-428.

Andersen, T. (Ed.). (1991). *The reflecting team: Dialogues and dialogue about the dialogues.* New York: W.W. Norton.

Anderson, H., & Goolishian, H.A. (1988). Human systems as linguistic systems: Preliminary and evolving ideas about the implications for clinical theory. *Family Process, 27*(4), 371-393.

Bell, J.M. (1995). The dysfunction of 'dysfunctional' [Editorial]. *Journal of Family Nursing, 1*(3), 235-237.

Bell, J. M. (1998). Rx for certainty in clinical work with families: Insatiable curiosity [Editorial]. *Journal of Family Nursing, 4*(2), 123-126.

Bell, J.M. (2000). Encouraging nurses and families to think interactionally: Revisiting the usefulness of the circular pattern diagram [Editorial]. *Journal of Family Nursing, 6*(3), 203-209.

Bell, J.M. (2009). Family Systems Nursing: Re-examined [Editorial]. *Journal of Family Nursing, 15*(2), 123-129.

Bohn, U., Wright, L.M., & Moules, N.J. (2003). A family systems nursing interview following a myocardial infarction: The power of commendations. *Journal of Family Nursing*, 9(2), 151-165.

Cecchin, G. (1987). Hypothesizing, circularity, and neutrality revisited: An invitation to curiosity. *Family Process, 25*(4), 405-413.

Duncan, B. L. (2005). *What's right with you: Debunking dysfunction and changing your life.* Deerfield Beach, FL: Health Communications.

Engel, G. (1980). The clinical application of the biopsychosocial model. *American Journal of Psychiatry, 137*, 535-544.

Feeley, N., & Gottlieb, L. N. (2000). Nursing approaches for working with family strengths and resources. *Journal of Family Nursing, 6*(1), 9-24.

Fisher, L. (2006). Research on the family and chronic disease among adults Major trends and directions. *Families, Systems, & Health, 24*(4), 373-380.

Fisher, L., & Weihs, K. L. (2000). Can addressing family relationships improve outcomes in chronic disease? *Journal of Family Practice, 49*, 561-566.

Hartman, A., & Laird, J. (1983). *Family-centered social work practice.* New York: Free Press.

Houger Limacher, L., & Wright, L.M. (2003). Commendations: Listening to the silent side of a family intervention. *Journal of Family Nursing*, 9(2), 130-135.

Houger Limacher, L., & Wright, L.M. (2006). Exploring the therapeutic family intervention of commendations: Insights from research. *Journal of Family Nursing, 12*, 307-331.

Houger Limacher, L. (2008). Locating relationships at the heart of commending practices. *Journal of Systemic Therapies, 27*(4), 90-105.

Kazak, A.E., Simms, S., & Rourke, M.T. (2002). Family systems practice in pediatric psychology. *Journal of Pediatric Psychology, 27*(2), 133-143.

Levac, A.M.C., Wright, L.M., & Leahey, M. (1997). Children and families: Models for assessment and intervention. In J.A. Fox (Ed.), *Primary health care of children* (pp. 3-13). New York: Mosby.

Maturana, H.R. (1998). *Biology of cognition and biology of love.* [Videotapes of a workshop presented at the Faculty of Nursing, University of Calgary in 1998]. (Available from www.janicembell.com)

Maturana, H.R., & Varela, F.J. (1992). *The tree of knowledge: The biological roots of human understanding* (rev. ed.). Boston: Shambhala.

McDaniel, S.H., Belar, C.D., Schroeder, C., Hargrove, D.S., & Freeman, E.L. (2002). A training curriculum for professional psychologists in primary care. *Professional Psychology, Research and Practice, 33*(1), 65-72.

McDaniel, S.H., Hepworth, J., & Doherty, W.J. (1992). *Medical family therapy: A biopsychosocial approach to families with health problems.* New York: Basic Books.

McGoldrick, M., Gerson, R., & Petry, S. (2008). *Genograms: Assessment and intervention* (3rd ed.). New York: W.W. Norton.

Rempel, G.R., Neufeld, A., & Kushner, K.E. (2007). Interactive use of genograms and ecomaps in family caregiving research. *Journal of Family Nursing, 13(*4), 403-419.

Robinson, C.A. (1998). Women, families, chronic illness, and nursing interventions: From burden to balance. *Journal of Family Nursing, 4*(3), 271-290.

Tapp, D.M. (2001). Conserving the vitality of suffering: Addressing family constraints to illness conversations. *Nursing Inquiry, 8*(4), 254-263.

Tomm, K. (1980). Towards a cybernetic systems approach to family therapy at the University of Calgary. In D.S. Freeman (Ed.), *Perspectives on family therapy* (pp. 3-18). Vancouver, British Columbia, Canada: Butterworth.

Walsh, F. (2002). Family resilience: A framework for clinical practice. *Family Process, 42*(1), 1-18.

Walsh, F. (2006). *Strengthening family resilience* (2nd ed.). New York: Guilford.

Weakland, J.H. (1977). Family "somatics"--a neglected edge. *Family Process, 16*(3), 263-272.

Weihs, K., Fisher, L., & Baird, M. (2002). Families, health, and behavior: A section of the Commissioned Report by the Committee on Health and Behavior: Research, Practice, and Policy, Division of Neuroscience and Behavioral

Health and Division of Health Promotion and Disease Prevention, Institute of Medicine, National Academy of Sciences. *Families, Systems, & Health, 20*(1), 7-46.

Wright, L.M., & Leahey, M. (1990). Trends in the nursing of families. *Journal of Advanced Nursing, 15*, 148-154.

Wright, L.M., & Leahey, M. (2009). *Nurses and families: A guide to family assessment and intervention* (5th ed.). Philadelphia: F.A. Davis.

Wright, L.M., & Levac, A.M. (1992). The non-existence of non-compliant families: The influence of Humberto Maturana. *Journal of Advanced Nursing, 17*, 913-917.

CHAPTER FOUR
Beliefs about Illness

"The more serious the illness, the more important it is for you to fight back, mobilizing all your resources—spiritual, emotional, intellectual, physical."
—Norman Cousins

Benj and Didi had been married for twenty-five years when Benj was unexpectedly diagnosed with colon cancer. "I believe my husband's cancer is due to his work life, working too many hours a week for too many years, and a refusal to talk about his problems or worries," Didi sighed. In this first meeting with their clinician, Dr. Lorraine M. Wright (LMW), the husband glared back at his wife and said: "You want this illness to be *my* fault! Well, it's just bad luck for three generations of men in my family. My father, grandfather, and now me have all had colon cancer. This illness was in my genes, Didi, and it would not have mattered if I retired at twenty-five years old, I still would have colon cancer." Benj had a dramatically different idea and belief about the etiology of his cancer—that it was due to a family history of colon cancer.

Sadly, the differences in their beliefs about etiology occupied all their conversations and determined the volume of their discussions. Their preoccupation about the cause of the illness dramatically interfered with their ability to move on to how they could unite as a couple to manage this illness. Didi's beliefs about the origin of the colon cancer implied that Benj could have done something to prevent the illness. Benj withdrew from this kind of blame and isolated himself by watching TV and working long hours out of town. Of course, the more he withdrew, the more Didi worried and expressed this worry through anger and frustration.

Later in the meeting, the clinician explored the husband's beliefs about his prognosis. Benj revealed that he had expressed his fears about his prognosis to his physician because he knew he would not be blamed. This disclosure escalated Didi's suffering as evidenced by her comment, "That makes me feel even more sad and frustrated. I, too, have fears, you know. Who do I have to talk to when you ignore me?"

This clinical vignette exemplifies well that what one believes about their illness contributes dramatically to how one experiences the illness and the effects on their relationships. In the *Illness Beliefs Model*, we assert that beliefs shape our experience with illness far more than the disease itself.

Benj and Didi were stuck in the "sin of certainty" about the etiology of the illness. There was no room for support, understanding, sharing of fears, and/or compassion. Each of their experiences of the illness was unfolding around their beliefs rather than around their relationship.

Even with the same disease, no two people have the same experience, whether it is the common cold or Crohn's disease. Two people with the same serious illness can have totally different experiences of that condition because their beliefs shape their perceptions and interpretations. For this reason, when discussing the impact of an illness on an individual and their relationships, we prefer to use the language of "experiencing an illness" rather than "having an illness." How persons experience an illness depends on the beliefs they have embraced prior to their illness experience, as well as the beliefs that evolve through the experience of the illness. The beliefs that family members hold are often reconstructed after the experience of an illness; conversely, family member beliefs influence and shape the processes, management, and outcomes of illness.

For example, how persons treat a cold depends on their beliefs concerning how they "caught" the cold in the first place. If you believe that a cold is due to inadequate rest and long working hours, you will probably treat the cold very differently than if you believe it is related to a recent loss. If you believe that the best remedy for a cold is to rest, drink plenty of fluids, and take vitamin C, you will probably follow that regime when experiencing a cold. But if the treatment remedy does not work, will you maintain your belief about the etiology? Will you be more or less open to other treatment remedies? Many factors influence what people consider treatment options when their original beliefs about the etiology and the treatment of an illness have been challenged. Benj and Didi's differences in the cause of the colon cancer prevented them from uniting around ideas for healing and treatment.

How families respond to a particular diagnosis also affects how the illness will be experienced. Rolland (1999) offers an example of what can inadvertently occur in a family if a patient's illness is seen as "his problem" versus "our challenge." If the condition becomes defined as the affected patient's problem, a fundamental split occurs between the patient, well partner, and other family members. This phenomena of a couple being divided when they do not view the problem as a "we" problem had certainly happened with Benj and Didi. They were not united at all in the illness being "our challenge."

By introducing the concept of "our challenge" early on, the health care provider "provides an opportunity for all family members to examine cultural and multigenerational beliefs about the rights and privileges of ill and well family members" (Rolland, 1999, p. 258). An alternate example of a positive coalition is when family members join together to help another family member stop smoking or stop drinking alcohol. They collectively voice their concerns to the individual and their intent to provide support and help. Therefore it can be useful for health care providers to embrace the belief that illness is a family affair and to offer this notion to individuals and families in their care.

Another influence on individual and family members' experience of illness is the health care providers' beliefs and how they play out as they offer their ideas of diagnosis, treatment, and healing. For example, with Benj and Didi, the clinician asked the couple whether it was important that they come to an agreement about the origin of the illness in order to move on. They adamantly said "yes" and then asked the clinician what she believed. These kinds of questions prove challenging to clinicians, but open a possibility for offering a more facilitating illness belief for the couple to consider. If LMW had aligned with one spouse's beliefs over another, it would have alienated the other spouse and reduced the therapeutic leverage of the clinician. Instead, the clinician cautiously offered the possibility that *both* the husband and wife's views and beliefs about the origin of the illness might be correct or possible. Surprisingly, they responded with "Why didn't we think of that?" The clinician was able to offer the couple a more facilitating belief that "both of you could be correct about the reasons" but then built on that facilitating belief by offering even another idea.

LMW noted from her previous clinical experience and the work of Karen Skerrett (2003) that "couples do better in managing their illness when they join together and view their illness as a 'we' experience than a 'solo' experience for each spouse." This couple opened space to the clinicians' beliefs and ideas, which proved to be a positive turning point in the first session. However, if the clinician had chosen to unite with one spouse, it may have resulted in a further escalation of the lack of support and isolation of these spouses in their experience of this illness.

Beliefs are also intricately intertwined with familial and socioeconomic contexts. The research of Corbet-Owen and Kruger (2001) found that the meaning pregnancy had for the women in their study not only determined the meaning of their pregnancy loss but also impacted their emotional needs at the time of the loss. For example, if a mother was very happy about being pregnant and felt devastated by her miscarriage, then her emotional needs would differ dramatically from those of another mother who didn't want to be pregnant and felt relieved by her miscarriage. Feelings about pregnancy loss ranged from feelings of devastation to relief.

The following figure presents the five beliefs about illness that we have embraced in our clinical practice. These beliefs enable more collaborative relationships with individuals and families and are guided by the *Illness Beliefs Model*.

⊛ **Figure 4. Illness Beliefs Model: Beliefs about Illness**

- **Health and illness are subjective judgments made by observers**

- **Illness beliefs and families are linked in a reciprocal relationship**

- **Illness narratives include stories of suffering that need to be told**

- **Increasing possibilities for managing illness increases possibilities for healing**

- **Illness arises and is influenced by interference with emotional dynamics in relationships**

Health and Illness are Subjective Judgments Made by Observers

Who decides when someone is well or ill? Health and illness are subjective judgments made by observers. Observers may include the ill person, family members, friends, and/or health care providers. The decision about health or illness is too often a unilateral decision made by health care providers, primarily physicians or nurses. A diagnosis is made using a combination of clinical expertise, medical science, and intuition; however, it becomes meaningful only when placed in a relational context, i.e., who offers the news about the diagnosis, who is present to receive the news, the experience of receiving the news, and the reactions of others when the news is shared.

It is also important to consider the professional context in which diagnoses are made. Health care providers may be exquisitely sensitive to selecting a diagnosis that is billable to third-party payers or that fits with current taxonomies for diagnostic assessment and illness classification such as the DSM IV TR (American Psychiatric Association, 2000). The context in which health care providers offer treatment, as well as their professional lens, may invite some to pronounce a particular diagnosis with regularity. For example, how is it that attention deficit hyperactivity disorder (ADHD) has become the diagnosis of choice for troubled children in certain areas of the country? Amundson (1998) has argued that an illness classification such as DSM IV TR "...is simply a collection of tales of suffering and complaint" (p. 3). However, it is interesting to note that the professional language of diagnosis does not often allow *illness suffering* to arise as a legitimate health concern.

A diagnosis is a social contract that occurs when one person (the medical or nursing expert) affixes a classification to another (the identified patient). At this point, the person pronounced with a diagnosis, his or her family members, and the health care providers enter into a "contract" regarding the diagnosis. The diagnosis implies that a cluster of signs and symptoms exists, places those manifestations in context, gives them meaning, and suggests a treatment.

As all health care providers know, however, it is difficult to have all parties in the contract agree on all aspects of the diagnosis. All diagnoses are subject, therefore, to negotiation and even disagreement. Initially, family members may accept a diagnosis of a myocardial infarction, but the patient may not. In other cases, family members may accept the label of the disease but disagree with the proposed treatment. Part of the social contract of the diagnosis requires family members to think of themselves in relationship to the illness. But what does it mean that a diagnosis becomes part of the family?

One family we worked with had an adolescent son diagnosed with a life-threatening illness. They explained their ability to cope by saying, "God knew that our family could handle it. Other families would have fallen apart." The meaning of the diagnosis to family members is important to determine. Some families perceive certain illnesses as a challenge, whereas other families consider the same illness a punishment or a threat. Some diagnoses unite families ("everyone in our family has hypertension"), whereas other diagnoses initially may estrange family members (i.e. sex addiction). It is this uniqueness that opens up possibilities for individuals who do not let their illnesses limit their world, but rather use their illnesses to connect with and inspire the world. The diversity of responses to and beliefs about diagnosis and treatment extends to health care providers, who rarely present a united voice regarding the management of an illness.

The difficulty of health care providers and family members coming to agreement on medical diagnoses is understandable, as there are many competing judgments, opinions, and beliefs. This is especially true in terms of agreeing on treatment because of the phenomenal impact of complementary or alternative health practices. Health care providers in Western culture are frequently critical of alternative or complementary treatments that do not fall within accepted beliefs about what is helpful. However, both family members and health care providers are adopting more complementary health practices for illness prevention and treatment.

Conventional medicine still gets top marks for dealing with trauma and infection. But for many other health problems, alternative and complementary health practices are gaining an overwhelming acceptance based on the belief that these practices take a more holistic approach to health and healing. Alternative health practices frequently offer more hope when the limits of more conservative medical treatment are exhausted. Beliefs about diagnosis and treatment vary, therefore. Many individuals use home remedies or complementary practices such as herbal medicines and acupuncture that they do not readily reveal to health care providers. One family reported to us that they would not tell their neurologist about acupuncture treatment to help with pain management of multiple sclerosis for fear the physician would be critical of this practice. What is deemed erroneous for one person may truly be a lifesaver for another.

Health and illness are distinctions that are brought forth through our relationships and languaging with each other. Distinctions such as health and illness are subjective judgments made by observers (i.e., individuals experiencing illness, family members, and health care providers). In the *Illness Beliefs Model*, the focus is not only on the beliefs held by a variety of observers but, most importantly, on whether there is agreement or disagreement between the beliefs of the major stakeholders who share a relational context.

The following verbatim transcript is from a telephone interview between Dr. Humberto Maturana (1988) and Dr. Lorraine Wright (LMW), illuminating Maturana's ideas about health and illness as distinctions of observers and how differences between observers can be mediated:

LMW: *Another question that we have been struggling with is that as nurses we encounter persons experiencing illness and we have been wondering if* *you perceive illness as a perturbation and also do you, when you say that nothing is an accident, do you also feel the same way about illness?*

MATURANA: *In illness there are several aspects. One is of course the assessment that there is illness. The assessment is made by someone, it could be a physician, or it could be the person him, or herself, it could be a nurse, someone must make the assessment for the illness to occur. That means that there is a situation which one considers an inadequate variance with respect to what one considers to be a normal or healthy flow. That, of course, puts the responsibility of the assessment on the person that makes it and the person that accepts it. Now, if the person who is considered to be ill accepts such assessment, then a conversation for treatment or whatever takes place about illness. Now, in the instant in which one makes the assessment of illness, one is claiming that the flow of structural coupling of this person within the domain in which one is assessing is inadequate, this person is flowing in a different domain of structural coupling. What one indeed does, is to claim that the person considered ill is flowing in a domain of structural coupling different from that which one considers should be the case.*

For example, let us suppose a tumor. I have a tumor and I live with it in perfect harmony; I am not ill. Somebody else can say, "Do something about this tumor. This is going to kill you." And I say, "Oh, no. Forget it. I mean it doesn't bother me. I'm quite all right with it. I do not even notice it." From my perspective there is no illness and from the perspective of the other person there is illness, but in the instant in which you make the assessment, you don't make the assessment in a vacuum. You make the assessment in a distinction of the structural dynamics of the person and so the assessment reveals you and the person assessed to the extent that you have adequately grasped the structure of the person and the domain of structural coupling in which you look at him or her. As one makes the distinction of an entity in a particular domain of existence, one brings forth implicitly its whole history of the person if one knows how to look at it. It's telling you how the structure of this entity is now and hence what kind of history this entity may have lived if it is an entity of this particular kind. Now, in human beings, it has particular significance because the flow of our body structure is not independent of how we live both materially and spiritually.

We human beings exist in cultures as networks of coordinations of languaging and emotions, so it is the manner we live in a culture that has certain consequences in the manner of our flow as it modulates or interlaces with its own internal structural dynamics. So, at any moment, one is an expression or revelation of how one has lived and how one feels in one's living. This is why a good clinical eye allows one to see much more than a particular symptom in a person. If one knows how to look, one can see almost in a glance the psychological and physiological history of a person, and that knowing must be learned.

LMW: *One of the things that we experience in nursing, once a particular illness has been assessed or diagnosed, is then trying to have patients comply to certain things that we think will make their life better in terms of their health. Patients aren't always willing to do the kinds of things that we ask them to do. This brings us to the notion of instructive interaction and we have been very curious about this as we have studied your ideas. How can we impart knowledge to patients about their health without getting into the trap of instructive interaction?*

MATURANA: *You cannot do instructive interactions. The most that you can do is to talk to the patient and seduce him or her to a reflection that will allow that person to accept or realize the validity of your assessment of illness, and see that there are certain things that can be done. At the same time there is a responsibility that the doctor or nurse must accept, since she or he will never convince another person to take a particular medicine if she or he is convinced or appears convinced of its value. Understanding cannot be forced.*

Illness Beliefs and Families are Linked in a Reciprocal Relationship

When illness arises, individuals and family members spend much time thinking about and formulating their beliefs about etiology, diagnosis, prognosis, and treatment of illness. The family members' responses to a diagnosis vary widely from shock to anger to sadness to relief. However, through our clinical practice, we have learned that more often the ill individual responds to their *family's* responses to the illness than to the condition itself. This idea has been powerfully demonstrated in a classic study by Reiss, Gonzalez, and Kramer (1986), who suggested that families experiencing end stage renal disease and are too emotionally close may inadvertently precipitate death in the sick family member. Death may represent an "arrangement" between the family and the patient: The patient dies so that the family may live. This is an extreme example, but perhaps the only "reasonable" response of the patient to the family's feelings of grief and burden.

Fekete, Stephens, Mickelson, and Druley (2007) point out the importance of circularity and reciprocity between illness and family functioning in their study of 243 women experiencing lupus flare-ups and their husbands. They found that more spousal emotional (empathic) support was interpreted as the husband's being more emotionally responsive, which in turn was associated with the wife's greater sense of wellbeing. In contrast, more problematic (minimizing) spousal support was interpreted as the husband's being less emotionally responsive, which in turn was associated with the wife's poorer sense of well-being. These findings have large implications of how beliefs and perceptions of family member's support or lack of it can directly affect the experience of illness.

Illness experiences can also invite closer family relationships, provide an opportunity to resolve old issues or conflicts, and promote healing. A couple in their mid-forties was interviewed about their experience of working with our clinical team in the Family Nursing Unit. The husband had experienced a life-threatening cardiac illness as a result of a congenital defect that had only become apparent four years previously. It was only after the husband had recuperated from numerous cardiac surgeries to stabilize his cardiac illness that his wife of fourteen years began to show signs of extreme weariness and decreased ability to cope. The couple was interviewed about the therapeutic conversations they had participated in together as a couple at the Family Nursing Unit. When asked about what was most helpful, the couple tearfully reported that they had never had a chance to talk about their lengthy illness experience together as a couple:

HUSBAND: *Like we would talk about it [the illness], but we never got too deep, you know.*

WIFE: *It was coming to the Family Nursing Unit because before we'd take little things out on each other because we were frustrated with the situation and not being able to emotionally deal with it and with each other. Coming to the Family Nursing Unit made me look at our relationship differently. We know we're going to be together forever, that's a given, but it's on a deeper level now than it was before we came to the Family Nursing Unit. We had always managed but on a surface level; somehow we coped day to day but when we went to the Family Nursing Unit, we saw how strong our relationship really is.*

Illness affects each family member, and family members in turn affect the healing process. Families adapt better when they possess or embrace facilitating beliefs about their illness experience. In our clinical work with families, therefore, we focus on understanding the reciprocal interactions between illness beliefs of family members and between family members' beliefs and health care providers' beliefs. Family members' beliefs, and subsequent reactions to illness, can significantly influence the decision to initiate or delay treatment, the perceptions of the seriousness of symptoms of the illness, treatment compliance, and satisfaction with the treatment outcome.

Consequently, we are always curious about what illness beliefs family members have about their health and illness and how they match with our beliefs as health care providers. As the family's, and our own, facilitating and constraining beliefs are drawn forth, we co-evolve new distinctions and new beliefs about health and illness. A health care provider's judgment or assessment of any family is not the "truth" about that family, but rather one subjective judgment from an observer perspective influenced by the clinician's core beliefs about illness and families.

Illness Narratives Include Stories of Suffering That Need to be Told

A family consisting of a 58-year-old mother and her 34-year-old daughter requested a clinical consultation at the Family Nursing Unit. They were seeking an opportunity to discuss their anguish related to their 72-year-old husband/father's life-threatening illness and their exhaustion as caregivers. The husband/father was too ill to be able to attend the outpatient clinic. The wife was the primary caregiver, but the daughter continued to live at home to assist her mother with this responsibility. Both women looked haggard, drawn, and beaten down. The clinician (LMW) invited the mother and daughter to tell their experience of this illness and the impact on their lives, marriage, mother-daughter and father-daughter relationships.

Their response to this invitation was a heart-wrenching telling of an illness story of devotion, exhaustion, guilt, and despair. At one moment in the interview, the clinician (LMW) reflected that their illness experience and long term care-giving entailed a lot of "suffering." The clinician then asked if this was an appropriate word to describe their illness experience. The daughter immediately responded that this was "the perfect word" to describe their experience. At the end of the consultation, the mother and daughter both looked visibly different, more animated and less drawn. They even sounded different by speaking in a more confident tone—no weepiness—and seemed to have brought forth a new resilience to return home and continue to care for their very ill husband/father.

They attributed that one major reason for this dramatic softening of their emotional suffering in just one session was due to being "really heard" and "understood" as they told their illness story. By the clinician inviting, witnessing, and validating their illness suffering, she triggered hope and healing for this devoted and loving mother and daughter.

This clinical example illustrates that illness frequently changes lives and relationships forever. Those who suffer from serious illness, loss, or disability need comfort, hope, and above all, the knowledge and reassurance that they are still cherished and that the life one is living and has lived is and has been worthwhile. These needs fuel the telling of one's illness narrative. Illness narratives include stories of suffering that need to be told, witnessed, and heard. In our clinical experience, however, we are astounded that families seem conditioned primarily to relate the medical narrative—stories of medications, diets, symptoms and surgeries—when speaking within the health care provider culture. The medical narrative of the disease is very different from the illness narrative of how this illness has affected their lives and relationships. Their inability or hesitancy to tell their illness narrative powerfully attests to the need of clinical work to provide opportunities to invite illness narratives.

When someone is newly diagnosed with diabetes, a chronic disease, much of the conversation between patient and health care providers focuses on symptoms, such as excessive thirst and frequency and urgency of urination. The hypothesis of diabetes is then confirmed by medical science through such tests as the fasting blood sugar. Following diagnosis by a physician, the conversation broadens to include other health care providers and switches to topics of diet, exercise, oral medication, and perhaps even insulin. These conversations are reasonable and necessary; however, following the diagnosis, patients and their families live predominantly within the domain of *illness* rather than disease or condition. To limit the therapeutic conversation to the aforementioned topics is to limit healing. Chronic illnesses are rarely cured, but they are managed through individual and family effort, resilience, diligence, and embracing facilitating beliefs.

Kleinman (1988), who is credited with the term illness narratives, offered a useful definition to describe a person's experience within the illness domain, in contrast to the domain of disease:

> By invoking the term illness, I mean to conjure up the innately human experience of symptoms and suffering. Illness refers to how the sick person and the members of the family or wider social network perceive, live with, and respond to symptoms and disability. (p. 3)

The illness experience is distinguished and drawn forth within the family and between the family and health care providers through conversations, both social and therapeutic. In the situation of a male, father, and husband with diabetes, the conversation would shift to how he and other family members experience his illness: What has been the biggest change in his life since the diagnosis of diabetes? How much does diabetes affect his sexual relationship with his wife? What response of his wife and children to the diabetes has been the most helpful? A focus on such issues broadens and shifts the conversation within the family and between the family and health care provider from the medical narrative to the illness narrative.

In the *Illness Beliefs Model*, we try to create a trusting environment for therapeutic conversations that invites open expression of family members' fears, anger, suffering, and sadness as well as their beliefs about their illness experiences (for more information see Chapter 7: Creating a Context for Changing Beliefs). Robinson's (1994) study examining the process and outcomes of interventions within our clinical practice in the Family Nursing Unit revealed that the clinicians' acts of bringing the family together and creating a sense of comfort and trust were the fundamental moves that enabled family members to convey their illness experiences. Providing the opportunity for each family member to talk about the impact of the illness on the family and, reciprocally, the influence of the family on the illness, gave validation and voice to their experiences. This conversation is different from limiting or constraining family stories to topics of symptoms, medication, and physical treatment, that is, to the medical narrative.

Inviting, listening to, acknowledging, witnessing, and documenting stories of illness suffering provides a powerful validation of an important human experience. By providing a context for the sharing among family members of their illness experiences, intense emotions are legitimized and illness beliefs are uncovered. Through the telling of the illness narrative, often the patient and family members can begin to make sense of illness suffering and draw forth new facilitating beliefs.

The goal of the *Illness Beliefs Model* is to soften or heal emotional, spiritual, and/or physical suffering. One beginning effort to soften suffering is to acknowledge that suffering exists and understand the beliefs that may invite suffering. Wright (2005, 2007, 2008), in an expanded understanding of the link between illness beliefs, suffering, and spirituality, developed the Trinity Model. She offers a useful definition of suffering:

> Physical, emotional, or spiritual anguish, pain, or distress. Experiences of suffering can include serious illness that alters one's life and relationships as one knew them; forced exclusion from everyday life; the strain of trying to endure; longing to love or be loved; acute or chronic pain; and conflict, anguish, or interference with love in relationships. (Wright, 2005, p. 3)

A discourse of illness suffering frequently opens up a discourse of spirituality (Wright, 2005). Positive responses and softening in emotional, spiritual, and physical suffering have convinced us of the necessity to invite family members to tell their illness narratives. This is accomplished by moving beyond social conversations with individuals and families about the illness to inviting purposeful therapeutic conversations. We direct the conversation, using the *Illness Beliefs Model*, in a manner that we hope will give voice to the human experiences of suffering, loss, and grief, as well as the beliefs that underpin these experiences.

Illness narratives, however, are not limited to only experiences of illness suffering. They also include the experiences of courage, hope, growth, and love. They also include stories of strength, tenacity, and tenderness. Health care providers are in a privileged position to hear and affirm illness narratives. By acknowledging illness narratives, we engage in the essential, ethical, and moral practice of recognizing the ill person and their family members as suffering others. In our clinical practice, we also want to open possibilities, through our therapeutic conversations, for recognizing the ill person and other family members as the heroic other, the joyful other, the giving other, the receiving other, the compassionate other, the passionate other, and the strengthened other. We want to open space for a breadth of human experiences with illness and the beliefs which shape these experiences to be spoken by each family member.

Increasing Possibilities for Managing Illness Increases Possibilities for Healing

As clinicians, it is important to examine our own beliefs about the place of power and control in illness. Some health care providers are strong proponents of assisting individuals and families to gain control, or mastery, over their illness. Health care providers even further assert that if one has control over one's life, one behaves differently by making choices instead of being the passive recipient of medical care or considering oneself the victim of bad luck or bad genes. Other health care providers take a slightly different stand on the issue of control, suggesting that most people do not appreciate how much our bodies heal themselves rather than by external controls such as doctors, drugs, or surgery.

Because we are aware of all these professional and personal beliefs about being in control, being out of control, external control, and internal control, we have found it useful in our clinical work using the *Illness Beliefs Model* to ask persons what their preferred goal is. Would they like to control, submit to, overcome, or live alongside their illness? Simply asking this question invites a reflection about beliefs, about control, and perhaps an awareness of greater possibilities for control. We have found that asking these types of questions often challenges a person's limiting beliefs about control and invites more facilitating beliefs that provide a way to escape the predominant societal belief that the only way to manage an illness is to control it.

The notion of controlling an illness is intertwined with the belief about what needs to be healed. Proponents of both conventional and complementary healing approaches have strong ideas about how healing occurs. One dominant belief is that the treatment of illness involves the restoring of the balance of power, either by weakening the power of the disease or by strengthening the victim's power. An example of strengthening the victim's power is provided by the case of a woman receiving chemotherapy for treatment of colon cancer. When she was asked what her beliefs were about her healing, she stated that she believed 40% of her healing was due to the medication (chemotherapy), 40% to what she and her friends and family were doing for her, 10% to interventions by nurses, and 10% to assistance by physicians.

We have experienced that the very act of inquiring about beliefs about healing draws awareness to the person of their own individual resources. One thing this woman experiencing colon cancer did to purposely assist her healing was to diminish external negative influences. She stopped watching or listening to the news on television or radio. Her belief was, "I cannot worry about global things because I have to put my energies into healing myself. I only have so much energy, and it has to go into getting well." She was focused on strengthening her own power and control.

The possibility of living alongside illness seems to be a more "collaborative" and manageable option than controlling illness. With many illnesses, living alongside takes less energy and is probably more effective than trying to overcome or completely control an illness. The crucial issue here, we believe, is to present possibilities to family members to help them decide how they would like to manage their illness. Perhaps the very act of presenting options, or possibilities, about how to manage illness is itself one way of increasing an individual's control.

Cultural and societal beliefs may influence how people manage illness.

One striking example of the influence of a belief about the management of illness in our culture is the paradigm of control. When illness is experienced, there is frequently an accompanying North American cultural belief that it's bad to be out of control and good to be in control. Frequently, we attribute catching a cold to a belief that our lives are "out of control" and therefore we are susceptible to illness. Commonly heard phrases about illness are "my diabetes is out of control" or "I'm going to get my cholesterol levels under control." Individuals describe how they are going to "fight and conquer the cancer," which is another way of languaging the belief about gaining control over disease.

What if someone is not able to endure the experience of illness and loses control? When the experience of illness becomes unbearable, behavioral manifestations of losing control include verbal and physical aggression. "Losing it" is considered unacceptable behavior; family and institutional sanctions are frequently brought against these individuals. Unfortunately, the issue of losing control is problematic for ill persons and their families because of the emphasis and demand placed on being in control, even during times of extreme suffering.

This predominant societal belief—that one must be in control—ignores the spiritual and subjective sides of the illness experience and limits possibilities for healing. We have found it useful to offer the additional possibilities of "living alongside illness" or "putting illness in its place" as other ways of dealing with illness, as opposed to the "control or eliminate" options.

Illness Arises and is Influenced by Interference with Emotional Dynamics in Relationships

We have all experienced that bad things can happen to good people. We are also well aware that there are people who breach every rule of good health but do not become seriously ill. Frequently, clinicians explain this by saying, "It will catch up with them one day," or "They must have good genes," or "They're just lucky." The particular structure of such an individual may be offset by other variables such as loving conversations, prayer, a sense of well-being, and genuine satisfaction and contentment with one's life. Furthermore, some individuals experience long standing conflictual relationships, dissatisfaction with their lives, and poor health habits, but nothing untoward happens to them. These situations invite health care providers to maintain their curiosity about what triggers illness and what makes symptoms and disease disappear, that is, what triggers healing.

Some health care providers believe that diseases are hard-wired; they just happen. At times our bodies act up, break down, refuse to function, and get sick without ever consulting us. Our bodies are susceptible to genetic diseases and prone to infection. We also believe that many diseases arise from or are influenced by particular kinds of interactions in which families engage over the course of numerous years that interfere with fundamental emotional dynamics (Maturana, 1988). Family members respond to such emotional interference based on their own bio-psychosocial-spiritual structures, which consist of their own unique genetic makeup (phylogenetic history) and history of interactions or past structural changes (ontogenetic history).

If someone with a genetic predisposition to a particular disease has been involved for numerous years with conversations containing criticisms and accusations (see Chapter 2), this combination may trigger a particular disease to occur. We emphasize, however, that we do not concur with representatives of health movements who purport that thinking more positively or being more hopeful can prevent or relieve illness. These ideas put undue pressure on ill people and can draw forth immense guilt when things go wrong despite efforts to be positive. The emergence of disease is not a sign of ethical, moral, or spiritual weakness. But it could be a sign that there has been interference with fundamental emotional dynamics in their relationships.

Humberto Maturana (1988) offered the idea in his phone conversation with Lorraine Wright that the basic emotion for health and healing is love: "The only thing that I know is that love is a fundamental emotion in human beings." Maturana further proposed that "most human diseases, most human suffering, arises from interference with these fundamental emotions". *Love* is defined as the ability to open space for the existence of another or acceptance of the other beside us in daily living (Maturana &Varela, 1992). Love is a biological dynamic with deep roots. The sixteenth-century physician Paracelsus offered, "the main reason for healing is love." The importance of love in the healing process is a complex notion that need not be trivialized by health care providers. Neither should sick people feel guilty in the name of love for not being well. It is instead important to appreciate the profound connection between emotions (particularly love) and biology and their influence on each other.

In the early 1950s, a sample of male undergraduate students was enrolled in the longitudinal Harvard Stress Mastery Study. Detailed medical records and psychological histories gathered thirty-five years later found that 91% of the men, who reported thirty-five years earlier the lack of a warm relationship with their mothers, had diagnosed illnesses in their lives (coronary artery disease, hypertension, duodenal ulcers, and alcoholism) compared with 45% who perceived warmth and closeness with their mothers. A similar association between the relationship with their fathers and future illnesses was also found (Russek & Schwartz, 1997).

The power of the presence or absence of love to change biology is legendary; it is built into folklore, country and western songs, everyday experience, and even research. John Gottman who conducted renowned marital interaction research for thirty-five years with over 3000 couples, found that women in ailing marriages experienced physiological arousal and subsequent illness when their husbands showed a pattern of stonewalling and withdrawal from marital conflict, or, in particular, showed contempt toward their wives. Gottman and his team also found that as marital interaction became aversive, the cascade of distance, isolation, and loneliness had a negative effect on the husbands' health (Gottman, 1999; Gottman & DeClaire, 2001).

There is a powerful and reciprocal connection between health and the nature of a person's long-term relationships (Post & Neimark, 2007). It is not just the length of a relationship that is important, but the quality of the relationship. One study found that a spouse who suppresses his or her anger when verbally attacked by the other has a higher risk of early death compared to spouses who express their anger (Harburg, Kaciroti, & Gleiberman, 2008).

In our own clinical work with families using the *Illness Beliefs Model*, we have been amazed at how physical and emotional symptoms diminish or disappear when familial conflict is reduced and when powerful loving conversations and emotions return. We believe that illness often appears to "strike" because we cannot see or know all that may have led up to its appearance. If we were able to peer into one another's organs or cells throughout our lifetimes, we could monitor the effects of our relationships and life experiences on the functioning of our organs and cells. Although we agree that disease can "just happen," we wonder if we would notice organs or cells malfunctioning when the emotional dynamics in our relationships were disturbed. Could a change in our biology be observed if we were able to open space to the existence of another, that is, if we were able to love? And what changes would be noted if we reciprocally experienced love from another?

A family sought help at the Family Nursing Unit to resolve long-standing marital conflict and resentment. The couple reported trying a marital separation and having several previous, unsatisfactory experiences with marital counseling in their attempts to resolve their conflict. The wife was suffering with terminal cancer and wanted to resolve these marital issues with her husband before she died. We wondered if she would be free to die following resolution of the emotional conflict and, therefore, wondered about the pace of therapy. If the couple resolved things quickly, would she die quickly? The wife's question to the clinician summarized her dilemma well: "Why had a relationship that started out so precious become so very destructive?" We saw this couple three times over three weeks. By the third session, the couple was reporting less conflict and increased ability to show caring to each other. The wife commented, "I feel like it's been very special…He's made a much bigger effort to listen." The wife died shortly after the third session. Did her husband's healing words "heal" her and set her free? The husband was seen alone a month later and reported that his wife had died peacefully. He reported that they had been able to forgive each other and had begun to write a new story for their relationship.

Another example (see genogram) of a significant change in the physical and emotional suffering of a family occurred with elderly parents and their 34-year-old son experiencing multiple sclerosis (MS). The parents had moved from Eastern to Western Canada to help care for their son in his home. The parents described much tension in the home, which they attributed to their own caregiver burden and lack of respite. They believed they needed their son's permission and initiation to take a break.

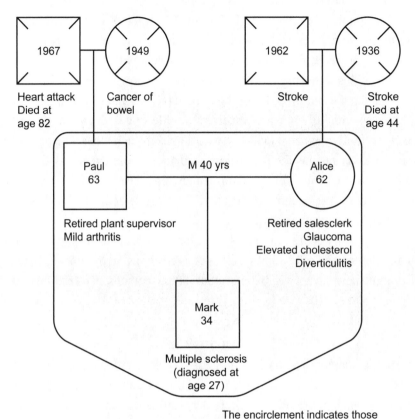

1967
1949
Heart attack
Died at
age 82
Cancer of
bowel

1962
1936
Stroke
Stroke
Died at
age 44

Paul
63
M 40 yrs
Alice
62

Retired plant supervisor
Mild arthritis

Retired salesclerk
Glaucoma
Elevated cholesterol
Diverticulitis

Mark
34

Multiple sclerosis
(diagnosed at
age 27)

The encirclement indicates those
family members who lived together

Figure 5. Genogram: Mark's Family

In her efforts to be helpful to the family, the clinician (LMW) encouraged all family members to tell their illness narratives. Specifically, she invited each family member to describe his or her story of illness suffering. Their narratives unfolded as the clinician conducted a purposeful inquiry through the asking of interventive questions: What has been the biggest surprise about your illness? Has any good come out of this illness? Do you have more influence over your illness, or does your illness have more influence over you? The clinician also highlighted the reciprocity between the illness and the family, that is, the effect of the illness on the family and the influence of the family on the illness. During the conversation, the son drew an important distinction between doing things "in spite of" the illness and "having influence over" the illness.

The clinician's purposeful drawing forth and distinguishing of the illness narratives in this family paved the way for a heart-to-heart conversation about the son's emotional suffering with MS. He had never spoken of his suffering to his parents. By acknowledging and thereby diminishing the emotional suffering of both parents and son, a context was created wherein all family members were able to talk openly about their need for family members to have a vacation from each other. The outcome was positive: respite for the parents and the son and reduced tensions and improved health for all family members. The MS was positively influenced by the occurrence of more loving interactions in the family members' conversations.

Our primary goal as clinicians, therefore, is to bring forth conversations of affirmation and affection as well as conversations of growth and change that invite new or renewed beliefs about illness, persons, and relationships.

Conclusion

In this chapter, we have highlighted that beliefs influence and shape the processes, management, and outcomes of illness. How families experience illness depends more on the beliefs they embrace than what disease has been diagnosed. Illness beliefs, illness suffering, and family functioning are exquisitely intertwined.

The *Illness Beliefs Model* offers core beliefs about illness that shape the therapeutic conversations that the clinician invites and facilitates. For example, a belief that illness is a subjective judgment made by observers invites the clinician to become curious about whether individuals and families believe the diagnoses they have been offered. Inviting individuals and families to tell their illness narratives provides an opportunity to inquire about their illness suffering and the beliefs associated with their suffering.

We believe individuals and family members are the experts on their illness experiences, whereas clinicians have expertise to offer for softening suffering and managing illness. The intertwining of these areas of expertise enables therapeutic change and healing to occur. Beliefs about therapeutic change will be examined next in Chapter 5.

References

American Psychiatric Association. (2000). *Diagnostic and Statistic Manual of Mental Disorders* (4th ed. Text Revision). Washington, DC: Author.

Amundson, J. (1998). Tales of suffering and complaint: Asking DSM IV to do more than it was intended for. *Journal of Systemic Therapies, 17*(3), 1-11.

Corbet-Owen, C., & Kruger, L. (2001). The health system and emotional care: Validating the many meanings of spontaneous pregnancy loss. *Families, Systems, & Health, 19*(4), 411–427.

Fekete, E.M., Stephens, M.A.P., Mickelson, K.D., & Druley, J.A. (2007). Couples' support provision during illness: The role of perceived emotional responsiveness. *Families, Systems, & Health, 25*(2), 204–217.

Gottman, J.M., (1999). *The marriage clinic.* New York: W.W. Norton.

Gottman, J.M., & DeClaire, J., (2001). *The relationship cure.* New York: Crown Publishing.

Harburg, E., Kaciroti, N., & Gleiberman, L. (2008). Marital pair anger coping types may act as an entity to affect mortality: Preliminary findings from a prospective study. *Journal of Family Communication, 8*(1), 44-61.

Kleinman, A. (1988). *The illness narratives: Suffering, healing, and the human condition.* New York: Basic Books

Maturana, H.R. (1988). *Telephone conversation: The Calgary/Chile coupling* [Phone conversation with Dr. Lorraine Wright and graduate students]. (Transcript available from www.lorrainewright.com)

Maturana, H.R., & Varela, F.J. (1992). *The tree of knowledge: The biological roots of human understanding* (rev. ed.). Boston: Shambhala.

Post, S., & Neimark, J. (2007). *Why good things happen to good people.* New York: Broadway Books.

Reiss, D., Gonzalez, S., & Kramer, M. (1986). Family process, chronic illness, and death: On the weakness of strong bonds. *Archives of General Psychiatry, 43*, 795-804.

Robinson, C.A. (1994). *Women, families, chronic illness and nursing interventions: From burden to balance.* Unpublished doctoral dissertation, University of Calgary, Alberta, Canada.

Rolland, J.S. (1999). Parental illness and disability: A family systems framework. *Journal of Family Therapy, 21*(3), 242–267.

Russek, L.G., & Schwartz, G.E. (1997). Feelings of parental caring predict health status in mid-life: A 35-year followup of the Harvard Stress Study. *Journal of Behavioral Health, 20*(1), 1-13.

Skerrett, K. (2003). Couple dialogues with illness: Expanding the "we". *Families, Systems, & Health, 21*(1), 69-81.

Wright, L.M. (2005). *Spirituality, suffering, and illness: Ideas for healing.* Philadelphia: F.A. Davis.

Wright, L.M. (Producer). (2007). *Spirituality, suffering, and illness: Conversations for healing.* [DVD]. (Available from: www.lorrainewright.com)

Wright, L.M. (2008). Softening suffering through spiritual care practices: One possibility for healing families. *Journal of Family Nursing, 14*(4), 394-411.

CHAPTER FIVE
Beliefs about Therapeutic Change

"Given the choice between changing one's mind and proving that change is not necessary, most people get busy on the proof."
—Professor John Kenneth Gailbraith

"The world will be different only if we live differently."
—Humberto Maturana and Francisco Varela

Our lives are filled with experiences that invite, encourage, request, and often require that we change our names, email addresses, weight, clothes, minds, beliefs, and sometimes our hearts. Just like beauty, change is in the eye of the beholder. But what triggers or invites change in clients and clinicians, and what does not? What conditions facilitate change; what constricts change from occurring? Health care providers are always in the business of change to ease the way to healing, yet we often do not understand the process, context, or nature of change. It is our hope that this chapter may illuminate some aspects of therapeutic change so that we can better pave the way for healing to occur.

Maturana and Varela (1992) offer that human beings are describers and observers, constantly observing ourselves and others and thus change: "Everything said is said by an observer to another observer that could be him- or herself" (Maturana, 1988b, p. 27). We not only observe each other's and our own change, we judge and critique it. If there is too much change, too frequently, one is judged as fickle; if there is too little change, too infrequently, one is "rigid." But always we need to ask—"according to whose beliefs is change valued as too much or too little?"

Our societal beliefs about change exist on a continuum. Some observe that change is not desired or is a hopeless pursuit: "Only a wet baby likes change," teases the bumper sticker. "The more things change, the more they stay the same" is a French proverb. Or "If the shoe doesn't fit, must we change the foot?" asks Gloria Steinem.

When we report the same complaint to a friend year after year; when we have the same resolutions every New Year's Eve; when the bathroom scales obnoxiously declare we are still fifteen pounds overweight; when the waiting rooms of outpatient mental health clinics are filled with the same patients week in and week out; when the ravages of wars continue despite our claims as humans to be more enlightened; we may wonder if there is such a thing as *change.* Yet our clinical experience tells us that people desire change, they do change, and more important, change is always occurring in ourselves and in our environment, whether we observe it or not.

The belief that change occurs and is essential to the therapeutic process is fundamental to all health professions, practice models, and healing rituals. A recent Google internet search revealed over 11.5 million entries under the topic of "Therapeutic Change!" Individuals and families experiencing serious illness desire a change in their physical, emotional, relational, and spiritual suffering—as do the clinicians privileged to work with them. The clinician's beliefs about therapeutic change are central to what the clinician, "sees", "says", and "does"—what assessment and intervention is offered as well as when it is offered, how it is offered, to whom it is offered, and perhaps even where it is offered. The beliefs of family members also influence therapeutic change—do they believe that the clinician can be helpful, is there agreement about what change is needed, and do they believe they are able to change (Hubble, Duncan, & Miller, 1999).

As clinicians, we want and desire individuals and families to experience therapeutic change because we believe that with change a shift will occur toward health and healing as well as toward more satisfying functioning and relationships. Sometimes change occurs suddenly and dramatically, with families reporting at the end of a therapeutic conversation that they are thinking and feeling very differently about their lives and relationships. Sometimes change seems to occur in a more gradual way, outside of the awareness of even the family members themselves.

Like a boiling frog, the frog in the pot does not sense the gradual rise in temperature until it is too late and it is cooked. We are often like frogs, sometimes unaware of the change in our beliefs, behaviors, and/ or affect until we are invited to observe and reflect about change in our lives and relationships. For families this may occur within the therapeutic conversation or sometime after; similarly, clinicians may be invited to a reflection about a change in their beliefs during a session with an individual or family, in the post session discussion, or perhaps as they document the clinical session. As clinicians we are curious and fascinated about how change happens in ourselves and in our clients (Heatherington, Friedlander, & Greenberg, 2005), and most importantly, how we can sustain therapeutic change that eases illness suffering.

When clinicians complete the sentence stem "change occurs..." a window is opened into their clinical practices and beliefs. Humberto Maturana and Francisco Varela, two Chilean biologists, offer compelling empirical evidence that cognition is a biological phenomenon. Maturana and Varela's Biology of Cognition (1992) influences not only how we view therapeutic change but influences what we think the clinician can and cannot do to help people change. In this chapter, we will discuss paradigms of therapeutic change, which have implications for the therapeutic stance of clinicians, and we conclude with guiding principles concerning therapeutic change. In so doing, we open the windows and doors of the *Illness Beliefs Model* to examine our beliefs as clinicians about therapeutic change. Let's begin with the radical notions about reality offered in the Biology of Cognition that are foundational to our beliefs about change.

WORLDVIEW: OBJECTIVITY-IN-PARENTHESES

"...the world everyone sees is not *the* world but *a* world
which we bring forth with others"
—Humberto Maturana and Francisco Varela

The *Illness Beliefs Model* has been influenced by Maturana and Varela's Biology of Cognition, which compels us to understand that everything an individual does—"smelling, seeing, building, preferring, rejecting, conversing—is a world brought forth in coexistence with other people" (Maturana & Bunnell, 1998, p. 3) through the phenomenon of explaining in language. The Biology of Cognition offers two explanatory paths to explain one's reality or experience: (a) the path of objectivity-without-parentheses and (b) the path of objectivity-in-parentheses.

The path of objectivity-without-parentheses leads to an explanation of experience where there is *one* objective reality that is independent of oneself as the observer and accessible through our nervous system. From the "objectivist" view, "a system and its components have a constancy and a stability that is independent of the observer that brings them forth" (Mendez, Coddou, & Maturana, 1988, p. 154). The beliefs undergirding an "objectivist" stance are certain: "what I see *is* reality" which leads one to conclude "there is one correct view and I have it!" These types of beliefs do not invite change in us or in others. Rather, they invite blame because if you do not see an "objective" reality the way that I see it, then one of us must be wrong—and it certainly is *not* me!

According to Maturana (1998), "emotional violence" is "holding an idea to be true such that another's idea is untrue and must change". I may become so entrenched in my "objective" view of the world as correct that I must convince you that you are not only wrong, but also in order for us to have a relationship, you *must* change. Maturana and Varela (1992) state:

> If we know that our world is necessarily the world we bring forth with others, every time we are in conflict with another human being with whom we want to remain in coexistence, we cannot affirm what for us is certain (an absolute truth) because that would negate the other person." (p. 245).

Professional "diagnoses," emotional conflict, and pride are some of the products of an "objective" view of reality. When clinicians adopt an "objectivist" view, they often behave like "experts" who know what is best for the "patient," bring forth pathology, demand particular change, and suppress healing (Tapp, 2000).

While working with individuals and families experiencing illness suffering, we have found that possibilities are opened up for change when a worldview of objectivity-in-parentheses is embraced. This explanatory path to understand reality or experience leads one to include oneself as observer and participant in what is being observed and therefore multiple realities are possible. "If we want to coexist with another person, we must see that his certainty—however undesirable it may seem to us—is as legitimate and valid as our own" (Maturana & Varela, 1992, p. 245). From a stance of objectivity-in-parentheses other individuals are experienced as having legitimate views, albeit different from my own. Respect, non-judgment curiosity, and responsibility follow.

The beliefs fitting with a stance of objectivity-in-parentheses include "I and the other person with whom I am interacting bring forth the world in our interaction with it" and "there are many equally legitimate views, although they are not equally desirable or pleasant to live in." Maturana (1988a) has stated, "one can live in hell or in heaven depending on what world one is bringing forth in coexistence with others". The only possibility for coexistence, Maturana and Varela (1992, p. 246) argue, is to "opt for a domain of existence in which both parties fit in the bringing forth of a common world...The knowledge of this knowledge constitutes the social imperative for a human-centered ethics."

Just as therapeutic curiosity about and respect for others and their views are among the products of objectivity-in-parentheses, so is love! According to Maturana (1998), love is a fundamental emotion in human beings. Love is the domain of actions that "lets us see the other person and open up for him room for existence beside us. This act is called love, or if we prefer a milder expression, the acceptance of the other person beside us in our daily living" (Maturana & Varela, 1992, p. 246). Love allows us to "open space" or "allows the other to arise as a legitimate other" (Maturana, 1998). Maturana and Varela (1992) stated the following:

> If we know that our world is necessarily the world we bring forth with others, every time we are in conflict with another human being with whom we want to remain in coexistence, we cannot affirm what for us is certain (an absolute truth) because that would negate the other person. If we want to coexist with

the other person, we must see that *his certainty—however undesirable it may seem to us—is as legitimate and valid as our own* because, like our own, that certainty expresses his conservation of structural coupling in a domain of existence—however undesirable it may seem to us. (pp. 245-246)

These two explanatory paths have implications not only for how we relate to others but also for how we as family clinicians listen. Maturana (1998) offers that in objectivity-without-parentheses, we "listen to see if what the other person says agrees with what we believe"; however, when we operate in the explanatory path of objectivity-in-parentheses, we "listen to make true what the other person is saying." We suspend the temptation to "listen to ourselves" and become judgmental as we compare our reality with what is being said; instead, we "listen to the other" and become insatiably and passionately curious about what he or she believes and where have those beliefs come from? In so doing, we resist the "sin of certainty" and are compelled "to see that the world will be different only if we live differently" (Maturana & Varela, 1992, p. 245).

PARADIGMS OF THERAPEUTIC CHANGE: STRUCTURAL DETERMINISM

Change is always occurring in each of us and in the environment we live within. Maturana and Varela offer another radical notion called structural determinism that offers, "the environment only triggers change…(it does not specify or direct change)" (1992, p. 75).

Changes that occur in a living system are determined by the present structure of that bio-psychosocial-spiritual system, which has a unique biological and social history, i.e., a unique genetic structure and a unique history of interactions in the world over time. We have found that when clinicians initially encounter the concept of "structural determinism"—that the structure of an organism determines every change it will undergo (Maturana & Varela, 1992)—the reactions vary from frustration to recognition. These varied reactions beautifully demonstrate the concept of structural determinism, because if change were not determined by structure, all clinicians would respond in exactly the same way to the same "stimulus." It is not the information from the environment that specifies how a person (a living system) will "respond" but rather the unique bio-psychosocial-spiritual structure of the person that determines what triggers will be selected by the individual that result in structural change.

In their seminal paper, "What the Frog's Eye Tells the Frog's Brain," Lettvin, Maturana, McCulloch, and Pitts (McCulloch, 1988) showed that the retina transforms, rather than transmits, the external image. Thus, perception is not a picture of the world coming in and recording on the frog's brain; rather, it is the frog's structure that determines what it sees.

Perhaps we should amend the words of one of Simon and Garfunkel's songs: "A man hears what he wants to hear and disregards the rest." We believe instead that "a man hears what he is currently structurally able to hear and doesn't know (is not able to regard) that he is disregarding the rest." Although less lyrical, it fits our view of perception influenced by Maturana and Varela's (1992) ideas that "we do not see *that* we do not see" (p. 19) and "we do not see *what* we do not see, and what we do not see does not exist" (p. 242).

The idea of structural determinism must be connected with Maturana's concepts of *plasticity* and *structural coupling*. The static-sounding notion of structural determinism can even sound like "pre-determinism" if one is operating from an "objective" stance; however, it is heard differently when one considers the structural coupling (discussed in a later section) and the plasticity of the systems involved.

Plasticity refers to the ability of an organism to make constant changes through its interactions with itself, its environment, and other structurally plastic systems (Leyland, 1988). This is no dismal, static view of change. It is vibrant, ever changing, and highly respectful, based on the view that "although the structure of the system determines how it will 'react' to a particular disturbance at a given instant, that interaction, in turn, leads to structural change which will alter the future behavior of the system" (Leyland, 1988, p. 362). New findings from neuroscience confirm the neuroplasticity of the brain and how our thoughts can actually change the structure and function of our brains (Doidge, 2007; Lipton, 2005).

Although we believe that changes that occur in a living system are governed by the structure of that system, we also believe that the systems with which we interact as clinicians are highly complex and, therefore, highly structurally plastic, or malleable, and richly coupled with other highly complex, structurally plastic systems. We believe that changes in a living system arise from the system's "internal structural dynamics and from the structural changes triggered in it through its interactions, or from the interplay of both" (Mendez et al., 1988, p.155).

PARADIGMS OF THERAPEUTIC CHANGE: STRUCTURAL COUPLING

Structural coupling is a term that describes the process through which the structural changes in living systems occur. Structural coupling involves two unities coming together in a medium. Through structural coupling, two distinct entities become less different from each other. "We speak of structural coupling whenever there is a history of recurrent interactions leading to the structural congruence between two (or more) systems" (Maturana & Varela, 1992, p. 75).

We believe that change involves changes in the bio-psychosocial-spiritual structures of the individual family members *and* the clinician. Change occurs as the structures of the clinician and the family members are triggered to change through the mutual perturbations arising from their recurrent interactions with each other; that is, through structural coupling. When family members and the clinician encounter each other in relational practice, the possibility for structural coupling exists (Maturana, 1988a).

When two distinct entities interact, each interaction triggers structural changes in both, and of course, the changes triggered are structurally dependent. Mutual triggering of structural changes (mutual perturbations) can lead to increasing structural congruence. They "fit" together. They are structurally coupled, like feet and shoes, or like two stones rubbed together, which increasingly "fit," changing congruently, changing in concert with the other (Maturana, 1988a). These structural changes can occur in the domain of positive or negative interactions (Maturana, 1988a).

Are parents' cautions of "I don't want you hanging out with that gang" expressions of fear of structural coupling and structural changes? Are fears that "You will become just like them" based on this biological principle? Do congruent changes arising from recurrent interactions explain why friends begin dressing alike and talking alike? Could structural coupling and structural changes explain why some couples over time often look alike? Do we grow to look like those we love? Is structural coupling the way we become more and more like those we admire and honor? Do we, through our recurrent interactions with someone, not only start looking like them, but start seeing them? Our structure determines what we see. And what has influenced our bio-psychosocial-spiritual structure? It is our interaction with others and our environment.

Families talk about these structural changes in terms such as, "I'm seeing things differently these days" or "His heart has softened toward our son." Structural changes involve actual bio-psychosocial-spiritual changes. Eyes change, hearts change, and cells change through structural coupling. Change involves transformation: structural change, change at the cellular level, and change at the "soulular" level.

We need to be mindful of our structural coupling and structural changes in our clinical work with families. Are we able to acknowledge how family members are influencing us in the process of our work with them? How are family members triggering perturbations in us in the process of our triggering of perturbations in them? With the worldview of objectivity-in-parentheses in mind, accompanied by an understanding of structural determinism and structural coupling, we set forth in the following section our beliefs about therapeutic change.

ILLNESS BELIEFS MODEL: BELIEFS ABOUT THERAPEUTIC CHANGE

Through years of clinical practice and clinical research, our beliefs about change have evolved. What we now offer are four core beliefs about therapeutic change that presently guide the *Illness Beliefs Model*. These beliefs that serve as guiding principles for therapeutic change are illustrated in Figure 6.

Figure 6. Illness Beliefs Model: Beliefs about Therapeutic Change

> •Therapeutic change occurs through the fit between the clinician's therapeutic offerings and the bio-psychosocial-spiritual structures of family members
>
> •Therapeutic change occurs as the core belief at the heart of the matter is distinguished, challenged, or strengthened
>
> •Change is inevitable, but the direction and pace of therapeutic change are unpredictable
>
> •Therapeutic change needs to be distinguished and languaged

Therapeutic Change Occurs Through the Fit Between the Clinician's Therapeutic Offerings and the Bio-Psychosocial-Spiritual Structures of Family Members.

The concept of "fit" arises from the theoretical underpinnings that change is structurally determined and that change involves structural coupling and a change in structure. It is each family member's structure, *not* the clinician's therapeutic offering, that determines whether the clinical intervention is selected as a perturbation that triggers change or not. Structural coupling between the clinician and the client can increase the possibility that the offering will be selected. However, what the specific structural changes will be are always unknown and unpredictable.

The concept of fit also meshes with the guiding principle that the clinician is not a change agent (see Chapter 6, Beliefs about Clinicians) but rather is one who, among other things, creates a context for change (see Chapter 7, Creating a Context for Changing Beliefs). Our clinical experience is that family members who *do* respond to particular therapeutic offerings do so because of the fit between their current bio-psychosocial-spiritual structures and the therapeutic intervention. In this instance, there is a fit and the intervention becomes a perturbation that creates change in the structure.

The concept of fit allows us to be non-blaming of clients and ourselves when "non-fit" and, therefore, "non-adherence" and non-follow-through occur. Clinicians, operating from a therapeutic stance appreciative of fit, are able to be highly curious about ways to increase the fit for *these* family members at *this* time. We also can scrutinize our therapeutic offerings for languaging, timing, and contextualizing to increase the likelihood that fit will occur. The need to be exquisitely sensitive to our clients' responses to our therapeutic moves is heightened as we look for opportunities to develop a "culture of feedback." The study of therapeutic change has led to a greater interest in obtaining client feedback to measure and track the clients' views of the therapeutic relationship and whether change is occurring and do so openly and directly within the therapeutic conversation (Duncan, Miller, & Hubble, 2007; Hill & Cox, 2009). This non-blaming, non-guilt-inducing stance, along with increased and persistent curiosity about the client's perspective, engenders therapeutic loving.

When the concept of fit is neglected, overlooked, or not appreciated, what happens between the clinician and family members? Therapeutic violence and certainty reign, reducing options and closing space for therapeutic conversations, curiosity, and collaboration. A tendency of clinicians to prescribe or lecture occurs when clients do not readily adopt their ideas or recommendations. As the discouragement of the clinician with him or herself and his or her clients increases, and vice versa, and when non-adherence to the therapeutic interventions occurs, there is no "fit". Without the conceptual lens of fit, health care providers label clients as noncompliant, not ready for change, resistant, or difficult.

Having been influenced by Maturana and Varela's Biology of Cognition, we make a seemingly outrageous claim that resistance is *not* a useful concept and is actually a *biological impossibility*! Lorraine Wright and Anne Marie Levac (1992) offer that noncompliant families are *nonexistent*! Sometimes in our work there simply is not a fit between what we offer family members and their current bio-psychosocial-spiritual structures. Not having a "fit" between a clinician's ideas and the persons in their care simply means the clinician needs to seek other ideas that might be helpful rather than blame oneself or the clients seeking assistance.

When clinicians are mindful of "fit," we open space for conversations about what family members want from therapeutic conversation and what they are experiencing in our work with them. We have called these "goodness-of-fit" conversations (for more information see Chapter 7, Creating a Context for Changing Beliefs). These conversations explore questions such as:

- How did you experience our work together today?
- What do you wish we had spent more or less time discussing?
- Are we moving faster or slower than you anticipated?
- Are you finding the sessions helpful or not?
- What were you hoping would happen in this meeting that did occur?
- Is this session, this topic and our work together, a fit for you?

Our responsibility as clinicians is not only to assess whether there is an overall fit in our work with family members, but also to be aware of the fit or non-fit of particular interventions for particular family members. Information, instruction, and interventions cannot be imported onto someone. They can only be offered as part of an interaction. How an individual responds is determined by his or her structure at that point in time. If living systems could be instructed, we would all respond in the same way to any given per' bation, from how to cook pasta to how to cope with an illness.

In light of the precedn concepts and consequences, our view of change leads us to re-phrase our belief about change: The *possibility* for therapeutic change is increased through an *increased fit* between the clinician's therapeutic offerings and the bio-psychosocial-spiritual structures of family members. Phrased this way, the belief sounds less linear and less imposing. It also opens space for clinicians to put their energies and abilities into assessing and increasing the fit between their ideas, opinions, and questions and the bio-psychosocial-spiritual structures of family members.

Therapeutic Change Occurs as the Core Belief at the Heart of the Matter is Distinguished, C' allenged, or Strengthened

Unique to the *Illness B< 'fs Model* is the notion of core beliefs. The experience of a core belief nce uncovered, is like saying, "Of course that's true, I don't even question it, and of course everyone else thinks that's true too!" However, as we have found in our clinical practice and daily lives, every belief pays rent—every belief has consequences. The focus of therapeutic change in the *Illness Beliefs Model* is to challenge and chip away at those limiting, constraining core beliefs that the clinician makes a professional judgment are enhancing suffering AND to strengthen facilitating core beliefs that diminish illness suffering. Family members' beliefs, the clinician's beliefs, the health care systems' beliefs, the societal and cultural beliefs, and the congruence between all of these beliefs are all under scrutiny in the therapeutic process. It is necessary to determine what shifts in which core beliefs will yield the greatest leverage for therapeutic change.

Families have taught us that *it is the belief about the problem that is the problem and increases suffering for families.* If a family is experiencing cancer, it is their beliefs about the cancer—where it came from, how it will affect their family's future, what treatment will be best—that invite suffering, *not* the cancer itself. In our clinical research, we have learned from families that beliefs have a profound influence on families' experiences with illness and their relationships.

Families have beliefs about all aspects of life, but our clinical exploration is focused on a purposeful inquiry about their beliefs about their illness. Within this exploration, we are seeking the beliefs that are at the heart of the matter: the core constraining belief(s) that is causing the family the greatest suffering and the core facilitating belief(s) that will invite healing.

The constraining belief that is at the heart of the matter is the belief that perpetuates and exacerbates the problem, the belief that constrains solutions, and increases suffering. Just as there are questions that clinicians can ask family members to begin to distinguish and "peel back the onion" about the belief at the heart of the matter (see Chapter 8, Distinguishing Illness Beliefs) we have formulated the following questions for clinicians to ask themselves to begin hypothesizing about the *core* belief:

- What are the illness beliefs of family member(s) or health care professional, or society?
- What belief underlies that illness belief?
- For this family experiencing this illness at this moment in

time, is the core belief constraining or facilitating?

- How might the core constraining belief perpetuate or increase illness suffering?
- How might suffering perpetuate the core constraining belief?
- What does the core constraining belief invite the family members to do and to feel?
- What does the core constraining belief hold family members back from doing and feeling?
- What core constraining belief invites problematic interactions between family members or between family members and health care professionals?
- What alternate core facilitating belief might soften illness suffering?
- How might the core facilitating belief diminish or soften illness suffering?
- What would the core facilitating belief invite family members to do or to feel differently?

To introduce clinicians to the idea of beliefs that matter, we ask them to think of a "family-of-origin motto", slogan, or saying. We ask them to identify the belief in that motto and to write about how that belief still influences their life today, personally or professionally. One favorite family-of-origin saying was "The work of the world is done by people who do not feel well." The belief is that good people who do not feel well still get their work done. How may that belief influence the person's life? For example, he may not be exquisitely attuned to his body and may work right through serious, even life-threatening, illness. Or he may rarely get ill because illness is not an excuse for not working. A problem may arise when that person becomes so ill that he cannot work. Now what happens to the belief that "good people who don't feel well still get their work done?" In the face of a life-threatening illness, when work is impossible, does this mean "I am not a good person because I cannot get my work done?" Is the view of oneself undermined rather than sustained at this point? Does this belief about work and illness stop working *for* the person and start working *against* him at this point? Does it shift from being facilitating to being constraining, even generating a problem?

How do we bring forth core beliefs, those beliefs at the heart of the matter? How do we distinguish them in order to challenge or solidify them, depending on whether they increase or soften suffering? Generally we agree that because we are often not aware of our beliefs, they need to be mined by listening closely to the stories people tell about their lives and relationships. Answers to the "One Question Question" (Duhamel, Dupuis & Wright, in press; Wright, 1989) may hint at what the belief at the heart of the matter may be or may be related to: "If you could have just one question answered in our work together, what would that question be?" This question invites family members to focus on their deepest concerns or suffering. Family members are often more ready to think about and reflect on their beliefs when suffering is present. Other questions can also invite reflections about one's beliefs:

- What have you come to believe about your son's strengths through our session today?
- What beliefs about yourself, your spouse, or your marriage will allow you to make the necessary changes you so desire?
- Are you the kind of man who believes_____?
- Some people in your situation would believe_____. Does that fit for you?

Asking questions in this manner enables family members to bring forth their more facilitating beliefs—their more loving and compassionate beliefs—about one another. Through these particular kinds of questions, the clinician is creating a particular "reality of goodness and compassion" amongst family members that is more likely to enable healing. If, however, the clinician were to bring forth a "reality of pathology and indifference", the questions would be more negative and judgmental, such as "Why do you think your husband does not support you?" or "Why do you keep nagging your wife when she is ill?"

We use a "both-and" approach when distinguishing the belief at the heart of the matter. Sometimes we need to begin to deduce information and possible beliefs from family members' statements during a clinical session. For example, a husband says to his wife in an emotionally explosive tone, "If she doesn't get off her fat butt and exercise, she is going to have problems with her diabetes and die." The belief at the heart of the matter may be, "If she loves me, she will change," or "A good husband protects his wife's health", or it may be, "I worry she will die and I will be left alone." Further exploration and embellishing of the core belief at the heart of the matter—the core of the marital conflict—needs to follow this palpable invitation from the husband (for more information, see Chapter 8, Distinguishing Illness Beliefs).

At other times we find that people initiate the offering of a core belief. A middle-aged couple sought assistance at the Family Nursing Unit after the husband experienced a stroke while receiving treatment for leukemia. While the leukemia was in remission, the effects of the stroke interfered with his ability to work, drive a car, and resume the activities of his life. In response to the "One Question Question," the following poignant interaction between the couple and a student clinician ensued:

HUSBAND: *I don't know whether to try or to give up...Am I beating myself against a wall? Should I accept it [debilitating effects of the stroke] but I have never been one to accept this...*

CLINICIAN: *So you are having these conversations with yourself around am I going to keep fighting, should I keep fighting, or should I accept that...*

WIFE: *This is as good as it gets.*

As the student clinician explores his illness suffering, she is invited by a phone-in from her faculty supervisor to ask about the couple's spiritual beliefs.

CLINICIAN: *The team is just wondering if you pray about what the future holds for you.*

HUSBAND: (nods*)...but there's no answers. I say "God, please show me the way," and nothing's come yet. You know I thank Him for my life, I don't want Him thinking that I don't appreciate, because I do, but there's got to be something more, but I'm not getting the answer about whether it's, like you don't expect Him to yell out what the answer is, but I still don't know,* *even if there's job opportunities or what, what my direction is. So yeah, I pray to God.*

CLINICIAN: *Since God hasn't kind of turned up with answers yet, what do you think His plan may be, or His answer is?*

HUSBAND: *I don't know. Because there's got to be something, because it's awfully traumatic what I went through and...maybe it's nothing. Like you say, maybe you're waiting for an answer, maybe there isn't an answer. I don't know.*

WIFE: *We believe that, that what we go through good or bad in our lives is a learning experience and that there's something that we had to learn by going though what we went through, we went through it together. And that everything good and bad is a learning experience, and that you had to learn something from this experience, that's going to affect what you're going to do. You didn't stick around to sit at home.*

HUSBAND: *I know, I know that.*

WIFE: *And do what you're doing, the path is there, you just have to be patient.*

HUSBAND: *It's hard to be patient.*

WIFE: *For it to come, and that's what I believe, that's what we believe in each lifetime, that we're here to learn more from all our experiences, that we learn from them, and we learned a lot about each other and...life through that experience. But I can't believe that He left you here just to sit at home and worry about what your future is.*

In this moving therapeutic conversation, the wife reveals her core belief about the meaning of this illness tragedy—that both bad and good events in life are opportunities for learning. While this core belief about meaning and purpose appears to be useful to her and perhaps even softens her suffering, her husband is more impatient for an answer and direction.

His suffering is about not being sure about the meaning and purpose of his life—should he push the limits, despite his stroke, or not?

Perpetual hypothesizing about the core belief transpires throughout a session as the clinician listens for cues and clues. This is a time of insatiable curiosity, which seeks specifics and brings forth the core belief. The therapeutic move of "bringing the belief to life" came to life for us through hermeneutic interpretation of a first session with a couple who were referred to the Family Nursing Unit by a cardiac research nurse. The husband had experienced two heart attacks during the previous year and was enrolled in an experimental cardiac drug trial. The wife experienced hypertension, arthritis, and neck and back problems. There was a strong history of heart disease in her family of origin. The couple wanted help to decrease their stress and marital conflict. Very early in the first session, the clinician (LMW) explored the beliefs about the prognosis and about how family members could influence the illness:

LMW: *Well, speaking about your life—if I can be so blunt—what have they told you about the future for yourself in terms of future heart attacks?*

Through the conversation, LMW uncovers the husband's belief that he can prevent further attacks. She brings the belief to life and deepens it:

LMW: *Are you a man that believes this? You are doing a lot of things to prevent another attack. So do you believe…?*

When the husband confirmed that he did believe his efforts could prevent a future coronary, instead of just rejoicing by saying "It's a wonderful belief," LMW shored up the husband's belief by offering a contrasting view:

LMW: *I've met some people that have had a coronary and they don't believe that if they exercise and do these things that it will make a difference.*

This counter-position invited the husband to elaborate the story of his former lifestyle, pointing out why he now believed as he did. His belief in his belief was deepened through this process. The husband's belief came to life, opening the door to his wife's belief, which was similar. She also believed she could influence her husband's future attacks. But her belief at the heart of the matter was that she could trigger an attack by bringing up stressful topics:

WIFE: *If we would fight or if I would create a stressful situation, he would get stress pain and then I would feel guilty as all get out.*

Her belief originated from being told by nurses not to visit her husband in the hospital if she could not keep her composure. When LMW asked her if she believed that keeping all that stress to herself could trigger a coronary for herself, the wife replied as follows:

WIFE: *Yes. My dad died of a coronary. I sat at my mother's bedside when she had two heart attacks; she had one in our home. And my brother had a heart attack this summer. So I believe it a lot!*

The wife believed that the behavior that was lifesaving for her husband—not talking about stressful things—was life threatening for her (keeping the stress inside could trigger a coronary for her). The belief at the heart of the heart attacks, past and potential, was the belief at the heart of the marital conflict. The core belief had been distinguished and brought to life, and it could now be challenged (for a further description of this clinical case, see Wright, Bell, Watson, & Tapp, 1995).

When we are able to distinguish the belief at the heart of the matter, opportunities for change open. How do you know when you are getting close to the belief at the heart of the matter? How can you tell when you are on the core belief? Experience has taught us that affective and physiological arousal are indicators that we are getting close.

The affective-physiological arousal can be on the part of family members, the clinician, or both. Affective leakage—analogical and paralinguistic showings of emotion such as tears, raised voice, sighing, or long silences—can point to the proximity of a bedrock belief. It would be an interesting research project to check heart rates, breathing rates, and hormonal secretions when asking questions or offering ideas that distinguish the core belief. As constraining beliefs are challenged and more facilitating beliefs are solidified, how do you measure change at the cellular and "soulular" level? How *does* a clinician measure a change of heart, a change of compassion, a change of goodness?

When we identify a core belief with family members, we want to make it real; we want to distinguish it. When our clinical team met with the young son (Mark) experiencing multiple sclerosis and his aging parents, the clinician (LMW) held the family members' attention when the belief at the heart of the matter was distinguished. Before moving on in the conversation, LMW persuasively stated: "No, wait. This is important. Do you believe him?" This, of course, is a judgment call by the clinician. The father and mother were then able to explore further their belief that they needed to have their son give them permission to take a holiday from care giving.

A core belief at the heart of the matter may include divergent beliefs about the etiology of the illness. This was the case with the couple described in our article "Osteophytes and Marital Fights" (Watson, Bell, & Wright, 1992). The husband's belief that his back pain was iatrogenically induced was vigorously countered by his wife's belief that the cause of the osteophytes was irrelevant. The spiraling symmetry in beliefs about the etiology of the illness was key to the exacerbation in the chronic pain both in the husband's back and in the couple's marriage.

Accessing the core belief (or beliefs) at the heart of the matter provides a glimpse of the internal structures of the family members. Beliefs are reflections of a person's structure; therefore, we believe a change in belief corresponds with a change in structure. Our clinical efforts are focused on challenging core beliefs at the heart of the matter once they are distinguished.

Maturana and Varela (1992) end their book *The Tree of Knowledge* with a story of island people who do not know how to swim and sail. When a student on the island approaches someone saying that he wants to learn to swim to another land but must take his ton of cabbages with him, he is told that the cabbages will prevent him from swimming.

"Then I can't learn how to swim," the student says. "You call my cabbages weight. I call them my basic food."

"Suppose," the islander, who knows how to swim tells him, "this were an allegory and, instead of talking about cabbages we talked about fixed ideas, presuppositions, or certainties?" (p. 250)

We believe that people's constraining beliefs are the cabbages they want to take with them as they learn to swim to a new land. The clinician's challenge is to distinguish which beliefs are cabbages and which may be floats or buoys: beliefs that would assist with the swimming rather than constrain it. Chapter 8 offers further ideas on how to distinguish constraining and facilitating beliefs; Chapter 9 offers ideas on how to challenge or alter constraining beliefs; and Chapter 10 provides our ideas on how to strengthen facilitating beliefs.

Change is Inevitable, but the Direction and Pace of Therapeutic Change are Unpredictable

What could be more compelling and challenging for a family clinician than these two beliefs about therapeutic change: (a) Change is always happening and inevitable and (b) the direction and pace of change are unpredictable. The juxtaposing of the *certainty* that change will happen with the *uncertainty* about what that change will be and when it will happen is the kind of conundrum that is liberating, not constraining.

When we are under the influence of the "temptation of certainty" (Maturana & Varela, 1992, p. 18), it is the "not-knowing" that invites worry, fear, and anxiety. "If I only knew…" commences many internal and external conversations, ranging from "If I only knew when my pain would stop" to "If I only knew what's going to happen next" or even more touching, "If I only knew how much longer my child will live."

In our personal lives, prognostications and predictions are sought and paid for, from those of the weatherman to those of the stockbroker. We want to know how things will turn out. Shall we plan that picnic for Wednesday? Shall we invest in that newest stock? In the professional sphere, many clinicians want to insert "Intervention A" and receive "Outcome B." However, family members experiencing difficulties with health problems are not *tabula rasae*. They are thinking, feeling, behaving, experiencing beings with histories and stories of those histories. Family members' bio-psychosocial-spiritual structures have been changed through those histories, and these changed structures determine how future interactions will influence family members and vice versa.

Because it is the current, unique structure of a person that determines what will be selected from the environmental perturbation, we cannot say a priori what a particular interaction with self, others, or the environment will "cause" a person to do. Clinicians do not know and cannot predict how family members will respond to an interaction because their response is determined by their present structures, not the clinician's ideas, plans, or recommendations. We cannot assume to know another person's structure. The question is always, "How will family members respond?" There is no family-outcome template we can lay on family members beforehand that will indicate how an individual or family will "be" following a therapeutic interaction.

Where does that leave clinicians, who are in the business of change? What is our "purpose?" We hope that leaves us in a more respectful place with individuals and families: non-oppressively passionate about change, non-impositional about "the next step" and "the right outcome." We want to be insatiably and intensely curious about what family members select from our therapeutic offerings and what the outcome of those perturbations will be. We are curious about the uniqueness of the family members, their current bio-psychosocial-spiritual structures, and their co-evolved relationships; we are curious about change; and we are curious about what family members will select from the therapeutic interactions. Clinical energy and ideas are put into efforts to understand family members' current structures, into the generation of creative, tenacious clinical moves to offer family members and their relationships, and into a heightened sensitivity in observing clients' responses to the therapeutic moves. Clinical energy and ideas are focused on increasing the structural coupling with and between family members and on increasing the likelihood that a move will be selected as a perturbation. Therapeutic moves are offered with therapeutic intent but without therapeutic predictions and prognosis.

Therapeutic Change Needs to be Distinguished and Languaged

Change needs to be distinguished and languaged to become real. Like other "realities," change is brought forth through the distinguishing of it. "The act of indicating any being, object, thing or unity involves making an act of distinction which distinguishes what has been indicated as separate from its background" (Maturana & Varela, 1992, p. 40).

Change has occurred when the observer who distinguished the problem no longer distinguishes the problem; that is, the person who was saying there was a problem no longer says there is a problem. Another way of conceptualizing therapeutic change is when the person who was suffering the most indicates a softening of their suffering. Maturana (1998) explained that "an explanation is not an explanation until it meets the criterion of the observer". The same is true for change: A change is not a change until it meets the criterion of the observer. When we say or hear that "something has changed" or "something is different," we need to ask questions: Who noticed it? Who distinguished it? Who is the observer of the change that has been distinguished? Who has distinguished a difference?

Because different observers have different criteria, change has been given many different names in the therapeutic world: first-order change, second-order change, continuous change, discontinuous change, paradoxical change, spontaneous change, and so on. We believe that without languaging change, change is not "real." Change that is not distinguished is diminished. The importance of distinguishing change through describing it and languaging it is reinforced through Maturana and Varela's (1992) words: "The experience of anything out there is validated in a special way by the human structure, which makes possible 'the thing' that arises in the description" (pp. 25-26). We want change to arise as a real thing. As we draw forth descriptions of change from the observers, change is brought forth. We also believe that the ability of clients to language the effects of perturbations can be evidence of a change in their bio-psychosocial-spiritual structure. We are passionate about our efforts to distinguish and language change in both our clients and in ourselves as clinicians (to learn about the specific ways to distinguish change in order to sustain it, see Chapter 10, Strengthening Facilitating Beliefs).

One of the questions we designed for the documentation of clinical sessions at the Family Nursing Unit involved asking the clinician to reflect on his or her changed beliefs as a result of participating in the therapeutic conversation. The student clinician who worked with the husband and wife, described earlier (who were enduring intense emotional and spiritual suffering) offered her reflections about her beliefs in her clinical documentation. "One belief of mine that was challenged, strengthened, or altered as a result of this therapeutic conversation was:"

1. Families are affected by illness in many different ways— some that create suffering among individuals and relationships, and some that create greater awareness and closeness in relationships and individuals.

2. Speaking the unspeakable is a valuable intervention because it opens up possibilities for family members to express concerns and have conversations that they have never been able to do before. This is valuable because it opens up further possibilities for healing and change.

3. Marriages can still be alive and full of love and passion even after twenty-five years and the intense suffering of serious illness.

These kind of reflections, whether by beginning or experienced clinicians, engender a particular kind of "goodness and compassion" in the reality that is brought forth in clinical work with individuals and families.

Conclusion

While there are many aspects of therapeutic change that still remain a mystery and a puzzle, the Biology of Cognition (Maturana & Varela, 1992) offers several worldviews and guiding principles that shape both the clinician's beliefs about change as well as the therapeutic conversation that ensues. By choosing objectivity-in-parentheses as a preferred explanatory path, the clinician becomes a particular kind of person with a deep respect for and intense curiosity about the client's experience of "fit". This client-directed, outcome-informed way of working (Miller & Duncan, 2000) with individuals and families is both satisfying and humbling, and offers the possibility of change in both the client and the clinician as well. Realities of goodness and compassion, brought forth in language between clinicians and clients, can then trump realities of pathology and indifference, thus enabling healing. More of our beliefs about the role and person of the clinician in the process of therapeutic change are offered in the next chapter.

References

Doidge, N. (2007). *The brain that changes itself: Stories of personal triumph from the frontiers of brain science.* New York: Viking Press.

Duhamel, F., Dupuis, F., & Wright, L.M. (in press). Families and nurses' responses to the 'One Question Question': Reflections for clinical practice, education, and research in family nursing. *Journal of Family Nursing.*

Duncan, B., Miller, S., & Hubble, M. (2007). How being bad can make you better. *Psychotherapy Networker, 31*(6), 36-45, 57.

Heatherington, L., Friedlander, M.L., & Greenberg, L. (2005). Change process research in couple and family therapy: Methodological challenges and opportunities. *Journal of Family Psychology, 19*(1), 18-27.

Hill, C.E., & Cox, S. (2009). Processing the therapeutic relationship. *Psychotherapy Research, 19*(1), 13-29.

Hubble, M.A., Duncan, B.L., & Miller, S.D. (Eds.). (1999). *The heart and soul of change: What works in therapy.* New York: American Psychological Association.

Leyland, M.L. (1988). An introduction to some of the ideas of Humberto Maturana. *Journal of Family Therapy, 10,* 357-374.

Lipton, B. (2005). *The biology of belief: Unleashing the power of consciousness, matter, and miracles.* Santa Rosa, CA: Elite Books.

Maturana, H.R. (1988b). *Telephone conversation: The Calgary/Chile coupling* [Phone conversation with Dr. Lorraine Wright and graduate students]. (Transcript available from www.lorrainewright.com)

Maturana, H.R. (1988b). Reality: The search for objectivity or the quest for a compelling argument. *The Irish Journal of Psychology, 9*(1), 25-83.

Maturana, H.R. (1998). *Biology of cognition and biology of love* (videotapes of workshop presented at the University of Calgary). Available from www.janicembell.com.

Maturana, H.R., & Bunnell, P. (1998, June). *Biosphere, homosphere, and robosphere: What has that to do with business?* Paper presented at the meeting of the Society for Organizational Learning Member's Meeting, Amherst, MA. Retrieved January 28, 1999 from http://www.solonline.org/res/wp/maturana/index.html

Maturana, H.R., & Varela, F.J. (1992). *The tree of knowledge: The biological roots of human understanding* (rev. ed.). Boston: Shambhala.

McCulloch, W. (1998). *Embodiments of mind.* Cambridge, MA: MIT Press.

Mendez, C.L., Coddou, F., & Maturana, H.R. (1988). The bringing forth of pathology. *Irish Journal of Psychology, 9*(1), 144-172.

Miller, S.D., & Duncan, B.L. (2000). Paradigm lost: From model-driven to client-directed, outcome-informed clinical work. *Journal of Systemic Therapies, 19*(1), 20-34.

Tapp, D.M. (2000). The ethics of relational stance in family nursing: Resisting the view of "nurse as expert". *Journal of Family Nursing, 6*(1), 69-91.

Watson, W.L., Bell, J.M., & Wright, L.M. (1992). Osteophytes and marital fights: A single case clinical research report of chronic pain. *Family Systems Medicine, 10,* 423-435.

Wright, L.M. (1989). When clients ask questions: Enriching the therapeutic conversation. *Family Therapy Networker, 13*(6), 15-16.

Wright, L.M., Bell, J.M., Watson, W.L., & Tapp, D. (1995). The influence of the beliefs of nurses: A clinical example of a post-myocardial-infarction couple. *Journal of Family Nursing, 1*(3), 238-256.

Wright, L.M., & Levac, A.M. (1992). The non-existence of non-compliant families: The influence of Humberto Maturana. *Journal of Advanced Nursing, 17,* 913-917.

CHAPTER SIX
Beliefs about Clinicians

"Compassion is sometimes the capacity for feeling what it is like to live inside somebody else's skin. It is the knowledge that there can never really be any peace and joy for me until there is peace and joy finally for you too."
—Frederick Buechner

According to Miller, Hubble, and Duncan (2007, p. 28), "*Who* provides the therapy is a much more important determinant of success than *what* treatment approach is provided." In the *Illness Beliefs Model*, the *who* is a particular kind of person, with a particular worldview, influenced by the Biology of Cognition that he or she brings to the therapeutic encounter with individuals and families. Our beliefs about clinicians flow primarily from Maturana and Varela's (1992) worldview of objectivity-in-parentheses as well as the ideas of structural determinism and structural coupling discussed in Chapter 5.

Following are seven beliefs that serve as guiding principles in the *Illness Beliefs Model* that influence the kind of person the clinician is and how a clinician offers healing through the medium of therapeutic conversations (see *Figure 7*).

⚜ Figure 7. Illness Beliefs Model: Beliefs about Clinicians

- The clinician offers love and compassion in the therapeutic relationship
- The clinician is a facilitator of change, not a change agent
- The clinician's preferred stance is relational and nonhierarchical
- The clinician and family members co-evolve therapeutic conversations
- The clinician offers invitations to reflection
- The clinician is not invested in a particular outcome
- The clinician is willing to change his or her own beliefs

The Clinician Offers Love and Compassion in the Therapeutic Relationship

"Compassion is that which makes the heart of the good move at the pain of others."
—The Buddha

Encountering illness suffering is a heartrending and profound human experience. Several publications have helped us understand more about illness suffering and how health care professionals can be helpful to individuals and families who suffer in their experience of illness—whether it is physical suffering, emotional suffering, spiritual suffering, or all three (Kleinman, 1988; Reed, 2003; Strong, 2002; Wright, 1997a, 1997b, 2001, 2005, 2008).

Our research team (Drs. Janice Bell, Nancy Moules, and Lorraine Wright) recently examined illness suffering conversations that occurred between family members and nurse clinicians in the Family Nursing Unit. In our hermeneutic interpretation of these moving clinical conversations, we uncovered that while we believe that suffering needs to be told, talked about, witnessed, and documented (Wright, 2005), illness suffering conversations are often very difficult and uncomfortable for clinicians to listen to and be fully present. Voices of pain, loneliness, fractured relationships, and loss of meaning and purpose in one's life have a gripping and oppressively heavy effect. As one young man with a rare form of muscular dystrophy told us, "Being ill and being sick is a very ugly thing when you're alone."

We found that, in a desire to "save" the person from their suffering or perhaps save ourselves from the difficult witnessing and listening, clinicians often fall into the trap of shifting the conversation to another topic, attempting to "cheer up" the client by focusing on the positive, or offering our own clichés and explanations about the meaning of suffering, hoping that this will soften the suffering.

Often health professionals will offer clichés that are advice or instructive oriented and therefore imply that the person or family is doing something wrong. For example, "You need to move on," or "you need to take more breaks, have more respite," or "you need to forgive and forget," or "you need to be strong for your child." Other times, the clinician may offer clichés that target emotions: "At least this illness is not life-threatening," or "at least she had a full life," or "things could be worse." Or the health professional shares his own emotions through clichés such as: "my heart goes out to you," or "I know how you feel." These kinds of clichés, although well intentioned, can often close down opportunities to be compassionate listeners and witnesses of illness suffering.

We believe that the skilled clinician needs to be willing and willful to step into illness suffering conversations, despite one's own discomfort and pain that often arises, and listen with deep compassion and intense curiosity to the "cries of the wounded" (a term borrowed from William James). Compassion is larger than just a willingness to understand another person's experience; it is a desire to alleviate suffering by listening fully and carefully regardless of how difficult it might be for the clinician to do so (Frank, 1998; Lee, 2008). The act of compassion begins with the clinician being fully present and "behind one's eyes" (Dr. Nancy J. Moules, personal communication, July 21, 1999) in the therapeutic moment, not preoccupied with multitasking or thinking ahead about all of the other responsibilities that must be accomplished or even thinking about plans for later in the day. It is important to rein in the "balloon of the mind" when our thinking and thoughts drift away from the therapeutic conversation. When clinicians are not fully present, the suffering of clients is enhanced due to their anguish not being fully registered or appreciated by the health provider.

Perhaps herein lays the link to Maturana and Varela's ideas about objectivity-in-parenthesis. When the clinician believes there are multiple realities (not all of them equally desirable or pleasant to live with), the clinician opens space for the existence of another. Love is the domain of actions that "lets us *see* the other person and open up for him room for existence beside us. This act is called *love*, or if we prefer a milder expression, the acceptance of the other person beside us in our daily living" (Maturana & Varela, 1992, p. 246). It is therefore likely not just courage or compassion, but these character traits fuelled by love, that allows the clinician to enter deeply into conversations of illness suffering that offer healing. "Deep listening is hard," Art Frank reminds us, "but it is a fundamental moral act" (Frank, 1995, p. 25).

The Clinician is a Facilitator of Change, Not a Change Agent

The term "change agent" implies a linear-positivist view of change and frequently a pejorative view of individuals and families. We believe that clinicians cannot and do not "change" anyone. Rather, we believe that clinicians facilitate change and invite healing in beliefs, in relationships, and in illness suffering.

Some may say, "What's in a name?" Just as different terms for the therapeutic process for ameliorating illness suffering cross disciplinary boundaries (Bell, Wright, & Watson, 1992; Wright & Watson, 1982) and perhaps open or close space for therapeutic change, what we call ourselves as clinicians also limits or facilitates the process of change. In a name are embedded assumptions, expectations, and permission to behave in certain ways. The term "change agent" can imply that the clinician is the only one in charge of change. It implies a linear relationship with change—"I change others"—inviting one to behave as an expert and forget or dismiss that families are also experts about their illness experiences and have preferences for living well in the world. Thinking of oneself as a change agent can invite a clinician to focus on the word "agent" and grow into the permission embodied in that term, which the Oxford dictionary defines as "one who exerts power or produces effect." This stance negates the ability of a family member to be a "free agent," that is, according to the dictionary, "one whose actions are not subject to another's control." Of course the only person the clinician can change in the consultation room is him or herself.

The term change agent can imply a one-up position: a stance of superiority and hierarchy. Predetermined hypotheses about how families should function, the laying on of goals, too frequent sessions, and a display of expert certainty can distance the clinician from family members and lead to therapeutic errors (Bell, 1999; Wright & Leahey, 2009). To invite and entice someone to a reflection about their beliefs, to offer someone a new belief, and to open space for solutions and a softening of illness suffering involves a humble and curious stance. We agree with Kierkegaard that "the helper must first humble himself under him he would help, and therewith must understand that to help does not mean to be a sovereign but to be a servant" (pp. 27-28). We believe that the clinician's strength is increased through humility, not hierarchy.

To say that we are not change agents does not mean we do not bring expertise to the therapeutic encounter. Graduate students studying relational practices and non-hierarchy have sometimes assumed that this means they have no expertise. The clinician possesses considerable expertise gained through clinical work with other families, life experience, research, and professional literature. However, the clinician's expertise is offered in a manner that recognizes and values the expertise of family members.

To say that we are not change agents does not mean we are not passionate about change. We are. We expect change. We embrace change. We are in the business of change. We believe that change is always occurring; therefore, if we do not find change in one place, we look in another. We tenaciously pursue avenues to invite change, but we are not passionate about change bringing about one particular outcome. We have a passion for change but not a passion to change others. We are passionate about helping, but not passionate about how family members will "be" after that help is offered. The role of the clinician is therefore not to change the family members but to draw forth their passion for change and living together with the challenges that life presents. This is the ultimate goal of an effective facilitator.

If clinicians do not change anyone, what do they do? Rather than saying that the clinician enables change to occur, our view is that change is constantly occurring from moment to moment. We see that part of our work is to clear away the obstacles that have been inhibiting a softening of suffering, change or solutions; distinguish constraining beliefs; challenge constraining beliefs; and affirm facilitating beliefs. (Chapters 7–10 elaborate on the four major therapeutic moves that constitute the *Illness Beliefs Model.*) Through these macromoves, the clinician invites, entices, and, as Maturana said, "seduces" the family members to a reflection. A reflection facilitates family members in seeing and softening their internal structure and beliefs. Another part of our work as clinicians, therefore, is to offer interventions and interactions that invite reflections. These have an increased likelihood of being selected as perturbations that reduce illness suffering.

The Clinician's Preferred Stance is Relational and Nonhierarchical

The relationship between the family and clinician frequently invites a traditional hierarchy to exist. The clinician is frequently perceived to be the only expert, in a one-up position; the family comes to the relationship needing help, a one-down position. The clinician often possesses power and control through knowledge, professional position, and skill; the family usually has exhausted its resources, and the members are looking for new ideas and solutions to soften their suffering. In many professional contexts, clinicians are offered money for their ideas, whereas clients most often have to pay for the clinicians' services.

Frequently, specific rules, albeit unspoken and implicit, govern a hierarchical relationship. Rules that perpetuate hierarchy include the following: "you are in a one-down position," "never comment directly about the rules that govern the relationship," and "never express dissatisfaction with the relationship nor raise problematic interactions of tension or mistrust." Family members frequently have a constraining belief that if they express their concerns, dissatisfactions, or frustrations directly, they might not receive adequate care or will be punished for challenging the health care professional's knowledge or authority.

When clinicians demand obedience to have a client follow a particular diabetic diet, take medication at a prescribed time, or stop nagging a spouse about his lack of exercise for his heart condition, they are under the influence of the belief that the knowledge and expertise of the health care provider is more correct than the ill individual or family about how to manage an illness. Health care providers who engage in these efforts of advice-giving or "instructive interaction," rather than inviting individuals to a reflection and engaging in collaborative interaction, typically operate from a worldview of objectivity-without-parentheses. A rule of many health care providers who prefer this worldview is as follows: "Label families as resistant and noncompliant if they do not follow your ideas and advice or are dissatisfied or distrustful." In doing so, health care providers do not have to share the responsibility of creating a context for therapeutic change nor examine their contribution to the interactional dilemmas that arise. By incorporating Maturana's notion of the impossibility of instructive interaction, however, it becomes clear that the distinction, or label, of "noncompliance" is not only not useful but is a biological impossibility (Wright & Levac, 1992).

Relational practice and non-hierarchy occurs when the beliefs and actions of the clinician, under the influence of Maturana and Varela's notions about love, (1992), turn these implicit rules and behaviors upside down. Possibilities for a different kind of relationship to exist between clinicians and families open up when the clinician is a particular kind of person who is able to open space for the existence of multiple viewpoints— frequently, viewpoints different from one's own. There is more than just unequal distribution of power in the therapeutic context, regardless of the steps that are taken by clinicians to make the context and relationship more egalitarian. There are also individual and family beliefs for managing and living with illness that are very different than the clinician's beliefs, which have been shaped by professional education, experience, and expertise. It is in these moments that the clinician strives to reduce the hierarchy by "opening space for another" as much as is professionally responsible and ethical.

An invitation to clinicians to behave in relational, nonhierarchical and collaborative ways with families was first offered in a new and unique way by the Milan team in the early 1980s. They proposed three unique guidelines for the systemic clinician to use in conducting a therapeutic conversation: hypothesizing, circularity, and neutrality (Selvini Palazzoli, Boscolo, Cecchin, & Prata, 1980). Hypothesizing refers to the clinician's perpetual effort to evolve different conceptualizations of the presenting problem and develop alternative explanations for family behavior. The clinician continually looks for new ways to understand the problem without getting stuck trying to find the one correct view, belief, or reality.

Circularity refers to the reciprocal influence between clinician and client and to the clinician's use of particular questions to understand family patterns of behavior and confirm or discard hypotheses (Loos & Bell, 1990; Tomm, 1988; Wright & Leahey, 2009).

Neutrality describes the clinician's attitude toward the family system, which constrains the clinician from taking sides or blaming family members. Neutrality, with respect to change and therapeutic outcome, is another level of neutrality shown by the clinician (Tomm, 1984). Cecchin (1987) later refined the ideas about neutrality by suggesting that the essence of neutrality is curiosity. Curiosity, he argued, "is the key element of therapeutic neutrality which invites the clinician to be constantly interested in alternative views and in inventing multiple punctuations of a behavior, interpretation, event, relationship, etc." (p. 407).

In seeking to understand a multiplicity of perspectives, the clinician avoids becoming trapped by one idea or one point of view about family members, about the illness or problem, or about solutions. The clinician's views are not more correct or more privileged than the family's views. In the process, clinicians become more respecting and more in awe of families' abilities and become more humble about their own ideas, however well conceptualized and informed they may be.

It is in this spirit of wonderment with a new lens and a new way of being with families that relational, collaborative, and nonhierarchical relationships with families are born. Greater equality and status are given to the family's expertise, which is drawn forth in the therapeutic conversation. The therapeutic relationship becomes more transparent. Family members are invited to comment on the therapeutic relationship in terms of what is useful to them and what is not useful. The family's ideas for the focus and direction of the session are invited and used.

Are clinicians to remain neutral and nonhierarchical when confronted with illegal or dangerous behaviors? We respect that each family functions in the way that they desire and in a way that they determine is most effective; however, being part of a larger system, clinicians are bound by moral, legal, cultural, and societal norms that require them to act in accordance with those norms regarding illegal or dangerous behavior. In these situations, clinicians may need to take a different position—one that is distinct from a nonhierarchical, collaborative stance. Confronted by illegal or suicidal behavior, a clinician has to abandon a curious, therapeutic manner and become a social control agent in order to conform to the moral or legal rules and their consequences. In other words, there are situations in which the clinician is required to behave within the domain of objectivity.

Our practice of offering family members a choice about how they would like to use the session is one way we operationalize the concept of relational, nonhierarchical, collaborative relationships with the families we work with. We frequently ask the following question at the beginning of a session: "How would you like to spend our time together so that the session will have been useful to you?" This question discards commencing with a preconceived idea about what this family should be talking about at this time. Although our graduate students are required to develop a pre-session presentation before commencing a therapeutic conversation we advise them to go to the session well prepared so that they can respond spontaneously to the surprises that family members may bring that day. Pre-session hypothesizing is viewed as a way to start focusing on the family, churning up the gray matter, making connections, and generating questions that the team would like to ask, rather than preparing an agenda for the session that is imposed on the family regardless of what the family members desire and despite changes that may have occurred since the last session. A nonhierarchical stance does not prohibit a clinician from bringing his or her own wonderings and unsettled issues from a previous session to the present session, however. He or she can ask the family members what stood out for them from the last session and also offer what stood out for him or her.

Nonhierarchy is also demonstrated in our relational practice through our use of closing letters. In the past, we followed the traditional format of providing a closing letter to the referring professional, which summarized our impressions of the family and the assistance provided to them. Over the past few years, we have experimented with a different format for the closing letter. It is still a summary of the clinical work, but it is written in a language that both family members and referring professionals can understand. Instead of addressing the letter to the referring professional, we address the letter to the family and send a copy to the referring professional. In the letter we summarize what the clinical team learned from the family and what we believe we offered the family. The following closing letter was sent to a family who was seen in our clinic:

Dear Julie and Robert:

Greetings from the Family Nursing Unit. Our clinical nursing team was happy to meet with you for four sessions. You initially consulted the Family Nursing Unit with concerns about sharing family responsibilities. In this letter summarizing our work with you, we will share our impressions of your family, what we learned from you, and some key ideas we offered.

What We Learned from You:

You taught us how a deeply caring couple, willing to work together as a team, can find ways to get their marriage back on track.

Julie, the team was impressed by your devotion as a caring and responsible mother and wife, and by your efforts to find ways to manage your exhaustion, both for the sake of yourself and that of your family. You helped us understand how your entire family is affected by Robert's heart attacks and chest pain. This knowledge will assist us in our work with other families.

Robert, you taught us that a person can overcome difficulties in his past and make challenging lifestyle changes. We were touched by your ability to express your love for Julie and your children, especially since you have said that it is difficult for you to talk about your feelings. We have also learned how parents cope with the stress of living with a child who is hyperactive.

What We Offered You:

The clinical nursing team agreed that your marriage was off track, and we offered ideas of how to help you get back on track, and to perhaps lessen the frequency of future derailments. We were impressed that even though the third session was difficult and painful for each of you, that you were both willing to open space to our ideas and some new ideas of your own of how to get back on track.

Some of the ideas included:
1. Try to spend time enjoying each other as a couple on a regular basis.
2. Plan regular consultation time as a way of supporting each other's efforts in managing areas of personal responsibility. We offered the idea of Julie being a Cardiac Consultant to Robert, and of Robert being a Tiredness Management Consultant to Julie.

We also offered ideas to each of you that may or may not have proven helpful. We look forward to our check-up session with you on June 1 at 2 p.m.

Approximately six months after our last session, a Research Assistant from the Family Nursing Unit will contact you to complete an outcome survey. Your assistance in participating in this study will allow us to evaluate the effectiveness our service offers to families. We send you our best wishes.

Sincerely,
Lorraine M. Wright, RN, PhD, and other members of the clinical nursing team

Another method we have used to flatten the family-clinician hierarchy is to invite families to co-author articles that describe our clinical work with them (e.g., Levac et al.,1998; NIFT Letter, 2006).

Therapeutic transparency is often cited as yet another way that clinicians operationalize the preferred stance of nonhierarchy. Therapeutic transparency involves talking out loud about the therapeutic process. For example, with the family to whom the letter was sent, the clinician (LMW) talks out loud about her dilemma in finding a focus for the first session (see genogram) At this point in the session, she has been speaking with the couple, Robert and Julie, for 1 hour and 10 minutes. The couple has described in great detail the difficulties they were experiencing. Listen to the clinician voicing her dilemma:

LMW: *Let me tell you what I'm feeling right now. I'm feeling like you've been very open with me and I've gotten a lot of information. But I feel like I should start on another whole session just to know about your stress—how have you dealt with stress, what have you tried in the past? I'm wondering if it would be premature for me to offer any ideas about stress until I know all the different things you've tried on your own before now.*

JULIE: *I've tried lots of things and meditated for a while.*

LMW: *Yes? You see, and that part, I don't know yet, do I? And so I need to be careful that I'm not plunging in and offering you ideas and then disappointing you because you've already tried that. And I'm sure you wouldn't be here if you hadn't tried and hadn't exhausted a lot of your own ideas already. So, let me take a break with the team. You know what I'm saying? It's been useful. I really needed to get all this part, but I'm wondering if maybe my assessment should really continue for another session, to be sure that I understand. I understand stress is a major problem. I understand some of the issues that are causing you stress. I don't think I have an assessment yet of the different things you've tried to reduce stress on your own, so that we don't just, simply say, "Try this and that," when you've already done it yourselves. So, that part probably we'll have to follow up on next time. But let me just take a little break with the team and see what ideas they have.*

Therapeutic transparency also includes admitting a mistake. An example occurred with a family our clinical team worked with in the Family Nursing Unit who was experiencing the chronic debilitating illness of muscular dystrophy. Following a second therapeutic conversation, our team was curious about the husband and wife's seeming lack of enthusiasm about the suggestions that had been offered to them during the session. They had reported that the husband's illness of muscular dystrophy and resulting cognitive changes were affecting their ability to parent well together. Our clinical team, guided by our therapeutic intentions to be helpful, had suggested that perhaps they might benefit from therapeutic conversations that would focus on strengthening their marriage (reprinted with permission from SAGE Publications: Bell, Moules, & Wright, 2009)

Example of a Family Nursing Unit Letter Admitting a Therapeutic Error

Dear Wilma and Tim:

Greetings from the Family Nursing Unit! Our clinical team learned a great deal from both of you during our conversation in January and we wanted to share our thoughts and impressions with you in a letter.

It was a pleasure to see both of you again during our second session. Once again we were grateful for your willingness to talk openly about the ways that the "intruder" of muscular dystrophy (MD) has impacted your lives. You two have been through a great deal together! We learned that you believe this illness has changed your relationship as a mother and father but has not changed your strong love for your children. We were impressed with the dedication you have shown in raising two children who have, at times, had their own struggles. We learned that because of the changes that MD has brought, you are finding it challenging to work as a team in your parenting roles.

This session was an opportunity for us to learn more about your relationship as husband and wife and the meaning it has brought to your lives. Wilma and Tim, you helped us understand that you are very proud to have created a satisfying marriage by building a strong foundation for your marriage through your love and commitment to each other and your shared hopes and dreams. It seems that MD has not only broken into your marriage relationship but has stolen away your hopes and dreams for the future and has robbed you of feeling intimate and connected as a husband and wife. In particular, we learned that you believe that it is not the physical changes of the illness but the cognitive changes that are eating away at the strong foundation of your marriage. This left us wondering whether it would be helpful for the two of you to create small moments of connection as husband and wife every day as a way to interrupt the belief that you are becoming only a "care giver" and "care receiver."

We made an assumption during our session that, because of the

*strong foundation you had built for your marriage, you both wished for
some ideas about how to reclaim your special relationship as husband
and wife from the influence of MD. Upon reviewing the videotapes of
the session, we realize that we did not check with each of you directly
about whether you agreed with this goal of strengthening your marital
connection in our work together. From comments you made at the end
of our session, Wilma, we wondered if perhaps we made an error by
not asking each of you if you believe that it is possible to reclaim your
marriage from illness. We believe there are many possible ways that
illness suffering can be reduced and perhaps we were too premature
to conclude that strengthening the good foundation of your marriage
was the best way to reduce the suffering and isolation you are both
experiencing. We now wonder if we need to challenge our team's belief
about the best way to help your family heal.*

*Throughout our conversations, we have learned that your family
believes that the illness of MD has caused you, Wilma, the most
suffering. We are very impressed with the dedication, perseverance, and
wisdom you have shown as a wife and mother in caring for everyone
in your family for many, many years. We believe we need to understand
more about your experience and where you have found the energy
and resources to endure this unexpected life where illness has been
so present in your relationships and daily routines. How do you make
sense that your life has been one of caring for your ill family members
[husband and daughter]? Where do you find support and respite from this
responsibility? What are your hopes and fears for the future?*

*We have learned from our work with families that family members
are affected by illness differently at different times and phases over the
long haul of chronic illness. Just as it was helpful to see you together as
a couple, perhaps it would now be useful to have an individual session
with you, Wilma, to learn more about how you find the energy to care so
deeply for your family. If this idea fits for you, we would be pleased to
meet with you alone at our next session. If you have other ideas about
who should attend the session or what the focus of our work should be,
please let us know.*

Kind regards,

*Lorraine Thirsk, RN, MN, Doctoral student
Colleen Cuthbert, RN, 1st year Master of Nursing student
Janice M. Bell, RN, PhD, Director, Family Nursing Unit
and other members of the clinical team*

The transparent processing of the therapeutic error through the letter was a very useful opportunity to further uncover the wife's belief that her husband's illness had progressed significantly enough that she no longer considered him capable of functioning as either a husband or a father, leaving her alone and abandoned in her role as sole caretaker of the family unit.

The Clinician and Family Members Co-evolve Therapeutic Conversations

The Latin *conversa* translates as "turning around together." To discuss the human phenomenon of conversations, it is useful to ask the question, "Why do we talk?" Because we frequently complain to one another, "We're just not communicating, I don't feel heard, you're interrupting me, you're not listening, or we just don't talk anymore." One might infer it would be better if we just didn't talk to one another. Certain groups and individuals have chosen to do just that. Members of some religious orders take an oath of silence and do not talk, and some individuals choose to live in the woods or the mountains far away from friends and family members to avoid talking. Individuals who remain among their family and friends yet choose not to speak are given the diagnosis of mutism. Frequently, clinicians working with adolescents and families become caught in the challenge of trying to get "mute" teenagers to talk.

It becomes readily evident that we value and even demand talk from one another, which brings us back to ponder the question, "Why do we talk?" Our answer is that we talk to exchange ourselves and to render ourselves human. Our conversations are the stories that we tell of our lives, relationships, and experiences. Our conversations make us human and enable us to love. In fact, the nineteenth-century German philosopher Nietzsche said that love is a long conversation.

All human life takes place in conversations (for more information about different types of conversations, see Chapter 2). To be human consists of being part of a network of conversations. In fact, the family may be best characterized as a network of conversations. Genograms and ecomaps are assessment tools that are useful for defining with whom we, as clinicians, have conversations.

125

Conversations are a medium for storytelling and story-listening, in which all participants are speakers and listeners at the same time. A conversation is a verbal exchange of beliefs, opinions, ideas, observations, and sentiments that are embodied in our stories and myths within our social and cultural domains.

The illness stories people live, as well as the stories about those stories, are all that a clinician has to work with. Within health care settings, the stories clinicians are most likely to hear usually focus on medical narratives and illness narratives (see Chapter 4, Beliefs about Illness). In the *Illness Beliefs Model*, the clinician is carefully listening for the beliefs embedded in the stories about health and illness, family relationships and illness, generational legacies of illness, and encounters with "good" health professionals as well as those who were disappointing. A core illness belief that is contributing to the family's present suffering is likely nested somewhere within these illness stories.

Therapeutic conversations describe the medium in which clinicians and families encounter each other and where changed beliefs, healing, and softening of suffering hopefully begins. Health care providers have a tendency to behave as though their influence on the client through therapeutic conversations is unidirectional: The clinician does to or for the client. The ideas of structural determinism and structural coupling help us appreciate the relational, bi-directional, co-evolving nature of the therapeutic conversation and of change.

Therapeutic conversations are interactional: The responses of the clinician are invited by the responses of the family, which in turn are invited by the responses of the clinician. The direction and focus of the therapeutic conversation are co-evolved—we "turn around" together. The clinician may experience structural changes in response to family members' ideas, just as family members may experience changes in their bio-psychosocial-spiritual structures in response to the clinician's ideas. Both end up in a different place.

In our work with student clinicians and families in the Family Nursing Unit, we have often discussed what we learned from the families with whom we worked. We honored this reciprocal learning in the formal clinical documentation by asking the clinician to complete these trigger questions: "One new learning for me was_____" and "If this is the final session, what have you learned from this family that will help you in your work with another family in the future?"

Dianne Tapp (2001) offers an eloquent description of the importance of this reciprocal learning from families:

> In our complicit participation in these [therapeutic] conversations, we recognize ourselves, we recognize our own families, and we recognize our own loved ones. 'In listening for the other, we listen for ourselves' (Frank 1995, 50). If we listen carefully, we hear ourselves and our own lives read back to us in these conversations of illness and suffering. We hear possibilities for our own future, and we would be wise to listen well and to learn from these experiences. We will need the courage and credible knowledges of these families to face our own futures [with illness suffering and death] (p. 262).

The Clinician Offers Invitations to Reflection

"The moment of reflection...is the moment when we become aware of that part of ourselves which we cannot see in any other way" (Maturana & Varela, 1992, p. 23). Maturana and Varela speak of this reflection as being a phenomenon that occurs when one looks in the mirror. They say it is the moment when we are aware of ourselves in a new way. We believe that people also become aware of others in a new way (and of others' views of others and of others' views of themselves) through the process of reflection. A reflection can be about the past, present, or future. It does not just mean looking back. Reflections on the present and future can be powerful influences as well.

> Reflection is a process of knowing how we know. It is an act of looking back upon ourselves. It is the only chance we have to discover our blindness and to recognize that the certainties and knowledge of others are, respectively, as overwhelming and tenuous as our own. (Maturana & Varela, 1992, p. 24)

It seems that in some manner the dizzying circularity increases the clarity of what is "seen." Comments of family members after or on reflection sound like the following:

- "I've never seen it like that before";
- "I have a new view";
- "I saw my son again for the first time";
- "I've never heard my husband say those things before—it was wonderful";
- "I felt so freed up to listen";
- "I had time to think."

Invitations to reflection allow time for "inner talks" and time to reflect on the inner talk. We believe that an important part of our work as family clinicians is to invite, entice, and encourage the family members to a reflection: "You will never be able to do instructive interaction. The most that you can do is to talk to the patient and invite this person to a reflection that will allow the realization that there is an illness…Understanding cannot be forced" (Maturana, 1988). Inviting reflections on our lives and relationships creates the possibility for new facilitating beliefs to be drawn forth.

Questions are often a very useful and effective way to invite reflection (Loos & Bell, 1990; Wright & Leahey, 2009). Reflexive questions have been developed and described by Tomm (1987, 1988). White's (1988) self-description question—"What do you think that says about you?"— is a simple yet elegant example of the doubling back on oneself with an invitation to reflect that is extended through therapeutic questions. Invitations to reflect come to us in day-to-day conversations through questions as well. We are invited to a reflection when a previous lover returns and asks, "How do you explain that it never worked for the two of us?" We are invited to reflect when a friend asks, "Why do you think our friendship has remained strong all these years?" Reflexive questions can be quite elaborate but may appear simple. In the following example, a simple, even linear, question is asked: "Do you know who I am?"

A wife visited her severely cognitively and physically impaired husband in the nursing home. As she sat to visit, she asked him, "James, do you know who I am?" Her husband studied her face for what seemed to be several minutes and then said, "No, but I know you're someone who loves me." Was something seen that had not been seen before? Did reflection occur? Although this man could not identify the person of his wife, he was able to reflect on other times and experiences of a loving face.

In addition to questions, we can invite others to a reflection by "creating a context for change; creating an environment in which persons change themselves; offering ideas, advice and suggestions that can serve as useful perturbations" (Wright & Levac, 1992, p. 916). The ideas, advice, and suggestions that may serve as perturbations are offered in a manner that appreciates objectivity-in-parentheses. Invitations to reflect are offered in a spirit of wonderment and tenacity. The invitations to reflect are laden with the clinician's belief that new ways of seeing may be awaiting family members as they participate in a reflection.

The invitation to reflect may be extended by the clinician to family members through the reflecting position, stories of other families, research findings, commendations, and therapeutic letters. (For further elaboration of these therapeutic offerings, see Chapter 9, Challenging Constraining Beliefs.) We are tenacious in discovering or uncovering ways to invite family members to a reflection because of our belief that interventions that involve reflection have an increased likelihood of being selected as perturbations and of triggering changes in the bio-psychosocial-spiritual structures of family members.

With invitations to a reflection, the challenging of constraining beliefs commences. Family members are moved from "seeing through a glass darkly" to seeing through a glass magnified. Through inviting family members to a reflection, the "truth" of their stance, which has constrained solutions, is gently challenged. It is now possible to offer, entice, and invite them to consider that what they believed was true was only an illusion—that it "appeared to be" that way because of their original constraining beliefs about themselves, others, and life. We cannot make people believe something. We cannot give them a new facilitating belief. It happens through the process of structural coupling and invitations to a reflection.

The Clinician is Not Invested in a Particular Outcome

As clinicians, we are in the business of change, yet we are not invested in a particular outcome. When we appreciate the uncertainty that arises when people select what fits for them on the basis of their own present structures, it becomes impossible to be invested in a particular outcome. People will select what fits for them. A person's selection of an idea is dependent on his or her current bio-psychosocial-spiritual structure, not a health care provider's passionate presentation.

The respect we have for others' structures leads us to put our energy into areas other than pushing a particular outcome. Our approach to therapeutic conversations is not a hopeless *que sera sera* stance, but rather an exciting, optimistic stance that invites continual curiosity and increasing humility and awe as we approach family members and stand in amazement at their ability to change and the direction and pace of those changes.

Our wonder and amazement about particular outcomes influence even the language we use when writing academic course outlines. We do not state, "Students will..." instead we write, "Students will be provided with an opportunity to..." We cannot say a priori what the student will learn. Any professor knows that any one seminar is experienced in as many ways as there are students in the class, plus one—the professor's!

Being invested in a particular outcome is an occupational hazard for those working in health care. Clinicians need to be aware that their healing ability consists mainly of influencing and inspiring individuals and families to move along the course of their own healing path.

When clinicians are too passionate about change occurring in one direction, we become imposing in our ideas and we close space for change. It is options and invitations to reflection that facilitate the co-evolution of change, not demands. We have come to believe that in the domain of clinical work with families experiencing illness, passion for a particular outcome is about instructions, and prescriptions interfere with progress!

Non-investment in a particular outcome does not mean we are not interested in what the outcome is for these particular family members at this particular time. We are extremely interested in the outcome with each family and want to know what has happened. We are curious about the continuing changes that are occurring. This interest in outcome is what prompted LMW, in her final session with the young man experiencing MS and his aging parents to show as much interest in the outcome of the respite trip for the parents as she previously had taken in the catastrophically demoralizing events that initially prompted the family to seek help. Details of the vacation buffet and bus ride were explored with as much therapeutic curiosity as the dilemmas of the devoted care giving parents and debilitated son had been, in the earlier sessions. Our interest in each family's particular outcome and our investment in outcome as a genuine issue are also evidenced by our practice of conducting an outcome follow-up interview with families. Six months after the last session in the Family Nursing Unit, families were invited to provide an evaluation of the services they received and to comment on the changes they experienced in their beliefs and behaviors.

We are not attached to any particular outcome, only to one that would soften the illness suffering that families are experiencing. What is the outcome the family wants? The "One Question Question" focuses the clinician's therapeutic efforts on the desired outcomes of family members: "If you could have just one question answered during our work together, what would that one question be?" (Duhamel, Dupuis, & Wright, in press; Wright, 1989). The answers to this question usually describe the family's deepest area of suffering, concerns, or problems.

Clinicians have desired outcomes, in a general way, for each session and for our overall therapeutic work with families. For us, a "good" family session may include creating the context for change, clearing away obstacles, opening space for conversations that may decrease suffering and increase healing, and other macro- and micro-moves described in Chapters 7–10.

Our therapeutic goal as clinicians is to challenge constraining beliefs: beliefs that prohibit, impede, constrain, restrain, restrict, and diminish family members' lives, relationships, and managing illness and instead invite suffering. We want to identify, offer, and affirm facilitating beliefs that bring forth the family members' ability and resilience to face the challenges of illness, disability, and/or loss. We are continuously curious about what facilitating beliefs promote healing.

The Clinician is Willing to Change His or Her Own Beliefs

To be effective, successful, and compassionate in clinical work, a clinician's greatest challenge is to recognize, acknowledge, and ultimately challenge his or her own beliefs when they are no longer useful. This is exquisitely true when our beliefs about illness are not compatible with our colleagues or the clients with whom we are working, and directly or unintentionally are fostering more suffering. In these situations, a clinical judgment needs to be made about whose beliefs facilitate solutions and soften suffering and whose do not. Of course it is always easier to recognize the follies or shortcomings of our colleagues' or clients' constraining beliefs than our own. Sometimes clinicians have held treasured illness beliefs for many years but simply believing something for a number of years does not make it true or useful.

One family experienced the tragic suicide of their 72-year-old sister, a sufferer of clinical depression for most of her life. One of the siblings, a 68-year-old sister who had been the closest to the deceased, was the most distraught over the suicide. When the clinician (LMW) began working with this family one year after the suicide, this loving sister held a constraining belief that she had failed her sister and could have done something more to save her life. She sobbed uncontrollably as she shared the story of her sister's depression and suicide. As the illness story unfolded, the clinician also began to fall into the trap of another constraining belief that the health providers had also failed this woman and could have saved her life. Plus, the clinician was also blaming the deceased sister for the grief she had caused her family. However, neither the family member's nor the clinician's beliefs softened the suffering of this client but rather fuelled it.

When the clinician invited herself to a reflection about her own beliefs about the reason for this suicide, she concluded that placing blame on others (family members, health providers, or the sister who committed suicide) certainly did not soften the suffering of the family members, especially the incredibly distraught sister. Instead, she challenged her belief and tried to honor the decision that the elderly sister had made about her life and offered an alternate, more facilitating belief to her client.

"Your sister and her husband came to stay with you during the last month of her life. I wonder if her visit to your home was her way of honoring your very close relationship all of those years and her thoughtful way of saying goodbye. Perhaps she knew that her own suffering and those of her loving family had become unbearable after so many years of depression and her untimely and tragic death was her gift to herself and to all the family. If you could come to believe that her death was an honorable departure, do you think you could honor her memory and your relationship more? Perhaps you could also move out of this awful space of suffering to one of grieving and honoring her memory."

132

This entirely new belief, new view, and new conceptualization of the sister's tragic death by suicide invited *both* the clinician and the client to challenge their constraining beliefs.

The client's response to this new view of her sister's death was dramatic and immediate. She stopped sobbing and looked at the clinician with wide eyes and said, *"I never thought about it that way. But you are right, I have not been honoring my sister; only blaming myself for her death."* The belief offered by the clinician that the deceased sister was giving a gift to the family was totally different from the usual societal beliefs that frequently call the suicide "the most selfish act" or "a terrible legacy to leave a family." Sometimes challenging our own beliefs requires courage to ride against the usual prevailing societal, cultural, and/or religious beliefs in order for healing to begin. But it was at this moment that the first healing in a year began for this devoted and loving sister.

It is in these moments of reflection, when clinicians are willing to challenge and change their beliefs, that the most productive collaborative and therapeutic work can evolve with clients.

In our clinical documentation at the Family Nursing Unit, we strategically invited graduate nursing students to a reflection about their beliefs by having them answer the following questions: "What belief of yours was challenged today in the session?" and "What belief of yours was more confirmed in today's session?" We have found this process of reflecting after the session on the clinician's constraining and facilitating beliefs to be incredibly freeing and useful in the development of clinical skills in novice clinicians.

Another method to identify any constraining or limiting beliefs of the clinician is to ask the following questions:

- What beliefs of mine might be stopping me from softening the suffering in this client-family?
- Where did this belief come from?
- Who gave me this belief?
- What does this belief do for me?
- What is this belief costing me?
- How might my clinical work with this client-family be different if I changed my belief?

The willingness of a clinician to change one's own beliefs can frequently be the ultimate difference in the journey of suffering for the clients and families entrusted in our care. Therefore, our illness beliefs are well worth exploring, understanding, and changing when no longer useful.

Conclusion

This chapter has provided an in-depth discussion of our beliefs about clinicians, influenced by the worldview of objectivity-in-parentheses. We have offered seven beliefs about clinicians that influence the manner in which we approach and assist families suffering with serious illness. At the core is our belief that objectivity-in-parentheses invites the clinician to become a particular kind of person where curiosity, courage, compassion, and love influence what the clinician says and does to soften illness suffering and promote healing.

References

Bell, J.M. (1999). Therapeutic failure: Exploring uncharted territory in family nursing [Editorial]. *Journal of Family Nursing, 5*(4), 371-373.

Bell, J.M., Moules, N.J., & Wright, L.M. (2009). Therapeutic letters and the Family Nursing Unit: A legacy of advanced nursing practice. *Journal of Family Nursing, 15*(1), 6-30.

Bell, J.M., Wright, L.M., & Watson, W.L. (1992). The medical map is not the territory; or, "Medical Family Therapy?" - Watch your language! *Family Systems Medicine, 10*(1), 35-39.

Cecchin, G. (1987). Hypothesizing, circularity, and neutrality revisited: An invitation to curiosity: *Family Process, 26,* 405-413.

Duhamel, F., Dupuis, F., & Wright, L.M. (in press). Families' and nurses' responses to the "One Question Question": Reflections for clinical practice, education, and research in family nursing. *Journal of Family Nursing.*

Frank, A.W. (1995). *The wounded storyteller*. Chicago: The University of Chicago Press.

Frank, A.W. (1998). Just listening: Narrative and deep illness. *Families, Systems, & Health, 16*, 197-212.

Kleinman, A. (1988). *The illness narratives: Suffering, healing, and the human condition.* New York: Basic Books.

Lee, L.L.W. (2008). On listening. *Canadian Medical Association Journal, 179*(6), 562-563.

Levac, A.M.C., McLean, S., Wright, L.M., Bell, J.M., "Ann" & "Fred". (1998). A "Reader's Theater" intervention to managing grief: Posttherapy reflections by a family and clinical team. *Journal of Marital and Family Therapy, 24*(1), 81-93.

Loos, F., & Bell, J.M. (1990). Circular questions: A family interviewing strategy. *Dimensions in Critical Care Nursing, 9*(1), 46-53.

Maturana, H.R., & Varela, F.J. (1992). *The tree of knowledge: The biological roots of human understanding* (rev. ed.). Boston: Shambhala.

Miller, S., Hubble, M., & Duncan, B. (2007). Supershrinks. Why do some therapists clearly stand out above the rest, consistently getting far better results than most of their colleagues? *Psychotherapy Networker, 31*(6), 26-35, 56.

NIFT Letter. (2006). A letter written by George and Linda Jensen. Available from: www.janicembell.com.

Reed, F.C. (2003). *Suffering and illness: Insights for caregivers.* Philadelphia: F.A. Davis.

Selvini Palazzoli, M., Boscolo, L., Cecchin, G., & Prata, G. (1980). Hypothesizing, circularity, and neutrality: Three guidelines for the conductor of the session. *Family Process, 19*, 3-12.

Strong, T. (2002). Poetic possibilities in conversations about suffering. *Contemporary Family Therapy, 24*(3), 457-473.

Tapp, D. (2001). Conserving the vitality of suffering: Addressing family constraints to illness conversations. *Nursing Inquiry, 8*(4), 254-263.

Tomm, K. (1984). One perspective of the Milan systemic approach: Part 2. Description of the session format, interviewing style and interventions. *Journal of Marital and Family Therapy, 10,* 253-271.

Tomm, K. (1987). Interventive interviewing: Part II. Reflexive questioning as a means to enable self-healing. *Family Process, 26*(2), 167-183.

Tomm, K. (1988). Interventive interviewing: Part III. Intending to ask lineal, circular, strategic, or reflexive questions? *Family Process, 27*(1), 1-15.

White, M. (1988). The process of questioning: A therapy of literary merit? *Dulwich Centre Newsletter, Winter,* 8-15.

Wright, L.M. (1989). When clients ask questions: Enriching the therapeutic conversation. *Family Therapy Networker, 13*(6), 15-16.

Wright, L.M. (1997a). Multiple sclerosis, beliefs and families: Professional and personal stories of suffering and strength. In S. McDaniel, J. Hepworth, & W.J. Doherty (Eds.), *The shared experience of illness: Stories of patients, families, and their therapists* (pp. 263-273). New York: Basic Books.

Wright, L.M. (1997b). Suffering and spirituality: The soul of clinical work with families [Guest Editorial]. *Journal of Family Nursing, 3*(1), 3-14.

Wright, L.M. (2001). Suffering and family nursing intervention research: A healing combination. *Japanese Journal of Family Nursing, 6*(2), 133-140.

Wright, L.M. (2005). *Spirituality, suffering, and illness: Ideas for healing.* Philadelphia: F.A. Davis.

Wright, L.M. (2008). Softening suffering through spiritual care practices: One possibility for healing families. *Journal of Family Nursing, 14*(4), 394-411.

Wright, L.M., & Leahey, M. (2009). *Nurses and families: A guide for family assessment and intervention.* Philadelphia: F.A. Davis.

Wright, L.M., & Levac, A.M. (1992). The non-existence of non-compliant families: The influence of Humberto Maturana. *Journal of Advanced Nursing, 17,* 913-917.

Wright, L.M., & Watson, W.L. (1982). What's in a name: Redefining family therapy. In A.Gurman (Ed.), *Questions and answers in the practice of family therapy* (Vol. 2, pp. 27-30). New York: Brunner/Mazel.

PART II

THE ILLNESS BELIEFS MODEL

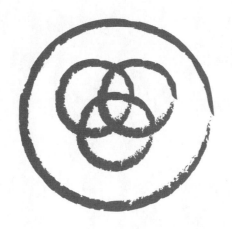

INTRODUCTION TO PART II

Intervention: c.1425, from
L.L. **interventionem** (nom. **interventio**) "an interposing,"
noun of action from pp. stem of L. **intervenire** "to come
between, interrupt," from **inter-** "between" + **venire** "come"
Online Etymology Dictionary

Move: change or cause to change from one state, opinion,
sphere, or activity to another; make progress; develop in a
particular manner or direction
(Macromoves and Micromoves)
Online Apple Dictionary

Part II of this book is the "how to" of the *Illness Beliefs Model*. The model comes to life through the medium of therapeutic conversations between a clinician and an individual or family. In the culture of health care, the word "intervention" has traditionally been used to describe the process that occurs between the clinician and client/patient. It is offered with the intention to heal and amplify wellness—whether that process is a laying on of hands (i.e., bed bath or dressing change), a procedure regulated by a machine (i.e., ultrasound or x-ray), or a talking cure (i.e., therapeutic conversation, psychotherapy, etc.).

The etymologic origin of the word "intervention" is explained as an "interposing; to come between; interrupt" (Online Etymology Dictionary). Interventions are offered to family members with the intent of effecting change and softening illness suffering (Wright, 2008; Wright & Leahey, 2009). Not all interventions accomplish this goal. We consider effective interventions to be those for which a fit exists between the intervention offered by the clinician and the bio-psychosocial-spiritual structure of the client-family member. The client's structure may be perturbed by the invitations to reflection offered by the clinician and vice versa. Through therapeutic conversations, the individual/family and clinician collaborate and co-evolve to discover the most useful fit. The central issue is one of fit.

A positive movement in the therapeutic process between clients and clinicians is the move away from deficit- or dysfunction-based family assessments to strengths- and resiliency-based interventions. The *Illness Beliefs Model* is a compassion, strengths, resiliency, and "goodness" based clinical approach.

The word intervention has recently come under scrutiny, particularly as it relates to the medium of therapeutic conversations (Houger Limacher, 2008). Do we "intervene" (see the etymology offered above) or do we collaborate with individuals and families? Is intervention a discrete act— it begins here and ends there—or embedded within the conversational process itself? Are there distinctions between assessment and intervention, or does assessment become intervention? Our working definition of the term intervention is:

> An intervention is any action or response of the clinician, which includes the clinician's overt therapeutic actions and internal cognitive-affective responses, that occurs in context of a clinician-client relationship offered to effect individual, family, or community functioning for which the clinician is accountable.

> We believe that clinical interventions are actualized only in a *relationship* between the clinician and the family members.

We find the term "intervention" or "micromove" useful when singling out a specific aspect of a therapeutic offering, such as a question, commendation, or suggestion, or the distinguishing of a temporal aspect, such as what is offered at the end of a clinical interview versus what is done at the beginning. However, we prefer the term "move" to account for the seamless flow of conversation between the clinician and family in face-to-face encounters and long after—all of which is intended to be interventional in softening illness suffering.

"Move" includes all of the conversational processes that involve change occurring between clinician and family members. This preferred language was developed through the hermeneutic interpretation of our clinical practice that occurred in a research project conducted by our team to examine the process of therapeutic change (Wright, Watson,

& Bell, 1996). Macromoves refer to the larger, major conversational processes; micromoves refer to the specific, particular components of each macromove.

The macromoves of the *Illness Beliefs Model* (discussed in Chapters 7–11) include:

- Creating a Context for Changing Beliefs
- Distinguishing Illness Beliefs
- Challenging Constraining Beliefs
- Strengthening Facilitating Beliefs

While these macromoves appear to be listed in sequential order, it would be misleading to think about them as occurring in a linear, step-wise process. While they guide the therapeutic conversation that may take place within one session or over time with several sessions, there is a back and forth movement between the macromoves as illness suffering is exposed, beliefs are examined, invitations to reflection are offered, and change and healing occur.

If you are a health care provider we hope the specific ideas for clinical work offered through these macromoves and micromoves of the *Illness Beliefs Model* will expand your knowledge and skills and increase your capacity for compassionately helping families experiencing illness. If you are a family member who is immersed in an illness experience, or as one family member explained, "encountering illness like a tornado ripping through a campground," we hope you may also benefit from the ideas for healing offered in this section of the book.

References

Houger Limacher, L. (2008). Locating relationships at the heart of commending practices. *Journal of Systemic Therapies, 27*(4), 90-105

Wright, L.M. (2008). Softening suffering through spiritual care practices: One possibility for healing families. *Journal of Family Nursing, 14*(4), 394-411.

Wright, L.M., & Leahey, M. (2009). *Nurses and families: A guide to family assessment and intervention* (5th ed.). Philadelphia: F.A. Davis.

Wright, L.M., Watson, W.L., & Bell, J.M. (1996). *Beliefs: The heart of healing in families and illness.* New York: Basic Books.

CHAPTER SEVEN
Creating a Context for Changing Beliefs

"Relationships are all there is. Everything in the universe only
exists because it is in relationship to everything else.
Nothing exists in isolation."
—Margaret Wheatley

Among the moves we identified in our Therapeutic Change
Research Project (Wright, Watson, & Bell, 1996), the macromove
we have come to call "Creating a Context for Changing Beliefs" constitutes
the central and enduring foundation of the *Illness Beliefs Model*. It is key
to the relationship between the clinician and the family members. It is
not just a necessary prerequisite to the process of therapeutic change; it *is*
therapeutic change in and of itself.

Through our research and clinical practice, we have come to understand
that a context for changing beliefs MUST be created and maintained if
healing is to occur. To honor the central importance of the therapeutic
relationship, this macromove cannot only be called "Creating a Context
for Change"; instead, we have deliberately named this move "Creating a
Context for Changing *Beliefs*." Beginning with the first clinician-family
contact, a relational context is established where suffering can be safely
shared and explored to more fully understand what experiences and beliefs
may be contributing to the illness suffering and what alternate beliefs may

lessen illness suffering. See *Figure 8* for the three micromoves of Creating a Context for Changing Beliefs.

(⊛) **Figure 8. Micromoves: Creating a Context for Changing Beliefs**

- **Creating a collaborative relationship**
- **Focusing the therapeutic conversation**
- **Removing obstacles to change**

To use a familiar metaphor, the clinician is like a gardener, carefully preparing the soil (through the creation of a clinician-family relationship that helps uncover those beliefs that invite suffering) and clearing away the obstacles to ensure that, as the seeds (the interventions) are planted, they will have the greatest possibility of growing and flourishing. Without the careful preparation and caretaking of the soil, there is no growth, no change, and no garden.

In the *Illness Beliefs Model*, a clinician's seeds may consist of interventions such as creating a therapeutic relationship or asking interventive questions or offering an opinion. The "relationship" interventions are no less important than the "opinion" interventions. One hopes that the soil will receive all the clinician's seeds in a manner that will result in growth. It is hoped that the interventions offered by the clinician will be experienced as perturbations by each family member's bio-psychosocial-spiritual structure. However, Humberto Maturana's ideas about structural determinism (see Chapter 3, Beliefs about Families) remind us that not all of the interventions offered by the clinician will fit with the family members' structures.

We have come to believe that when a context for change has been successfully created, there is increased likelihood that the interventions will fit. More seeds seem to fall on receptive, fertile soil when the ground has been carefully prepared and continuously maintained through the process of creating a context for changing beliefs. It is important to note that the term *intervention* is not limited to the therapeutic conversations that happen after a context for change has been created. Skilled interventions include *all* of the ways the clinician begins and maintains a collaborative relationship with family members.

The therapeutic relationship is not a one-way street. In the process of preparing and maintaining the soil, not only does the ground undergo change, but also the gardener changes. Maturana and Varela (1992) referred to this phenomenon as "structural coupling" (for elaboration of this concept, see Chapter 5, Beliefs about Therapeutic Change). Tapp (2001) reminds us that in the process of understanding the illness suffering of others, we learn important life lessons that instruct and humble us—making us more compassionate and skilled in conversations with families and perhaps more wise when we encounter our own illness experiences.

Micromove: Creating a Collaborative Relationship

In this first micromove of Creating a Collaborative Relationship, there is a special but often taken-for-granted process of developing a collaborative relationship that occurs in the first meeting between the clinician and the family members. Within as little as the first three seconds of interaction, the first, and long-lasting, impressions are formed (Gladwell, 2005). Subsequently, each additional encounter provides further opportunities to renew the connection and reassess the strength of the partnership. The notion of partnership implies a nonhierarchical relationship with synergism between two parties who both come with expertise: the expertise of family members about the experience of illness and the expertise of the clinician about managing illness.

The process of developing and maintaining a collaborative relationship is not immediately tangible. It is invisibly embedded in the relationship that develops between the clinician and the family. It becomes obvious only through its absence. Clinical literature has referred to this relational process using a variety of terms such as *engagement, joining,* and *therapeutic alliance.* So important is the process of developing and maintaining a respectful, collaborative relationship between the clinician and the family that research about therapeutic alliance has found that it is one of the best predictors of success and therapeutic change (Garfield, 2004; Martin, Garske, & Davis, 2000; Hubble, Duncan, & Miller, 1999).

In a deliberate first step, the clinician begins preparing the ground for the relationship in the first meeting by attending to several important rituals of welcome and setting the tone:

- greeting the family by introducing him or herself
- offering a handshake, using eye contact and facial expressions to convey interest (i.e., if this is compatible with the culture)
- explaining the setting and nature of the work (e.g., "I am interested in learning how I can be most helpful to you with the challenges your family is experiencing…")
- offering an agenda or plan for the therapeutic conversation
- offering parameters about the duration and scope of the therapeutic relationship such as the frequency of meetings, etc.

The provision of structure reduces the fear of the unknown, making people who are strangers feel more comfortable, and is a first, concrete step in developing a collaborative relationship. Wright and Leahey (2009) remind us that these first rituals of welcome and showing "good manners" are often overlooked or taken for granted by busy health care providers and require as much attention or even more attention to detail as the more sophisticated interventions that health care providers can offer. Without attention to this careful work of entering into a collaborative relationship, the interventions offered by the clinician will likely not fall on fertile ground.

Early in the process of developing a collaborative relationship, the family is routinely asked three questions:

- Have you previously sought help from another health care provider with this problem/illness? If so, who did you seek help from and what was the nature of your consultation with them?
- What is the worst advice that you have been offered by a health care provider?
- What is the best advice that you have been offered by a health care provider?

Answers to these questions provide useful clues about what the clinician needs to consider in working effectively with this individual or family. The clinician does not want to be redundant with other professional help the family may already be receiving and will need to carefully distinguish how the present therapeutic relationship and focus with the family will be different. The clinician will not want to repeat the mistakes made by others and will want to frame suggestions and ideas in a way that will be a fit for the family members' bio-psychosocial-spiritual structures.

One useful tool in preparing the ground during the first meeting using the *Illness Beliefs Model* is the genogram (McGoldrick, Gerson, & Petry, 2008; Rempel, Neufeld, & Kushner, 2007; Wright & Leahey, 2009). The genogram works as a vehicle to begin a purposeful therapeutic conversation and elicit information about the family's illness experience in a non-threatening manner. Through the seemingly simple and highly structured process of the genogram, which begins with asking about the names, ages, occupations, and health concerns of all family members, a great deal of useful information can be obtained from family members, while also providing information to family members about themselves. For example, the following two questions could provide the clinician with a useful thumbnail sketch about each family member early in the genogram interview and also providing "new" news about themselves:

- What is one characteristic that best describes your dad?
- What have you come to appreciate most about your brother since his illness began?

The genogram questions are focused on understanding the family's current structure, development, and function in the context of the illness against the backdrop of the family's history and generational links of illness experiences. The clinician remains intensely curious about which of these elements of family structure, development, and function have changed since the illness began (for more information see Calgary Family Assessment Model [Wright & Leahey, 2009]. What resources or lack of resources does the family bring to this illness experience? What special knowledge and expertise do family members bring because of previous experiences with illness from their families of origin? Other questions that we routinely ask in our clinical practice when completing a genogram include:

- Who do you count on most for support these days?
- Is there anyone else who is important and that you consider like "family"?
- Does anyone in your family have difficulties with alcohol, drugs, or any other addiction now or in the past?
- Are there any particular religious or spiritual beliefs that have been helpful to you, or not helpful to you, in your illness experience?
- Has your illness created any financial concerns for your family?
- In your family, is there/or has there been any problems with physical or sexual abuse?

These kinds of questions, when asked as a matter of course within the safety of the genogram, prepare the ground for later elaboration and exploration of other sensitive topics (for more information about other useful genogram questions see: Frame, 2000 and Hodge, 2001, for assessing spirituality; and Keiley et al., 2002, for assessing cultural issues).

Once the genogram is completed, we often provide an opportunity for the family to view the genogram and we ask, "What stands out for you as you look at this map or picture of your family?" For many families, this is the first time they have had an opportunity to see their family diagrammed in this way. They are often invited to a reflection about their present illness experience against a backdrop of beliefs and behaviors in their larger family system: "I didn't realize our family has had so many suicides," "I have a renewed appreciation of all of the strong women in our family who have survived so many challenges," "My grandfather really taught me a lot about how to live with a life-shortening illness."

The clinician uses the family's language to make the explanations and questions palatable to all family members. For example, the clinician might use humor if it fits with the family, or use more casual, less formal language when talking with adolescents and children. Even within the first few minutes of conversation, the clinician looks for opportunities to make connections among the pieces of data elicited through the genogram in a manner that may be new information to the family. These observations are offered as "trial balloons" and passing comments, without any need on the part of the clinician to persuade the family or for the family to agree. In the following example, the clinician (LMW), through the process of collecting genogram data, noted the possible connection between the numerous challenges the family was dealing with and the health problem:

LMW: *Okay, let's just go back and finish up* [referring to the genogram, which elicited information about marital tension that existed around stepfamily parenting and concern about the health of another family member]. *That was very helpful to me because it is an important aspect of your family life and other challenges you have in addition to your health problems. Sometimes these issues can affect your health problems, sometimes not. Would you guess that these issues affect your health problems?*

CONNIE: *Hard to say, because it's been like that for so long, I don't know.*

LMW: *It's like the old chicken and the egg; we don't know which comes first. Your family problems get exacerbated or become worse because of health problems, or do the health problems become worse because of family problems?*

The clinician senses she may have stumbled onto something here: the client's beliefs about the etiology of her health problems. By offering the possible connection between the stresses in the family and the mother's cardiac illness and anxiety attacks, the clinician brings into awareness an issue that may be new information for this client. The connection is deliberately offered in a tenuous manner. Without needing to convince the client of the correctness of this idea, the clinician watches to see how the mother responds to the idea that health problems and family stress may be connected in a recursive manner.

From the beginning of the first meeting, the clinician chooses to make a clear distinction between a social conversation and a therapeutic conversation (see Chapter 2, Understanding Beliefs). Although there is initially an element of social conversation in the meeting and greeting, the ground is carefully prepared for a therapeutic conversation to occur. This includes deliberately breaking the strongly sanctioned, unwritten rules of social conversation. Being insatiably curious, which is enacted through the asking of questions (particularly questions such as those concerning the experience of violence; alcohol, or substance abuse; financial concerns; death of family members, etc.), the clinician breaks the rules of social conversation. Speaking the unspeakable, such as commenting on strong affect in the room as soon as it is noticed (e.g., "You look really unhappy about being here"), invites conversations that are outside the social domain.

A powerful belief that is challenged throughout the process of developing a collaborative relationship is the belief that health care relationships are hierarchical: the clinician is the expert and maintains a one-up position; the client-family, less expert and in a one-down position, must "obey" the expert clinician or be labeled as noncompliant (refer to Chapter 6, Beliefs About Clinicians). In a hierarchical relationship, there is an unspoken rule that the person in a one-down position must never speak aloud about the relationship or about the process. One question the clinician can ask that encourages families to break this relationship rule and enter into a more nonhierarchical relationship is, "I have asked you a number of questions today; is there anything you would like to ask me?" (Wright, 1989, p. 15).

One of the most useful ways to continually challenge the limiting belief that a good clinician-family relationship is a hierarchical relationship is for the clinician to model and invite transparency in speaking about the therapeutic relationship (Hill & Knox, 2009). We call these "goodness of fit" conversations between the clinician and family. These conversations are about taking the temperature of the therapeutic relationship, and just as vital signs are monitored frequently in health care, so is the therapeutic relationship. Questions that we have found useful to check the temperature of the collaborative relationship include:

- Have you had a chance to tell your story?
- How did you experience our session today? Was it useful?
- Does this way of working fit for you?
- Are we meeting your expectations and needs?

- Is there anything you need more or less of in our work together?

These questions invite commentary about the relationship, the therapeutic process, and send the message that the family's expertise and experience matters and is respected. Close attention is paid to the family member's early perceptions and reactions to the therapeutic relationship to avoid early termination, dropouts, and no-shows. Equally important is the careful monitoring of the relationship over time. Draper and Hannah (2008) offer other useful reflexive questions to invite reflection about the therapeutic conversation.

As important as it is for the family to feel comfortable or "engaged" with the clinician, engagement and therapeutic alliance is not all the skilled clinician offers in order to reduce illness suffering. The second micromove of creating a context for changing beliefs is the process of identifying the specific problem with which the family desires assistance and identifying what the illness suffering is about.

Micromove: Focusing the Therapeutic Conversation

Clarifying the illness problems/challenges that the family is currently facing and choosing the focus of the therapeutic conversation is the second micromove within the macromove of Creating a Context for Changing Beliefs.

While the language of "problem" might sound like pathologizing discourse, we recognize that families generally seek assistance from health care providers when they are feeling stuck, discouraged, oppressed, or overwhelmed by illness suffering. We believe that careful mining for the family's perception of the challenges they are experiencing, linking these to their illness narrative, and taking the opportunity to learn more about their illness suffering are all important for this phase of the therapeutic work. Cecchin (1987) warns clinicians to accept neither their own nor the client's definition of the problem too quickly, and Maturana and Varela (1992) encourage clinicians to adopt an attitude of permanent vigilance against the temptation of certainty. By remaining curious (Cecchin, 1987), a clinician has a greater chance of escaping the sin of certainty: the sin of being too invested in one's own opinions and beliefs.

Once an understanding of the illness suffering has been co-constructed by family members and clinician, the therapeutic process, guided by the *Illness Beliefs Model*, shifts to understanding beliefs and particularly core beliefs that are connected to the illness suffering (for more information see Chapter 8, Distinguishing Illness Beliefs). Definitions of the "problem" will widen and expand as beliefs that support, maintain, and sustain illness suffering are brought to the fore. We are concerned with two levels of conceptualization: the illness suffering and the beliefs that are connected to the suffering. Although both are important, we believe that family members' beliefs about their suffering are more illuminating and central to treatment and healing.

A series of questions have been helpful to us in clarifying the focus of the therapeutic work:

- What is happening in your family that invited you to seek help at this time (or be referred for assistance for your family)?
- How are you hoping that we can be most helpful to you?
- What is causing you the biggest challenge these days?
- What were you hoping we could talk about today?
- Who in your family is suffering the most?

These are followed by questions that begin to uncover those beliefs that contribute to the suffering and those which seem to diminish the suffering (for further elaboration about uncovering and distinguishing beliefs, see Chapter 8, Distinguishing Illness Beliefs). One of the most effective questions we use in the *Illness Beliefs Model* to distinguish the preferred focus of the therapeutic conversation is the "One Question Question" (Duhamel, Dupuis, & Wright, in press; Wright, 1989):

- If you could have just one question answered in our work together, what would that one question be?

The "One Question Question" uncovers the family's most pressing concern or greatest suffering. We have experienced the focusing power of this question, such as when the family's answer to the question is different, sometimes dramatically so, from "the problem" that has unfolded to that point in the therapeutic conversation.

In another example, the use of the "One Question Question" with Connie, who was experiencing angina and panic attacks, illustrates the way this question is used not only to clarify the beliefs about her suffering but also to clarify her beliefs about the solution.

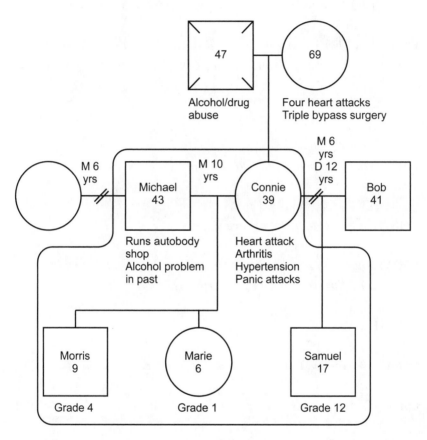

Figure 9. Genogram: Connie's Family

LMW: *Well, I guess that brings me to a question that we always like to ask in our first meetings with people we see here at the Family Nursing Unit. If there was just one question that you could have answered during our work together, what would that one question be? What is the question that you would most like to try to get some help with or to get answered?*

CONNIE: *Ah...*

LMW: *What is the question that you would have for myself or the team to try and help answer for you in our work together?*

CONNIE: *How I can either get over this or how can you help me deal with it [*panic attacks*]? Like put it in perspective or something.*

LMW: *Well that's a very important distinction, isn't it? Is your question, "how can I get over it," which means getting total control of it, or "how can I deal with it?"*

CONNIE: *Well...*

LMW: *Which do you want? Do you want to be totally over it or do you want...*

CONNIE: *I want to be totally over it.*

LMW: *You want to be totally over it. So, you don't want to just learn how to live with it like you do with your arthritis?*

CONNIE: *No.*

LMW: *No, you don't want that. For this, you want to be rid of it?*

CONNIE: *Yes.*

The "One Question Question" is an example of asking a question that is more than a question. It invites the client to narrow the field and uncover the most serious concern at the heart of the matter. In this process, the clinician is invited to a deeper level of understanding about the suffering of the family. Note the persistence and the tracking involved in making the distinction between living alongside a problem versus getting past a problem. The family member is invited to reflect on her beliefs about the problem and the solution: what is the main concern and what does she most want from the therapeutic encounter? Knowing the client's preferences has implications for treatment; the question provides a deliberate opportunity for the client to be clear about the focus of the therapeutic conversation that would be most useful to her.

Other questions that we have also found useful in this micromove of focusing the therapeutic conversation have to do with being curious about expected change:

- What do you want to change? What do you want to remain the same?
- Suppose…while you are sleeping, a miracle happens and, the problems that brought you here are solved, just like that! But this happens while you are sleeping, so you cannot know that it has happened. Once you wake up in the morning, a) how will you go about discovering that this miracle has happened to you? OR, b) how will your best friend [or your family member] know that this miracle happened to you? (deShazer, n.d.)

Micromove: Removing Obstacles to Change

The action-packed movie *Indiana Jones and the Last Crusade* portrays the undaunted, tenacious hero, Indiana Jones, in his arduous quest for the Holy Grail. There is a striking similarity between the experiences of Indiana Jones and the work of the clinician in creating a context for changing beliefs. When Indiana Jones finally, after many adventures, locates the cave and proceeds toward the Holy Grail, he has a belief that his search has been successful. Like Indiana Jones, the clinician may feel good about how the therapeutic relationship is evolving—a collaborative relationship has been established, a useful focus for the therapeutic conversation has been decided, and now change should likely begin to happen.

However, Indiana Jones, to his surprise, encounters several unexpected obstacles that constrain his progress: crisscrossing knives, uncertain stepping-stones, and unexpected chasms. He is required to discover the clue to defusing each new obstacle to continue his progress toward his goal. The clinician's role is similar. While offering a collaborative relationship and focusing the therapeutic conversation, a variety of obstacles may constrain change, from a dissatisfied, angry family member to conflicting involvement of multiple health care providers. No further interventions can be offered until these obstacles are cleared away. No ideas or questions chosen to alter, challenge, or modify constraining beliefs are useful until the context for changing beliefs has been fully prepared.

In our team's research about therapeutic failure (Bell, 1999; Wright & Leahey, 2009), we chose to examine our clinical work with families who reported in a follow-up outcome interview that there was no change in their presenting concerns, that they were dissatisfied with the services they had received, or they terminated the therapeutic relationship prematurely. It was disturbing research to conduct as we witnessed errors of omission in the videotaped therapeutic conversations that we studied (interventions characteristic of our clinical practice with families were not offered) and errors of commission (interventions were offered but were not useful, given the data available).

In one disheartening example, our clinical team seemed to be convinced of the rightness of our beliefs about etiology: that the difficult behavior the parents reported of their son diagnosed with ADHD had more to do with the father's parenting practices than with other factors. This blinded both the student clinician and the faculty supervisor from being curious and asking for a systemic description of the reciprocal impact of the son's behavior on all family members, and instead invited a linear, judgmental conversation almost solely with the father about his parenting skills. It also blinded us from asking about the family's illness suffering or their beliefs about their suffering. The mother's frequently voiced concern, "But what can we do about the fighting between the children?" was virtually ignored. This family terminated after two sessions and reported in the outcome interview that the family's suffering was "not understood" by the clinician or the clinical team.

From this research, we learned that therapeutic change had not happened in these families primarily because a context for creating change in beliefs had failed to occur. Either a collaborative relationship had not been formed, the illness suffering had not been fully distinguished before interventions were offered prematurely, or obstacles to change had not been addressed directly or sufficiently. Wright and Leahey (2005, 2009) have expanded on these ideas in, "How to avoid the three most common errors in family nursing."

The Institute of Therapeutic Change (www.talkingcure.com) has begun an ambitious project of tracking the outcomes of thousands of psychotherapists in North America and Europe based on tens of thousands of assessments by clients (Duncan, Miller, & Hubble, 2007; Duncan, Miller, & Sparks, 2004). These researchers have developed two brief standardized instruments for: 1) tracking therapeutic change (Outcome Rating Scale); and 2) monitoring the therapeutic relationship (Session Rating Scale) (Duncan et al., 2007). Their findings suggest that the best clinicians do not differ from the worst clinicians in experience, training, theoretical orientation, or gender. Nor is there a difference in the clients they treat in terms of diagnosis, age, or gender. What makes the difference between the effective clinician and the not-as-effective clinician? Attention to client engagement! "They're [the effective clinicians] more likely to ask for and receive negative feedback about the quality of the work and their contribution to the [therapeutic] alliance" (Miller, Hubble, & Duncan, 2007, p. 33). The excellent clinicians (those in the top 25% of treatment outcomes) report lower therapeutic alliance scores at the beginning of the therapeutic relationship:

> ... perhaps because they're most persistent or are more believable when assuring clients that they want honest answers—enabling them to address potential problems in the working relationship. Median therapists, by contrast, commonly receive negative feedback later in treatment, at a time when clients have already disengaged and are at heightened risk for dropping out." (p. 33)

From this body of research and from our own clinical experience using the *Illness Beliefs Model*, it is important to be exceptionally alert to the therapeutic relationship and be able to "speak the unspeakable" promptly when obstacles are encountered. A high level of therapeutic transparency is necessary for removing obstacles to change. The clinician needs to be open to feedback and be curious to ask directly for feedback, even probing for negative feedback (Hill & Knox, 2009).

Examples of obstacles to change that we have seen in clinical work include a family member who does not want to be present or attends the session under duress, a family member who is dissatisfied about progress in the therapeutic work, unclear expectations of the therapeutic relationship, previous negative experiences with health care professionals, simultaneous involvement with multiple health care providers, and unrealistic or unknown expectations of the referring person about treatment. Clinical examples are provided in the next section to demonstrate how the skilled clinician deals with these obstacles in the process of creating a context for changing beliefs.

Obstacle: A Family Member Who Does Not Want to be Present or Attends the Sessions Under Duress

One of the hallmarks of our clinical approach is the ability of the skilled clinician to "speak the unspeakable": to raise issues that are implicit and outside the norms of social conversation. One such issue is the family member who shows, usually nonverbally, a disinterest in the session or resentment or even anger at having been coerced to attend. In a social conversation, particularly in the early stages, one would normally feel constrained from commenting on nonverbal communication or inquiring about affect that is impeding a relationship. In a therapeutic conversation, if a clinician feels socially constrained, it is usually a sign that he or she needs to act contrary to social graces by acknowledging the socially non-sanctioned issue and raising it for discussion.

In a clinical family referred to the Family Nursing Unit by a nurse, the intake information indicated the mother suffered from several chronic illnesses and was living with a male partner and her 13-year-old son. In the process of obtaining the genogram information, the graduate student clinician learned that the male partner was not the mother's common-law husband, but a roommate. His resentment at being present for the session was evident as he relayed, with an irritated tone of voice, the story of the referral: "I have no idea what kind of information you were given. The only information we were given is that we had no choice but to come here. We had no choice. We were told we had to show up, otherwise all of Jane's [the mother's] rights and privileges would be taken away by homecare... None of us are here willingly. We were forced to come by homecare."

Having learned this information, the graduate student clinician had several options. It was tempting to try to define the problem by exploring the family's perception of why the homecare nurse had coerced the family into seeking help. It was more important, however, to deal first with the obstacles of coercion, disinterest, and resentment. The clinical supervisor

(LMW), observing behind a one-way mirror, phoned into the session and quickly instructed the student to redirect the therapeutic conversation:

LMW: *Before we move forward, we must first deal with the larger issue of them being here under duress and . . . validate that this is not a fun way to be here. We don't see people under duress, so we're wondering if we should even proceed at this point. Would they be willing to stay if we could change the idea that they're here because they have to be, or should we end the session right now and talk to the nurse who referred them? I would just like to get their opinion on that, because I would like to tell them we have a very strong belief that we do not see people here who are required to be here. We don't believe in that.*

A further supervisory suggestion was phoned into the graduate student clinician to put her pen and paper down and clearly say to the family;

STUDENT: *We are [not going] to proceed as if this is a clinical session because we need to talk about what we should do with a situation of a homecare nurse who wants you to be here more than you want to be here. So what should we do about this?*

The focus of the conversation was purposefully redirected from talking with the family about their illness experience to helping them deal with the nurse who had made the requisite referral. The dilemma of what to do about the nurse invited a humorous, playful element into the formerly oppressive, tense conversation. Should the family come for "pretend therapy" or should they tell the nurse they did not need therapy? Several possibilities were explored. Note that the therapeutic conversation centered on how to deal with the coercion experienced by the family members from the directive of the referring nurse. This is in contrast to distinguishing the problem or assessing the need for the family to be in therapy. To do otherwise would fail to clear away a major obstacle to facilitating change—that of the family being at the Family Nursing Unit under duress.

The clinical team's end-of-session intervention consisted of suggesting four options in response to the family's and clinician's dilemma:

1. Pretend therapy—the clinical team could have social tea parties with the family, exchanging cookies and engaging in social chitchat;
2. Homecare therapy—the clinical team could send a letter to the nurse about the problems of a coercive referral;
3. Archaeology therapy—the clinical team could "dig" for problems and assess whether there were any problems or challenges the family was confronted with in managing the mother's chronic illness; and
4. Research therapy—the clinical team could learn from this family what was working well for them in managing a chronic illness and use the clinical videotapes as teaching tapes for other families.

The family was asked their opinion of which option would be most helpful and whether they had other ideas that might work even better.

The adolescent son chose a combination of talking about problems and talking about what was going well, as long as cookies accompanied the discussion! Both the mother and the roommate agreed that an integration of the four options would be useful, with the family bringing the cookies the first time. The whole mood changed from one of antagonism toward the clinician and the therapeutic process to one of collaboration on how the therapeutic process would be defined. Defining the nature of therapeutic conversation rather than defining the presenting problem cleared away the obstacle of coercion in a respectful and focused manner. A context for change was co-created, without which, the dramatic positive outcomes would not have occurred. These outcomes, that the family later reported, included less conflict between the mother and son and greater control for the mother over her illness.

Obstacle: A Family Member Who is Dissatisfied About Progress

Another form of speaking the unspeakable has to do with acknowledging and talking about "strong affect" in the session, be it anger, sadness, or other intense emotions. Any strong affect is a priority that demands immediate attention. This guideline is especially relevant when the affect is due to dissatisfaction with the progress of therapeutic work.

For example, a couple was seen for five sessions over a period of eight weeks. The couple, Julie and Robert, presented with concerns about their ability to cope with stress related to the husband's cardiac illness (see genogram). In the first few minutes of the third session with the couple, Julie showed sadness and began crying. "The only reason we are here is because I'm screwed up…We're not getting anywhere, nothing is changing," she said. This statement was surprising, definitely a major difference, seeing as the couple had responded positively to the first two sessions.

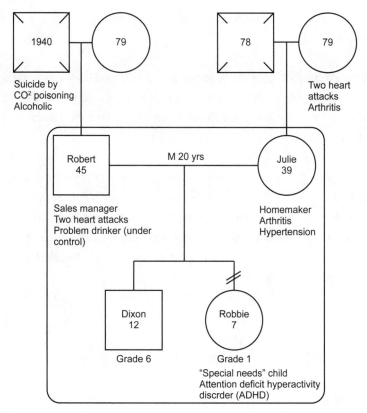

Figure 10. Genogram: Julie and Robert's Family

Notice the clinician's (LMW) immediate exploration and insatiable curiosity about Julie's affect:

LMW: *I'd be interested in knowing what's troubling you today?*

JULIE: [sighs] *I don't know where to begin or how to talk about it. I just feel like he's [Robert] trying, but things aren't getting better.* Julie continues, still crying, *I basically feel like just giving up. Like things just keep happening...*

She describes a variety of stressful situations she has been dealing with in between sessions as an explanation for her discouragement. However, the clinician does not get caught in the explanations. She persists.

LMW: *Okay. But I'm still trying to understand how come you're so troubled today?*

Julie suggests that Robert looks like the "good guy." She provides examples of his behavior that show he was trying to be supportive of her, but contends that these are not the complete story of what has been going on at home.

LMW: *You feel that through the story he [Robert] presented here that somehow I'm getting the idea that he's a good guy and you're the bad guy? So when you said the comment to me right when we started this session that "we're here because of me," and you said it in a certain tone, that somehow you're worried that I'm getting the perception that you're at fault, that you're to blame?*

JULIE: *Yes!*

LMW: *Really! Is there anything that I've been doing to give you that impression?*

This question shows the importance of inviting and facilitating the client's ability to speak the unspeakable about the clinician's behavior. What is the origin of the wife's belief that she is the "bad guy" and to blame? The clinician shows curiosity and an openness to facilitate speaking the unspeakable—that perhaps the clinician's behavior has contributed to the wife's belief. The clinician flattens the hierarchy by transparently talking out loud about the therapeutic relationship in a non-threatened and non-threatening manner.

JULIE: *No, it's just, I don't see a lot of positive coming out of it* [therapy*]*.

LMW: *And if there were more... ?*

JULIE: *The first time* [first session] *I did. And I went home last time, and I felt really good because I felt we were being really honest and open. But I felt really angry because I remember Robert saying things, like the one I just brought up, where he took all that time off,* she continues to cry, *so that I could get away, and he gets to be the hero. And I get to be the unappreciative bitch.* Julie laughs a little. *And I don't think, maybe that's right, maybe that's the way it is. I don't know, but that's not certainly the way I want it to be.*

LMW: *Well, I've got a lot of things I want to say to you, but first of all I want to tell you, I in no way perceive him as the "good guy" and you as the "bad guy." I want to be real clear about that. I see my job here to be an advocate for your relationship. I'm not trying to be more on one side than on another person's side. If I do that, then I don't feel I'm doing my job.*

JULIE: *I don't feel that you're doing that, but I was really afraid to say what I just said because I know it's going to make him angry. And yet that's what I see happening. I didn't come in here to say he's a "bad guy" and he did this and he did that, but unless I do some of that, I'm not giving you a clear picture of how I feel either.*

LMW: *Well, I'm trying to understand what would constrain you from getting your anger out.*

JULIE: *Well, first, I don't want to make him mad. I don't want to hurt him.*

LMW: *So what would be wrong with getting him mad? So what? So he gets mad.*

JULIE: *It's really unpleasant when he's mad.*

LMW: *Oh, it's unpleasant. Well, that's different then. So, you're saying if you come in here and tell me some not nice stories about your husband, that you don't want him to get mad. But now you're saying, it's not just that you don't want him to get mad—he's not nice when he's mad. Is that right? So what's the worst thing he does when he's mad?*

There's a long pause in the conversation.

JULIE: *He loses his, loses control.*

The persistence to understand the wife's suffering uncovers the belief that the wife thinks the clinician is allied more closely with the husband. Through the explicit discussion of the therapeutic alliance, the clinician shows a willingness to speak the unspeakable and process strong affect. Her declaration of neutrality to persons and advocacy for the marital relationship draws forth the significant news of a difference: the news of violence in this couple's relationship. The wife is caught in a bind. Her catastrophic fear is that if she makes her husband mad or upset, he will lose control and possibly have another heart attack. However, if she constrains her feelings, she becomes stressed and angry. Could it be that the open, frank discussion of the therapeutic relationship between the clinician and wife allowed the wife to speak the unspeakable about violence? We believe this is what enabled the wife to be so open.

Obstacle: Unclear Expectations About the Therapeutic Conversation

How can the clinician move toward challenging constraining beliefs and strengthening facilitating beliefs when the client's beliefs and expectations about the therapeutic process are unclear? One way the clinician can inquire about expectations of the therapeutic process is by asking the family about prior "best and worst advice" they have received from health professionals: "What is the best and what is the worst advice you've been given in terms of trying to get a handle on these panic attacks?" This allows the clinician to know what has fit for the family in the past and what has not fit or not been palatable for them. It prevents the clinician from falling into the trap of offering ideas similar in content or process to past offerings or advice the family has previously experienced as not helpful.

Another move that lends clarity to expectations about treatment is "distinguishing the solution." For example, the clinician might ask, "If you saw something positive happening, what would you be seeing that would be different?" These questions allow for opportunities to explore the specifics about what the family members would like to see changed in the future and how they might be helped to achieve the future vision.

The clinician can also inquire about what the family has already tried in their attempts to solve the problem. The question may be phrased, "What have you been doing to try to deal with this problem?" Again, this information is critical for the clinician in learning about the family's expectations of therapeutic conversations. By learning what the family has tried in the past, the family's resourcefulness is drawn forth and may be admired by the clinician and the family. Knowledge about past efforts also guides the clinician's efforts to offer interventions that may be "news of a difference" rather than more of the same.

The clinician needs to assess the family's goals for the therapeutic relationship. In the first session with Connie, she described her experience of angina and panic attacks. The client's beliefs about the treatment were explored:

LMW: *Is that important to you to find out why it's* [the panic attacks] *happening?*

CONNIE: *No, I just want to get rid of it.*

LMW: *You just want to get rid of it? Okay...*

CONNIE: *I just want to get back to normal.*

LMW: *Okay, that's helpful for me to know because some people I meet,* *they want to know why they have a problem. It's like a search, and they're not going to be happy until they know why. And then there are other people, like you, that don't care why they have it, they just want to get rid of it.*

CONNIE: *I just want to get rid of it.*

LMW: *So that helps me to know.*

An important distinction is made about the client's expectations of treatment. Is it more important for this client to understand why she has a problem (the etiology of the panic attacks) or more important to get rid of the problem (the cure)? This is an extremely important distinction because it will direct the treatment focus the clinician offers. Because the clinician has clarified the client's beliefs about treatment, the clinician and client can work together on the same agenda and goals. Through the invitation to reflect on the treatment goals, the client may also develop a new understanding of the problem or the solution.

Obstacle: Previous Negative Experiences with Health Care Providers.

It is important to learn about the family's previous experiences with the health care system. This knowledge allows the clinician to learn more about what kind of relationships have worked for the family in the past, what their beliefs about health professionals are, and where the pitfalls lie. A family presented in their first session with concerns about Chronic Fatigue Syndrome experienced by the youngest daughter, Sarah, who also experienced diabetes (see genogram). Thirty minutes into the first session, during the completion of the genogram, the clinician explored the origin of the belief about the diagnosis of Chronic Fatigue Syndrome. This initiated a discussion about the family physician, in which the family indicated that they were changing doctors. Notice the clinician's (LMW) immediate curiosity about the reason for the change and the way she inquires about all of the family members' experiences with the physician. (C1= eldest daughter, C2 = youngest daughter.)

LMW: *Okay, and who made the diagnosis of Chronic Fatigue Syndrome,* *do you know?*

FATHER: *Dr. D.*

LMW: *But you said you're changing* [doctors] *right now?*

MOTHER: *We're changing our family doctor.*

LMW: *You're changing your family doctor. And the reason for changing?*

C1: *Whenever we're sick, she doesn't really buy it. She thinks we're just wasting her time and that we're hypochondriacs, me and my sister.*

LMW: *How did you get that idea that she thinks these things?*

C1: *Well, every time I go in, she goes, "What seems to be the problem this time?"* The daughter mimics the doctor's speech, elongating the word "seems." *And she was really rude.*

LMW: *Does she say it in that tone to you?*

C1: *Yes, and whenever I'm sick, she always does tests, and if there's nothing major wrong, she thinks I'm faking it, even though I'm coughing, I sound like I have a cold, or I feel lousy, she . . .*

LMW: *But does she ever say to you, "I think you're faking," or is this sort of something you're picking up?*

C1: *No, it's something I pick up because she'll say, "Okay, I'll give you a prescription for this, but I don't really think you need it," and stuff like this, and she thinks I should go to school even if I'm feeling really sick and stuff like that.*

LMW: *Does she doubt anybody else in the family besides you?*

C1: *Yes, Sarah too. Because with this* [the Chronic Fatigue Syndrome], *she* *thought my sister was faking. The only reason she didn't quite believe she was faking was because she was going to the doctor.*

LMW: [to C2] *What do you think? How does she treat you?*

C2: *Well, I don't think she really acts like I'm faking it, but she's just kind of, she's really a textbook doctor, everything has to be black or white, you know, and she just seems like you can't talk to her. She's not a very good listener, but that's my impression.*

LMW: *Okay, so you came to a decision to stop going to her.* LMW then speaks to the parents, *Have you been going to her as well?*

MOTHER: *Yes.*

LMW: *Do ever get this impression that she doesn't believe. That she thinks that you're faking things?*

MOTHER: *My impression was that I felt that whenever I asked a lot of questions, because I want to know the answer, I felt that she was very defensive whenever I would do that.* The mother relates several other instances when she was dissatisfied with the physician. *We were definitely not on the same wavelength at all.*

LMW: *It doesn't sound like it's a fit for you. I mean we all have to figure out what fits for us, and I'd like you to think the same way about us. That if you feel after today or another session that this is a fit, that's great, we should continue working together. But if you go home and say, "You know, this isn't a fit for us, those things they're telling us don't fit," then I'd really like you to tell us that and let's talk it through, because I don't want you to feel you have to stay with us if it's not fitting. I admire you, because, you know, we give doctors a lot of status in our society, and I admire you for being able to say, "Gee, if it doesn't fit for us, we'd rather go somewhere else."*

MOTHER: *That's for sure.*

LMW: *I'm really glad you've taken responsibility for that ...*

The clinician responds to the family's disparaging language of the physician by calling it a "lack of fit." She uses this information about fit in a therapeutic manner to legitimize the family's assessment of the present relationship with her and the clinical team regardless of whether the family's assessment is positive or negative. She commends the family for their ability to know what fits for them in spite of society's beliefs about appropriate conduct with doctors, which would normally silence the family. The clinician confirms the family's ability to know and recognize a fit or non-fit with professionals; that is, the family members are "one-up" to professionals who usually put them "one-down." The clinician voices not only that she expects the family to be evaluating the goodness of fit with the present clinical team, but also her belief that the decision to continue or discontinue with treatment necessarily falls to the family. A spirit of collaboration and nonhierarchy is modeled, with the clinician again speaking the unspeakable: that the family may not wish to continue the therapeutic relationship and are invited, even expected, to say so, because *they* are experts on their experiences with "experts."

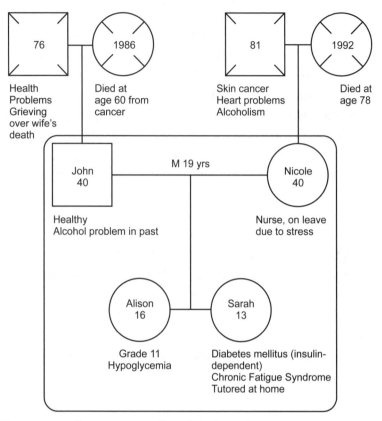

Figure II. Genogram: Sarah's Family

Obstacle: Simultaneous Involvement With Multiple Health Care Providers

When many health care providers are involved with a family concurrently, it may be difficult to distinguish the problem that should be addressed in the present therapeutic relationship or determine the boundaries of concerns dealt with by the different clinicians. Until these issues are sorted out, the clinical work cannot proceed.

In one clinical family, the single parent mother and her adolescent daughter reported multiple, chronic health problems. In the process of understanding what was involved in the family's health care, the clinical team learned that there were physiotherapists, a Chronic Fatigue specialist, and an immunologist providing health care at the time. In addition, both the mother and daughter were receiving individual counseling and the daughter was also taking antidepressant medication under the supervision of a psychiatrist.

The clinician immediately raised the question, "How can we be helpful to you in a manner that is different than the other health care providers?" An opportunity to hear ideas of the reflecting team (see Chapter 9, Challenging Constraining Beliefs) was offered to the family, during which two issues were raised: (a) the pros and cons of having so many health care providers in the family members' lives and (b) ideas for how the family might deal with conflicting advice. Family members were encouraged to remember the importance of their own voices and ideas by deciding which opinions offered by health professionals fit best for them.

Several authors have concurred that understanding the other, larger systems with which the family is involved and the nature of those relationships is an important issue to be assessed early in the therapeutic relationship (Imber-Black, 1988, 1991; Robinson, 1996; Thorne & Robinson, 1989). A context for change is difficult to create if larger system issues have not been acknowledged and discussed with the family.

Obstacle: Unrealistic or Unknown Expectations of the Referring Person about Treatment

The challenges posed by the expectations of the referring person have been addressed in a classic article by Selvini Palazzoli, Boscolo, Cecchin, and Prata (1980). Our response to the referral of a family by a health care provider is to have the referring professional request that the family contact our clinic directly for an initial appointment. Using this model of referral by health professionals serves two purposes. First, it requires that health professionals explain to families *their* reasons and expected benefits of a referral. This removes the confusion or anger families can experience when referred to another health professional or agency.

Second, it provides an opportunity for the family, rather than the referring professional, to respond to our questions regarding initial intake information, i.e., genogram of the nuclear family and description of the presenting concern. In this way, information about the family, from the family's perspective, is privileged over that of the referring professional. The following example illustrates how the clinical team dealt with the unrealistic expectations of a referring professional for a clinical family.

The family consisted of a single parent mother and her four children, ranging in age from 9–24 years. The mother indicated that she wished for help with the stress of her chronic degenerative disc disease, which made her wheelchair-bound; she was also concerned about her daughter's school truancy. The family's welfare caseworker and the family physician referred them to the Family Nursing Unit.

The letter of referral from the family physician described many health and social concerns including chronic illness, codependency, alcoholism, school truancy, depression, developmental delays, sexual assault, economic difficulties, and chronic pain. The physician requested help from the Family Nursing Unit to "get us out of what seems to be a treadmill of disasters in this family and their treatment." The family was "the worst and most chronic" the physician had seen in his practice. The physician and the caseworker were discouraged in their attempts to assist this family: "In summary there exists a variety of maladaptive dynamics that will delay or sabotage any progress." The physician's letter concluded by saying, "Considering the severe noncompliance of this family . . . I am hoping that your service can provide at least an overview of the family dynamics in order that we can plan some 'damage control' over the next few years and maximize their potential."

One of the obstacles to creating a context for change was the temptation of the clinician and clinical team to join isomorphically in the discouraging, problem-saturated view of the referring physician about the family. The family was seen for four sessions over six weeks. After meeting with the family for two sessions to understand their concerns, the following letter was sent to the physician:

Dear Dr. Smith:

Greetings from the Family Nursing Unit! Thank you very much for your referral letter regarding this family. As you know, we have now seen them on two occasions, and found it very helpful to have your impressions. Our team was struck by your obvious interest and concern for this family, as reflected in the care and time you took to write to us.

We appreciate your perspective of this family's numerous problems, and acknowledge that it can often be quite challenging to avoid the trap of becoming discouraged and overwhelmed by the magnitude of their problems, and the degree of suffering experienced by them. In our work with families, we also find we have to resist the temptation of becoming disheartened about families who face multiple challenges/problems. It is our belief that in focusing on the family's strengths and resources, rather than only their problems, we can help them to open space to new solutions, and a new view for family members of themselves as competent, capable individuals, who are able to survive despite the many adversities they face.

In our conversations with the family, the mother described a sense of feeling overwhelmed by their situation, and felt she could only manage to survive by living day to day. We have found the mother's belief an extremely facilitating one for her. We invited the family to continue working on one issue at a time, in order to punctuate their strengths and abilities, and gain a sense of mastery over their lives.

As you know, the Family Nursing Unit has a collaborative relationship with families, in which mutuality and reciprocity are integral components of our approach. In keeping with this philosophy, we have offered the family a copy of this letter.

Sincerely,
Lorraine M. Wright, RN, PhD and members of the Family Nursing Unit clinical nursing team

The letter to the referring physician helped create a context for changing beliefs on several levels. First, it was an opportunity for the clinical team to declare their beliefs about the resourcefulness of the family (which had been drawn forth and co-evolved with the family) rather than getting trapped into only seeing pathology. By providing a copy of the letter to the family, a further opportunity was provided to emphasize their strengths and resources. The clinician read the letter to the family members prior to mailing a copy to the referring physician and asked if they would like to change or add anything. They did not, but they seemed pleased as well as surprised that this opportunity was provided for them to comment.

In sending the letter to the referring professional, it expanded the audience and made the commendations of the family even more public, thereby solidifying them. Finally, the letter may have been a useful perturbation to the physician. The letter both communicated respect and understanding for his view and offered an alternative view of the family and their problems. Perhaps it opened space for a different family-physician relationship to co-evolve.

All of the examples provided above about the micromove of Removing Obstacles to Change focus on the tough challenges of Creating a Context for Changing Beliefs. These are the ones that make or break the collaborative relationship. While it may be difficult to ask for feedback about the therapeutic alliance for fear it will be negative or uncover a lack of fit with the treatment approach, new research findings suggest that negative feedback has the potential to actually strengthen the therapeutic alliance and is associated with better treatment outcomes (Duncan et al., 2007).

Conclusion

How does the clinician know that a context for changing beliefs has been created? Expert clinicians talk about "knowing the moment" that a context for change has been created, just as they talk about sensing that a context has not yet been created. Some of the signposts that a context for change has been created are that the family is engaged, structural coupling has occurred through a collaborative relationship, the problem and illness suffering has been clearly defined, and the customers for change have been identified. A family may move from feeling resentful about being coerced into a therapeutic conversation to wanting a chance to talk about their illness experience; a wife may disclose the existence of violence in her marriage because she feels safe in the therapeutic relationship and that her voice has credibility. There is a sense that the hard work of clearing away the obstacles is over for the moment, that a focus for the therapeutic conversation has been carefully negotiated, and that a readiness and openness to new beliefs and ideas for managing illness exists.

When this macromove of Creating a Context for Changing Beliefs is successfully navigated, therapeutic change is not about to happen; it has already begun. This provides the foundation for the macromoves of Distinguishing Illness Beliefs, Challenging Constraining Beliefs, and Strengthening Facilitating Beliefs. The skilled clinician moves back and forth between these interventions in a fluid rather than linear fashion and continues to create and maintain a context for changing beliefs throughout the duration of the clinical work, constantly attentive to taking the temperature of the relationship and monitoring the progress of the therapeutic conversation frequently.

References

Bell, J.M. (1999). Therapeutic failure: Exploring uncharted territory in family nursing [Editorial]. *Journal of Family Nursing, 5*(4), 371-373.

Cecchin, G. (1987). Hypothesizing, circularity, and neutrality revisited: An invitation to curiosity. *Family Process, 25*(4), 405-413.

deShazer, S. *Miracle question* (n.d.). Brief Family Therapy Center. Retrieved on March 1, 2009 from: http://www.netzwerk-ost.at/publikationen/pdf/miracle_question.pdf

Draper, A., & Hannah, C. (2008). Enabling new understandings: Therapeutic conversations with the terminally ill and their families. *Journal of Systemic Therapies, 27*(2), 20-32.

Duhamel, F., Dupuis, F., Wright, L.M. (in press). Families' and nurses' responses to the "One Question Question": Reflections for clinical practice, education, and research in family nursing. *Journal of Family Nursing.*

Duncan, B., Miller, S., & Hubble, M. (2007). How can being bad make you better? Developing a culture of feedback in your practice. *Psychotherapy Networker, 31*(6), 36-45, 57.

Duncan, B.I., Miller, S.D., & Sparks, J. (2004). *The heroic client: A revolutionary way to improve effectiveness through client-directed, outome-informed therapy* (rev. ed.). San Francisco: Jossey-Bass.

Frame, M.W. (2000). The spiritual genogram in family therapy. *Journal of Marital & Family Therapy, 26*(2), 211-216

Garfield, R. (2004). The therapeutic alliance in couples therapy: Clinical considerations. *Family Process, 43*(4), 457-465.

Gladwell, M. (2005). *Blink: The power of thinking without thinking.* New York: Little, Brown.

Hill, C.E., & Knox, S. (2009). Processing the therapeutic relationship. *Psychotherapy Research, 19*(1), 13-39.

Hodge, D.R. (2001). Spiritual genograms: A generational approach to assessing spirituality. *Families in Society, 82*(1), 35-48.

Hubble, M.A., Duncan, B.L., & Miller, S.D. (1999). *The heart and soul of change.* Washington, DC: American Psychological Association.

Imber-Black, E. (1988). *Families and larger systems: A family therapist's guide through the labyrinth.* New York: Guilford.

Imber-Black, E. (1991). The family-larger-system perspective. *Family Systems Medicine, 9*, 371-396.

Keiley, M.K., Dolbin, M., Hill, J., Karuppaswamy, N., Liu, T., Natrajan, R., Poulsen, S., Robbins, N., & Robinson, P. (2002). The cultural genogram: Experiences from within a marriage and family therapy training program. *Journal of Marital & Family Therapy, 28*(2), 165-178.

Martin, D.J., Garske, J.P., & Davis, K.M. (2000). Relation of the therapeutic alliance with outcome and other variables: A meta-analytic review. *Journal of Consulting and Clinical Psychology, 68*, 438-450.

Maturana, H.R., & Varela, F.J. (1992). *The tree of knowledge: The biological roots of human understanding* (rev. ed.). Boston: Shambhala.

McGoldrick, M., Gerson, R., & Petry, S. (2008). *Genograms: Assessment and intervention* (3rd ed.). New York: W.W. Norton.

McLeod, D.L. & Wright, L.M. (2008). Living the as-yet unanswered: Spiritual care practices in family systems nursing. *Journal of Family Nursing, 14(1),* 118-141.

Miller, S., Hubble, M., & Duncan, B. (2007). Supershrinks: Why do some therapists clearly stand out above the rest, consistently getting far better results than most of their colleagues? *Psychotherapy Networker, 31*(6), 26-35, 56.

Rempel, G.R., Neufeld, A., & Kushner, K.E. (2007). Interactive use of genograms and ecomaps in family care-giving research. *Journal of Family Nursing, 13*(4), 403-419.

Robinson, C.A. (1996). Health care relationships revisited. *Journal of Family Nursing. 2*(2), 152 - 173.

Selvini Palazzoli, M., Boscolo, L., Cecchin, G., & Prata, G. (1980). The problem of the referring person. *Journal of Marital and Family Therapy, 6,* 3-9.

Tapp, D. (2001). Conserving the vitality of suffering: Addressing family constraints to illness conversations. *Nursing Inquiry, 8*(4), 254-263.

Thorne, S., A. & Robinson, C.A. (1989). Guarded alliance: Health care relationships in chronic illness. *Image: The Journal of Nursing Scholarship, 21*(3), 153-157.

Wright, L.M. (1989). When clients ask questions: Enriching the therapeutic conversation. *Family Therapy Networker, 13*(6), 15-16.

Wright, L.M., & Leahey, M. (2005). The three most common errors in family nursing: How to avoid or side-step. *Journal of Family Nursing, 11*(2), 90-101.

Wright, L.M., & Leahey, M. (2009). *Nurses and families: A guide to family assessment and intervention* (5ᵗʰ ed.). Philadelphia: F.A. Davis.

Wright, L.M., Watson, W.L., & Bell, J.M. (1996). *Beliefs: The heart of healing in families and illness.* New York: Basic Books.

CHAPTER EIGHT
Distinguishing Illness Beliefs

"In spite of illness, in spite even of the archenemy of sorrow, one can remain alive long past the usual date of disintegration if one is unafraid of change, insatiable in intellectual curiosity, interested in big things, and happy in small ways."
—Edith Wharton

Our illness beliefs can be found embedded and grounded in the stories we tell of our struggles and suffering when serious illness arises in our lives. To bring forth illness beliefs, the clinician must know what illness beliefs are most relevant to distinguish. We prefer the word "distinguish" to describe the activity and behavior of the clinician to discern and identify particular illness beliefs. Certain illness beliefs are very useful in providing an understanding of how the family experiences the illness. This enables the clinician to learn if any of the illness beliefs may be generating suffering and impeding solutions to managing their illness more successfully. As health care providers, we have an ethical mandate to invite, listen, and be a witness to illness narratives but also to uncover, distinguish, and make a clinical judgment about which beliefs will foster healing and which beliefs are holding family members captive in their illness suffering.

If you are a family member reading this book, our list of the most useful illness beliefs and the questions you may ask yourself to examine your illness beliefs are also included in this chapter.

Distinguishing Congruence and Compatibility of Illness Beliefs between Various Systems Levels

Before a clinician can confidently distinguish and explore the illness beliefs of the clients they encounter, he or she needs to understand the importance of obtaining congruence and compatibility between a number of beliefs: the beliefs of the individual experiencing the illness; beliefs between family members; beliefs between the individual/family members and health care providers; and beliefs between the individual/family members/health care providers and society/culture/religion.

For example, if there is no congruence between what family members believe is the "accurate" diagnosis, conflict will inevitably arise about the best approaches for healing and treatment. Suffering can also arise if there is no compatibility about the beliefs of healing and treatment between family members and health care providers. It is at this intersection of beliefs that clinical dilemmas arise and suffering may be enhanced. If differences do exist in the beliefs between health care providers and individuals/families, the health care providers take the initiative to embrace compromise and collaboration. This will avert unnecessary suffering and nurture healing. The specific micromoves of Distinguishing Illness Beliefs will be presented next.

Distinguishing and Exploring Illness Beliefs

Which illness beliefs are the most useful to distinguish and explore? What are the most useful questions that could be asked to bring forth illness beliefs? There are numerous illness beliefs that could be explored, but we have found eight specific illness beliefs to be the most worthwhile and productive. This list of micromoves for Distinguishing Illness Beliefs is not meant to be exhaustive, but simply the beliefs we have found to be most useful in our clinical work with individuals and families (see *Figure 12*).

Figure 12. Micromoves: Distinguishing Illness Beliefs

- Beliefs about illness suffering
- Beliefs about diagnosis
- Beliefs about etiology
- Beliefs about healing and treatment
- Beliefs about mastery, control, and influence
- Beliefs about prognosis
- Beliefs about religion/spirituality
- Beliefs about the place of illness in lives and relationships

In this chapter, we offer specific ideas and clinical examples related to the "how to" of exploring these important illness beliefs. We also offer interpretations from our team's research project that focused on exploring the process of therapeutic change in therapeutic conversations with families (Wright, Watson, & Bell, 1996).

Other beliefs that may be helpful for the clinician to explore include beliefs about the role of family members when illness arises and beliefs about the role of health care professionals. To illustrate, we offer a poignant illness narrative from a reader of our first publication, *Beliefs: The Heart of Healing in Families and Illness* (1996). Following this illness narrative, we will offer our clinical judgment about what illness beliefs were embedded in this story, which ones served this family well, and which ones did not.

At the age of twenty-five, my family fractured nearly to the breaking point. My parents had separated in the same way they had lived all the years of their marriage—fighting, unrelenting fighting. For all the years of my life, I had heard people say of my parents that their relationship would collapse if they ever had to spend more than a month together—and they turned out to be right. My father had spent his entire career traveling. My mother, a holistic healer and medical intuitive, ran the house. There was a constant power struggle between my parents every time they were under the same roof. They fought as passionately as they loved each other. It was neither abusive nor violent, just loud, and we always knew it would end as quickly as it had erupted.

They did their very best to raise us, my sister and me. Our childhood, in amongst the tension they seemed to feed off of, was filled with idyllic moments and real love. There was, however, always a line. A small fissure was created down the middle of our foursome, carving out two ever-so-subtle teams. On one side there was Mom and my sister. On the other there was Dad and I. The teams were never spoken about. We didn't have jerseys or team colors. They just were. Dad and I shared the same sense of humor, similar personalities and beliefs. Susan and mom were exactly like each other, and completely different from us.

The divorce solidified and widened that line to previously unimaginable dimensions—especially between my mother and I. My sister, her husband, son, and I all remained close at the core, but we could see our beliefs no longer matched up the way they used to. There became things we simply didn't talk about anymore. There was space between my sister and I that had never been there before.

For five years we all worked to tape the remnants of our family back together as best we could. The fights continued through their divorce, through the aftermath, and threatened to separate my mother and I permanently. As a holistic healer, my mother had been my spiritual teacher as a child. In my adulthood, I began questioning the beliefs she had instilled in me. Through the divorce, I began setting them aside completely. For her, it wasn't just a change in my faith; it was a rejection of her as my mother. The scotch tape holding us together seemed to be growing weaker by the day, losing its stick, its ability to bind us.

Then the grenade landed in my hand. At the age of thirty, having just finished moving in with the love of my life, Joseph, the week before, I lost the feeling in my legs. It was nearing Christmas time and the closer the season came, the less sensation I had. Within a week, I started losing control of the muscles. "Multiple Sclerosis," the neurologist in the Emergency Room (ER) said, as though it happened every day.

The noise of the busy ER seemed to fade all around me. I looked to Joseph and was relieved to see he was asking questions and taking notes. All I could think about was what this would do to my family. Do I tell them before Christmas? Afterwards? How will they take it? What will they be the most mad about?

The MRI followed quickly and three days before Christmas I had a firm diagnosis. Relapsing Remitting Multiple Sclerosis. Joseph and I were in the truck on our way to a Christmas in the mountains with my dad, ironically he had booked us a ski vacation as our gift.

"There are numerous scars, black holes, showing on your scans," the doctor said. "Try to have a good holiday. No skiing. When you get back, you'll be referred to the MS Clinic..." there was more, I'm sure there was more, but I couldn't hear it. I knew right then, as I stole a glance at my father's stoic face, that I held the grenade in my hand.

I had told Dad it [MS] was a possibility; there was no way around it with the vacation planned and the amount he would be seeing me in the days leading up to the trip. Upon confirmation, his initial response was what I should have expected. "You didn't get it from me. There's no MS on my side of the family, just cancer and diabetes."

I knew, without saying a word, that my mother's response would be the exact same, and it was. I called her the day we returned from vacation. Her immediate reaction was to take the blame away from her side of the gene pool. I tried to make it clear that I wasn't calling to blame her or Dad. There was no blame, yet their fingers were pointed directly at each other.

Her secondary reaction was to set out a plan of action, through a string of alternative-medical practitioners to cure me. While she encouraged me to begin taking traditional medications and to listen to my doctors, she also believed, beyond a shadow of a doubt, that she could heal me, if I would just give her the chance.

I had a choice. Denounce her beliefs, which I no longer held to be entirely true, and outright and permanently sever our relationship, or try to explain where my own beliefs were then residing. At that point, although I'd had a few days to think things through, I was still confused, scared, and not ready to make any decisions.

My sister's first question upon hearing the news was, "Are you going to use traditional medicine or alternative?" It was also her husband's first question. When I said I didn't know, they looked stunned. As though I was so stupid I couldn't see the obvious choice in front of me. They were shocked that I wasn't busy popping vitamins and getting on with being cured.

I pleaded for time. Made no promises either way and asked for time to sort it all through. I'd only had a week at that point to take in the diagnosis myself. It seemed like everyone I told expected me to have a game plan. Friends were emailing advertisements for exclusive spas promising cures through meditation, my doctor was busy explaining medication options, there were rounds of steroids, needles to figure out, and my head was spinning. "My only goal right now," I explained to all of them, "is to regain my mobility and keep it as long as possible."

Then the silence ensued. Suddenly, my entire family stopped talking about it. In fact, they went to great lengths to avoid the topic altogether. It was as though we were all holding our breath. Would I throw the grenade? Would I choose traditional Western medicine over my sister and mother's core beliefs of a holistic cure? That's what it all came down to.

I knew what my mother had on the line; not only our relationship, but her professional reputation as well. If she missed diagnosing her own daughter, how could she help her clients? They would begin to wonder. If her own daughter couldn't be cured, what did that say about her abilities?

For more than three months, we walked around each other in awkward silence. Never daring to actually talk about it. Finally,

Chapter 8: Distinguishing Illness Beliefs

I knew I had to decide. I knew my sister and her husband were angry. They believed that I was turning my back on getting better. That I was becoming a victim of MS. "We don't want to be forced to think of you as handicapped," my brother-in-law explained.

"But I am," I told him, looking them both straight in the eye. "You have to understand that me having this disease is not a choice. That part is fact. I have MS. No matter how I choose to manage the disease and the symptoms, that will always be fact. I have MS. I will live with it all my life."

"If it were me," he said in a last ditch effort to save his side of the argument, "I'd be trying everything I could..."

"And if it were you, I'd support that. But this is me. My only goal is to maintain my mobility as long as I possibly can. I can't focus on more than that. You have to allow me to focus on that."

In a split second, as my words sunk in, the tension between the three of us evaporated. For the first time since learning of my illness, they could see the new reality of me, of my life. I was now sharing it with MS, whether they liked it or not. I wasn't choosing it over them. It just was.

For my mother, I decided not to have 'the talk.' I realized that the only thing she had to hold on to, for the sake of our relationship and her reputation, was the fact that I wasn't willing to discuss the options she had for me. As time went by, this allowed her to stand firm in her beliefs, while it gave me the freedom to manage my disease the way I needed to. Her own story of her daughter's illness could then be, "I want to help heal her, but I can only do that if she invites me to." It takes all the pressure off her and puts it on me—something that's easy for me to carry, since I don't travel in the same circles as she does.

Allowing my mother to save face has also allowed us to redefine our relationship and our roles in each other's lives. She's no longer responsible for my spirituality or for the course of my illness. She's free to just be my mom. I'm allowed to be her daughter, who's coping with MS the best she can. While we may never be as close as we once were, we've settled into the new roles quite easily.

My father still doesn't talk about my disease with me. He talks to his friends, gets advice, then passes it on to me as something like, "Pat was saying that her niece has MS and she's doing just fine..."

"I am, too, Dad. I'm managing just fine. Work sure is keeping me busy," I reassure him. He believes that as long as I'm not 'sick' I'll be fine. He talks around my disease, knowing it's there but terrified to stir it up. All he needs to know is that I'm doing everything I can and that I'm not sick. As long as those criteria are met, he's happy to accept whatever course of action I choose now or in the future.

And Joseph? Well, he's still taking notes and asking questions. He's there to support me no matter what happens, how I choose to deal with the effects of MS, or what course it takes. He's stayed right by my side, accepted my illness, and made the decision to live alongside it, as well as me. He'd made that decision before we even left the Emergency Room.

This beautifully written illness narrative by a very brave and insightful young woman highlights the power and influence of illness beliefs: how they can contribute to suffering; how they affect ideas about etiology, diagnosis, and prognosis; how they affect decisions about healing and treatment; and the impact they have on family relationships. The attachments and coalitions in this family's structure following the family divorce (i.e., mother and sister; father and daughter/sister experiencing MS) became even more entrenched when the unannounced and unexpected serious illness of MS came into the family. Fortunately, a more balanced and supportive response occurred with her partner, Joseph, who was not trying to influence or challenge her illness beliefs but rather to be a "fact finder" about the illness and to stand by her side and live alongside the illness.

From the moment of diagnosis, this young woman was concerned about the impact that this diagnosis would have on her family. Consciously or not, she knew that illness is a family affair. Both parents wanting to "divorce" themselves from any genetic responsibility also played out in the shock and awe of this frightening diagnosis. They embraced the belief that their side of the family could not have contributed or been responsible for this illness diagnosis. The young woman experiencing the illness did not focus so much on the beliefs about etiology but rather moved to accept the diagnosis: "I have MS. I will live with it all my life."

The mother's beliefs about healing and treatment were embellished by her role and status in the family of being an alternative medical healer. Here was an opportunity for the mother to play a starring role by implementing her alternative practices to provide healing (she believed) for her daughter. However, this path of healing and treatment by the mother was not compatible with her daughter's beliefs about preferred traditional treatment. However, to preserve their relationship, the daughter very cleverly enabled her mother to retain her beliefs about treatment. She freed her mother of this huge responsibility to heal and/or cure the illness by no longer being "responsible for my spirituality or the course of illness. She's just free to be my mom." In this way, unnecessary mother-daughter relationship suffering was removed, which may have hampered healing.

Joseph and his partner experiencing MS have embraced the belief of living alongside MS. Her father seems to not want to live alongside the illness but rather wishes to "cure" the illness. He has chosen not to speak directly about the illness to his daughter but rather to offer advice for treatment that he has gleaned from others. Perhaps this is a useful way for him to soften his own suffering about his daughter's illness. No doubt all family members have suffered with this illness diagnosis of their daughter, sister, sister-in-law, and partner. Each family member's beliefs about the illness softens or enhances their own suffering and may contribute to the suffering of their family member afflicted with MS. Reciprocally, the ill family member can enhance or diminish the suffering of other family members. However, this young woman has managed her upsetting diagnosis and future treatment with much grace in addition to her thoughtful, reflective, and brilliant insights into how to manage her family's beliefs and ultimately, her own beliefs about and responses to her illness.

It is unknown if this young woman and her family were offered assistance from health care professionals to deal with the impact of this illness on their lives and relationships. If a compassionate and competent health care provider had been involved with this family from the moment of diagnosis, perhaps much of their illness suffering could have been averted or at least softened. The responsibility that fell on the shoulders of this young woman to manage her family's reactions and responses also could have been lightened through competent and caring therapeutic conversations. In so doing, she could have focused her energies on her own healing rather than also having to deal with the reactions and responses of her family members to her illness, and the tension of the incongruent beliefs within the family, which we believe may have temporarily interfered with moving forward in her healing and treatment.

Micromove: Beliefs about Illness Suffering

A necessary component of the therapeutic conversation is to distinguish beliefs about illness suffering. At our clinic, we had the privilege and opportunity to soften the suffering of a 34-year-old man experiencing multiple sclerosis (MS). LMW began the therapeutic conversation with the question, "What is the toughest part about managing multiple sclerosis every day and coping with it?" So began an extremely moving and useful therapeutic conversation between the clinician and the young man about his experience with MS.

The ensuing therapeutic conversation was not about symptoms, medication, or treatment, but rather about the young man's beliefs about his illness experience— in particular, how this illness had affected his life and relationships. What he found the most difficult to manage brought forth his emotional suffering. This question invited both the client and the clinician to move away from the medical narrative and to draw forth the illness narrative. This brave but sorrowful young man (Mark) responded with a profound expression of his emotional illness suffering:

MARK: *I don't know, just those things that seemed so trivial, I can't really do anymore.*

LMW: *Yes?*

MARK: *They're not really important things, but everyone does them.*

This client helped us to learn and remember that many of the daily tasks and routines that are normally out of our awareness and taken for granted are now *out* of his capabilities yet very much *in* his awareness in the context of illness. These moments of being aware that daily tasks and routines were no longer possible triggered his emotional illness suffering.

Illness suffering invites many questions about why this illness has occurred and how it can be endured. The questions that we ask ourselves about our illness can indicate our beliefs about illness suffering. For example, if one asks, "Why has this illness happened to me?" an underlying core belief might be: "I have been a good person all my life and do not deserve this illness." However, if one believes that "suffering is part of life", then their question might be: "Why not me?" These questions center on how we try to make sense of our illness suffering.

There are also many beliefs and ideas that exist about the lessons and purposes of suffering. One belief about the benefits or lessons of suffering is frequently offered through religious or theological explanations. Theological beliefs and perspectives suggest that suffering has redemptive and transformative qualities. In the traditional Christian outlook, both clients and their health professionals regard suffering as a consequence of one's own acts or as part of God's plan, and are therefore to be endured. In clinical practice, one family offered the belief that, "God knew we needed to become closer as a family and this illness was His way of helping us learn that." However, another family believed that their ill family member "was suffering due to his choices in life and that having HIV/AIDS was his 'punishment from God.'"

An alternate philosophical belief often offered to those who are suffering is that of downward comparison with others: "Life could be worse." This belief is offered to provide comfort and encouragement, but can inadvertently enhance suffering. One elderly woman, suffering from a neurological disease that caused a loss of speech, did not find this kind of belief helpful. She wrote on a pad of paper: "I know life could be worse. I could not be able to walk. But those philosophies or beliefs do not get rid of my fears, my frustrations, my tears of not being able to talk and the isolation that it brings." These responses caution us that each person's suffering is unique and that attempting to have persons "count their blessings" can inadvertently trivialize suffering from illness (Wright, 2005).

Anne Morrow Lindbergh (1973) offers another alternate belief about what lessons can be learned from suffering:

> I do not believe that sheer suffering teaches. If suffering alone taught, all the world would be wise, since everyone suffers. To suffering must be added mourning, understanding, patience, love, openness and the willingness to remain vulnerable. (p. 3)

When individuals and families are suffering, they frequently ask themselves a lot of questions to try to understand their suffering and to make sense of it (Wright, 2005). Therefore, it is useful to inquire about the questions they ask themselves to learn where the greatest suffering lies. When suffering lessens, the individual and family ask fewer questions of themselves about their illness experience.

Useful Questions to Distinguish Beliefs about Illness Suffering:

- How do you make sense of why this illness has happened to you?
- How do you understand why this illness has happened to your family?
- How do you answer the question, "Why me? Why us?"
- Who in your family is suffering the most?
- Is the suffering physical, emotional, relational, spiritual, or all three?
- What gives your life meaning and purpose these days [with illness present]?

Micromove: Beliefs about Diagnosis

Family members' beliefs about diagnosis influence how open they will be to various ideas about healing and treatment. Part of exploring beliefs about diagnosis is to learn whose ears are privileged to hear the diagnosis as well as whose voice is the privileged voice of authority about the diagnosis (for more information, see Chapter 4 Beliefs about Illness). Some cultures, such as the Japanese, believe that knowledge of a life-threatening diagnosis will cause a patient to lose hope and the illness to become worse, which often leads to collusion between health care providers and family members to avoid informing a patient of the diagnosis.

In our clinical work with a woman who was suffering from panic attacks, the clinician (LMW) distinguished the client's (Connie's) experience of the illness and what she believed about the diagnosis by accessing the questions that the client had been asking herself.

LMW: *You know when you have fears like this, or anxiety, you have a lot of conversations with yourself. We also have conversations like you and I are having with each other right now, but we have a lot of internal conversations with ourselves. What kinds of conversations have you been having with yourself? Like what kinds of questions do you ask yourself in a day?*

CONNIE: *Well, I get up in the morning and I think to myself, "Now, am I going to be able to get through today?" Or, "Is this* [anxiety] *going to start?" And sure enough, fifteen minutes after I'm up,* Connie begins to cry, *I get that gut feeling in my stomach and I'm trembling inside and I'm trembling outside. I'm past the stage of feeling like I might be having a stroke because the physical symptoms are so strange...*

LMW: *Mmm.*

CONNIE: *...that you just wonder what's going to happen, eh? I've been to the doctor and that's what he thinks it is.*

LMW: *So you ask yourself the question, "Am I going to get through the day?"*

CONNIE: *Like, "Am I normal today . . ."*

LMW: *Or, "Am I going to be normal today?" Okay, and then I'm sorry I didn't catch the last part of what you said. When you went to the doctor.*

CONNIE: *Well, he said he thinks it's anxiety too.*

LMW: *Yes? And you thought that's what it was? Did you believe that before you went to see him?*

CONNIE: *No, I didn't know what it was.*

LMW: *You didn't know what it was. Okay, so he gave you this idea.*

In this conversation, the clinician explores the belief about the diagnosis and the origin of this belief by drawing a distinction: Was the diagnosis her idea or was it "given" to her? It is also an effort to determine whose voice about the diagnosis is being privileged.

In another family, a 13-year-old younger sister, Sarah, of two (C2) was experiencing Chronic Fatigue Syndrome (CFS). Beliefs about the diagnosis of CFS were explored, and in the process, another diagnosis, "chronic uncertainty syndrome," was uncovered.

LMW: *And what do you think about your doctor's diagnosis of Chronic Fatigue Syndrome?*

C2: *I think it's right...*

LMW: *Is he on the money or . . .?*

C2: *Everybody thinks that's what I have.*

LMW: *Yes, but what do you believe? Do you think he's accurate and on the money here?*

C2: *Sure.*

LMW: *Okay. So, what advice has he given you so far to manage this?*

C2: *He's saying to, "do what you can. Don't overexert yourself. Try to get your schoolwork done." That's probably the most important thing.*

LMW: *And what does he say to you about how long he thinks this CFS is going to last? Does he give you any idea?*

C2: *No, it's indeterminate; it could last for like five years or two months. They don't know. Nobody knows.*

In this session, the clinician is exploring the young girl's beliefs about her diagnosis. She offers an interesting distinction: she believes her diagnosis but does not believe that anyone knows how long it will last. This is a facilitating belief. It offers the option that if nobody knows when her Chronic Fatigue will end, perhaps she can learn some strategies to maintain–and improve her health. An alternative diagnosis of "chronic uncertainty syndrome" was co-created.

Useful Questions to Distinguish Beliefs about Diagnosis

- What has your family been told about the diagnosis?
- Which family members have been told? By whom?
- Do you believe the diagnosis you have been given?
- Who in your family agrees most with the diagnosis you have been given?
- Is there anyone in your family who disagrees with the diagnosis?

Micromove: Beliefs about Etiology

It is imperative to draw forth and understand family members' explanations of why they are encountering a particular illness experience in their lives at this time. Everyone gives themselves an explanation about major unusual or unexpected events in their lives. Beliefs about the etiology of illness are as varied as family members and can range from assuming personal responsibility (e.g., my hypertension is due to my obesity), to giving others responsibility (e.g., I have diabetes because my mother gave us too much sugar when we were kids), to blaming external forces (e.g., my life on a farm contributed to my respiratory condition).

Family members almost always have beliefs about the cause(s) of an illness. The Greek root from which the word *etiology* (the study of causes) is derived means not only "cause" but also "responsibility" and "blame." Many "causes" have been interpreted as explaining illness: supernatural; physical-biological; external societal, such as severe poverty and community disorganization; traumatic life events; and family system processes.

What family members believe about the cause of an illness influences how open or closed they will be to various approaches for healing and treatment. In the following segment, Mark was asked a "difference question" (Selvini Palazzoli, Boscolo, Cecchin, Prata; 1980; Tomm 1988; Wright & Leahey, 2009) to draw forth his beliefs about how MS had affected his life. Note that this one question immediately drew forth intense affect as this young man's silent tears gave evidence of his suffering about his illness. In this important discussion about his explanation of his illness, his beliefs about etiology were revealed.

LMW: *What's been the thing that's been the biggest surprise to you about it all?*

MARK: [sniffs] *I don't know. It's kind of hard to believe you could have twenty-nine,* Mark continues to cry silently, *twenty-nine good years . . .* He takes a long pause.

LMW: *And now some not-so-good years.* The clinician nods her head. *Yes? Do you see these as not good years?*

MARK: [crying] *Yes.*

LMW: *Well, it's like I've said, you've been dealt a challenge and a blow in your life, Mark, most people do not have to face. And I can appreciate that must be a real struggle for you. How do you make sense out of that for yourself? What thoughts do you have about why you and not other people? How come other people haven't been faced with this challenge in their life? How have you answered that for yourself?*

MARK: *There's not really any logical explanation for it. It's just the odds* *or the luck of the draw or whatever.*

LMW: *Always one of the things that people really struggle with, I find, especially young people when they have been diagnosed with a serious illness and experience a serious chronic illness...*

MARK: *Yes.*

LMW: *... is trying to make sense out of it for themselves, you know, trying to understand, and they have many different beliefs about it. I'm wondering what your belief is about how it is that you have MS?*

MARK: *There's not really any explanation, I guess. No one in our family has it.*

FATHER: *No.*

MARK speaks directly to his parents: *On either side of your families?*

FATHER: *That's right.*

LMW: *So how do you explain it? The luck of the draw? You had a stroke of bad luck? Is that what you say to yourself? Anything else you say to yourself about it?*

MARK: *Not really.* [pause] *I can't really rationalize . . .*

The clinician validated Mark's suffering by making a connection that his grief was tied to his beliefs about the cause or etiology of his illness. It could be speculated that Mark's belief that it is "the luck of the draw" caused him more grief, because this belief places MS out of his control. This is a different explanation from that of his parents, who believed that the MS was the result of a virus or measles when he was a boy.

Useful Questions to Distinguish Beliefs about Etiology

- All people give themselves an explanation about why they have an illness—what is your explanation about why your son has... asthma?
- How do you make sense that your family is experiencing... cancer?
- How do you explain what has caused the illness?
- Where do you believe this illness came from?

Micromove: Beliefs about Healing and Treatment

We hold a strong belief that eliciting, discussing, and expressing one's illness suffering can potentially foster and pave the way for healing. Specifically, we believe that talking is healing. Families have often remarked in our clinical practice how they have appreciated the opportunity to talk with one another about the effect of illness on their lives and relationships, and that it resulted in softening their suffering.

Families have even remarked that they felt better physically or had a reduction in symptoms following a therapeutic conversation about their illness suffering (Wright, 2005). Robinson (1994) studied clinical practice at the Family Nursing Unit offered to families experiencing chronic illness. She found that one of the most useful interventions reported by families was the opportunity to engage in meaningful conversation with clinicians about the impact of illness and the experience of illness suffering on their lives.

Although it is never easy to listen to stories of suffering, the capacity of clinicians to be "witnesses" to these stories of patients and families is central to providing care; it is frequently the genesis of healing. A heart-to-heart conversation between the clinician and Mark later proved to be a turning point in this young man's healing from his intense emotional suffering. In the final session, his parents reported that they believed one of the most useful aspects of the sessions was having their son talk about his illness experience, something they claimed he had never done before. The intense affective sharing began with the clinician drawing a distinction about possible affective responses to illness, specifically anger versus sadness.

LMW: *I see you get sad about your MS. Do you ever get angry about having MS?* Mark nods yes. *Which emotion is more common for you to feel about your MS? Do you feel sadder or angrier about it?*

MARK: *Sad.*

LMW: *At this moment?*

MARK: *Sad.*

LMW: *More sad about it. And which one is easier for you to deal with? Which emotion do you feel more comfortable with? Is it easier to be sad about it or to be angry about it?*

MARK: *Angry.*

LMW: *Easier to be angry. The sadness is harder? Can you tell me about that?*

MARK: *Well, it's just letting off steam; it's easier than feeling bad about it.*

LMW looks at Mother and Father: *Do you agree with that? Do you think it's easier? Do you notice that it's easier for him to be angry than to be sad?*

MOTHER AND FATHER: *Yes, oh yes.*

LMW: *That's a harder emotion. What about for you? What's the harder one for you to see your son experiencing, sadness or...*

FATHER: *Sadness.*

LMW: *...or anger? Sadness.*

FATHER: *I'm glad when he's angry and shouts and screams and lets it out; then he's good for a while. But when he's sad and sits there and we ask, "What's the matter, Mark?" he says, "Nothing"...*

MOTHER: *Doesn't say anything, just sits . . .*

FATHER: *No conversation, just watches TV.*

LMW: *Actually, in some ways it probably takes more strength to be sad, doesn't it, than to be angry? Because, like you say, when you're angry, it's over.*

MOTHER: *Oh yes, it's over.*

LMW: *But it takes a lot of strength to be sad. When you're sad, do you cry on the inside or do you cry on the outside, Mark?*

MARK: *Both, I guess,* he says softly.

MOTHER: *Sometimes he cries.*

FATHER: *Oh yes, he has incidents of crying...*

LMW: *Because I've had other patients with MS and other illnesses tell me that crying on the inside takes more energy. They find when they cry on the outside and let the tears come, that it doesn't take as much energy. Do you find that?*

MARK: *Yes.*

LMW: *It's harder, and it seems like it saps your energy more if you just cry on the inside? So sometimes you allow yourself to cry on the outside?*

MARK: *Yes.*

LMW: *Good. That's good. Do you understand what I mean?*

MOTHER AND FATHER*: Oh yes. I wish he would do it that way all the time.*

LMW: *That he cries on the outside.*

FATHER: *Have a darn good cry and then...*

LMW: *Just like anger then, it's out, doesn't take as much energy, but being sad all the time on the inside, you're always being angry on the inside...*

FATHER: *It's eating away...*

LMW: *It saps your energy, doesn't it?*

FATHER: *Oh, yes, it's hard, yes.*

LMW: *Do you ever hold back or cry on the inside because you're afraid it might upset your mom and dad?* She pauses. *Would you ever hold it back because you're...*

FATHER: *I hope he doesn't. I wish, if he wants to cry, let him cry.*

MARK: *I don't think I purposely do.*

In this short yet intense focus on affect, the clinician draws a distinction between anger and sadness, exploring which affect is easier for the son to experience and which is easier for his parents to observe. From the family members' responses, family beliefs that were drawn forth were (a) it is okay to be angry, (b) it is not okay to be sad, and (c) it is weak to cry and weak to be sad. The clinician embeds the suggestion that sadness—a difficult emotion for this family—takes more strength and courage, and she counters societal beliefs about sadness: "Actually, in some ways it probably takes more strength to be sad, doesn't it, than to be angry?" As the parents hear the clinician explore these issues with their son, they are hearing the previously unspeakable (their son's sadness) being spoken in front of them.

The facilitating distinction between "crying on the inside" and "crying on the outside"—learned from our clinical work with other families—led to further understanding about the son's experience of illness. The clinician combines an exploration of affect with an exploration of cognition and behavior. Note that the use of the words *sad* and *sadness* in this segment of the therapeutic conversation opened possibilities for the family to make room for the expression of sadness in ways they had not previously been able to. The clinician also had an intense affective experience of sadness while listening to this young man and, for a few moments, suffered with him as well as being a "witness" to his suffering.

Useful Questions to Distinguish Beliefs about Healing and Treatment

- What do you believe is the best way to heal from this illness?
- Do you believe that talking can be healing?
- Who would like to talk about this illness experience?
- Does anyone in the family believe that talking about the illness might make things worse?
- Who in your family is most supportive of your choices for treatment? Who in your family disagrees with your treatment choice?
- Do you believe in alternative methods for healing? If so, do you practice any?
- Do you believe in prayer to help your illness?

Micromove: Beliefs about Mastery, Control, and Influence

An in-depth discussion about our beliefs about controlling and managing illness is offered in Chapter 4, Beliefs about Illness. We credit our ideas about mastery, control, and influence to the work of the late Michael White (1988/1989, 2007; White & Epston, 1990) and his ideas about Narrative Therapy and the particular intervention known as externalizing. His ideas have influenced our clinical practice of exploring beliefs about mastery, control, and influence to more fully uncover illness suffering.

The following clinical examples illuminate these illness beliefs and how to explore and distinguish them. The move of introducing temporal boundaries in the management of chronic illness is one way of offering the idea that persons can have an effect not only on their experience of illness but even on the duration of their illness. In so doing, hope is offered to a family that they can influence their illness. A clinical example is presented next about offering this micromove to a family member, the youngest daughter, Sarah (C2), who is experiencing Chronic Fatigue Syndrome (CFS). C1 is her older sister. (refer to the Sarah's Family genogram on page 171).

LMW: *I'm a real believer that people often know how long their illness is going to last. Do you have a best guess of what you think?*

C2: *I have no idea.*

LMW: *Like if you were to guess, would you say six months, a year, three years?*

C2: *I don't know. I can't tell.*

LMW: So, *you're just playing it by ear right now, are you?*

C2: *I have "off" days and "on" days, so it's really hard to tell. Like some days I'm feeling fine, and other days I feel really bad.*

LMW: *So, you've been struggling with this for about three months now?*

C2: *Yes.*

LMW: *Is that about right? So would you say you're better, the same, or worse than when the symptoms first started?*

C2: *It depends on the day.*

LMW: *It depends on the day whether you're better, worse, or the same.*

Do you have any days that are absolutely worse than what you first had?

C2: *Oh, yes.*

LMW: And *do you have any days that are really better?*

C2: *Yes.*

LMW: *So when you have a good day, what do you do then?*

C2: *Well, I'm not supposed to work too hard on a day that I am feeling good, because then I could fall back for the rest of the day.*

LMW: *Really, and do you find that? That has been given to you as advice, eh? And have you experimented with that, to see if that's so?*

C2: *Yes*, she laughs.

LMW: *And if you go at it too hard on a good day, then you pay for it the next day? Do you?*

C2: *Yes, that's right.*

LMW: *Okay. And on a not so good day, what kinds of things do you do then?*

C2: *I do my homework.*

LMW: *Right. Can you get together with friends or go out?*

C2: *My friends are not really dealing with this very well.*

LMW: *What are they doing?*

C2: *Well, they're scared to come and see me because they don't know what I have and they're kind of...*

C1: *They probably think they're going to get it, and it's contagious and stuff like that.*

LMW: *Oh really. So have you missed seeing them?*

Of course, the amount of influence varies depending on the disease. For example, MS is not anticipated to improve over time, whereas with CFS, little is known about the length of the illness; it's as if the illness has no boundaries and therefore the client has little control over it.

Regardless, the clinician explores a significant belief about how long the illness will last in an attempt to define Sarah's perception of the temporal boundaries of the illness. The clinician offers her belief that clients often possess expert knowledge about the duration of an illness and invites the client, Sarah, through a "best guess" to declare her belief about the length of her illness: "I'm a real believer that people often know how long their illness is going to last. Do you have a best guess of what you think?" When the client claims that she does not know or cannot tell, the clinician persists by offering options of time (six months, one year, or three years) and thus sends a powerful implicit message that "your experience is credible; you are the expert on your experience." The clinician's question about the length of illness drew forth Sarah's experience of "good days" and "not so good days." Exploring the Sarah's experience with different kinds of days pursued this distinction: "What kinds of things do you do on good days?"

Throughout this process, the clinician shows that she is interested in both kinds of days. For example, she says, "And on a not so good day, what kinds of things do you do then?" A significant micromove occurs when the clinician suggests that Sarah is disagreeing with the experts— that the client is challenging the beliefs of the experts about the length of time of the illness precisely by the fact that Sarah cannot guess how long CFS will last. The experts say two months to five years, but the clinician counters that notion with "But you know your own body best, how long do you think it will last?" This inquiry begins to put a "chink" in the armor of the chronic question mark of CFS. Sarah's belief is challenged, providing evidence that assessment may also be intervention. To expand the small opening, the clinician attempts to augment with perspectives of the sister and mother. This challenges the beliefs that CFS is interminable and that health care providers are more expert than the client and the family.

One useful way to distinguish illness beliefs about mastery, control, and influence is to invite family members into the role of experts about their illness experience and the effect of their illness on their lives and relationships. In a further session with Mark and his elderly parents, the clinician (LMW) invited questions from the son about his MS. The clinician invited Mark into the expert role by suggesting that there might be things that she could learn from him.

LMW: *Can I shift a bit and ask if there is anything else you want to ask me, Mark?*

MARK: *No, I don't think so.*

LMW: *Okay, is there anything else about experiencing MS that you think would help me to understand better? Anything else you want to tell me about your experience that you think would...*

MARK: *Well, it's just very frustrating to deal with.*

LMW: *Yes. Do you feel like it rules your life at this point, or do you feel like you are able to rule MS sometimes?*

MARK: *Well, a lot of things I don't do because of it.*

LMW: *Yes. Are there any ways that you think you influence MS, that you have an influence over it?*

MARK: *Yes.*

LMW: *Yes? Terrific, can you tell me what those are? What ways do you think you influence the MS?*

MARK: *Well, not really influence, things that I do in spite of it.*

The dominant theme in this therapeutic conversation with the son, in the presence of his parents, was distinguishing his illness experience as a real entity. Various distinctions were drawn through questions exploring such things as the toughest part of the illness and relative influence over the illness. These types of questions are asked on the basis of our belief that beliefs arise out of distinctions that are drawn. This manner of questioning embeds the clinician's beliefs into the therapeutic conversation and clarifies the young man's beliefs. Many different paths of questioning could have been taken. For example, the son responded to the question "Anything else you want to tell me about your experience...?" with "Well, it's just very frustrating to deal with." Although exploration could have been attempted for further understanding of his frustration, the clinician instead confirmed his experience with a simple yes and then moved on to ask a relative influence question (White 1988/1989): "Do you feel like it rules your life at this point, or do you feel you are able to rule MS sometimes?" This type of inquiry moves away from examining more of Mark's suffering to distinguishing his beliefs about his competence in managing and influencing MS.

Emphasizing this young man's competence, influence, and expertise about his illness enables a story of determination and courage to be expressed as he tells of doing things "in spite of" MS. It was this response that helped LMW better understand Mark's experience of MS and introduced the clinician to a new illness paradigm. Mark's admission that he did not consider that he influences his illness but rather does things "in spite of it" lifts the illness experience out of the control paradigm, which the line of inquiry about relative influence is based on, and moves it into the "in spite of illness" paradigm (for further elaboration of the "control paradigm" concept see Chapter 2, Understanding Beliefs).

An extremely useful facilitating belief had been distinguished: "I can do things in spite of MS." The "in spite of illness" paradigm versus the "control paradigm" has continued to be a useful distinction and has influenced our clinical work with other families. Drawing forth this distinction is not used as a therapeutic technique but rather as a powerful alternative way to conceptualize influencing and managing illness.

The clinician's questions were based on a belief about the importance of exploring the illness experience from every direction to obtain a richer understanding of the expertise of this young man in his experience of illness. The clinician's view of the client's expertise was embedded in the shift from asking questions to inviting questions and further explanations from the client. In so doing, the clinician stepped out of the expert role of "I know what to ask," opening space for the client to step into the expert role.

From the therapeutic conversation, the clinician learned that the toughest part for Mark was dealing with everyday "trivial" things and that the notion of influence over illness was not a fit for him because he preferred to think of "doing things in spite of the MS." Following Mark's intense affective sharing, the relationship between him and the clinician became much less hierarchical. Both clinician and client had their expertise acknowledged: the clinician's expertise about ideas and possibilities for softening emotional, relational, physical, and spiritual suffering, and the client's expertise of the experience, mastery, control, and influence of the illness on his life and relationships.

Useful Questions to Distinguish Beliefs about Mastery, Control, and Influence

- What is your preference for dealing with your illness?
- Are you the kind of person/family that believes that you should fight/control the illness (or overcome your illness, etc.) or would you prefer to learn to live alongside it?
- What degree of influence do you (or your family) have over your illness?
- What degree of influence does your illness have over you (or your family)?
- What degree of influence would you (or your family) prefer to have?

Micromove: Beliefs about Prognosis

Family members' beliefs about prognosis provide a glimpse of the future: What do family members anticipate the future trajectory of the illness will look like? Are they hopeful or pessimistic about the outcome of the illness? Is there agreement or disagreement between family members about the prognosis or between family members and health care providers?

Norman Cousins (1989) suggested that our beliefs about prognosis affect our physiology, stating, "beliefs become biology." He proposed that a healthy disregard for prognoses pronounced by "experts" might indeed be life giving, even in the face of life-shortening diagnoses.

The following segment is from the first session with a family. The youngest daughter, Sarah, (C2) experiencing CFS, confidently and repeatedly states her belief that "I will get better." This is in stark contrast to the beliefs of other family members, particularly her older sister (C1).

LMW: *All right, so your primary hope for coming here is getting some ideas—see if I've got this right—you would prefer some coping mechanisms to provide support and to help the family to pull together.*

MOTHER: *Yes, because in my work* [nursing] *and just in my own experience, I found that even the diabetes was a real strain for a while until we could get a handle on it. I think that part of this is so long term; it just indefinitely knows that if we don't pull together, we may not make it through as a whole.*

C1: *I think it's hard on the rest of us because we have to deal with the fact that she may never get better, and I think it's hard for us to see her like that. Like we don't want to see her tired all the time.*

LMW: *So in terms of her prognosis, you're saying, because it's unknown, you're saying she may never get better?*

C1: *Exactly.*

C2: *I will get better,* she states in a very determined tone.

LMW: *Does anybody else believe she* [youngest daughter] *will get better? Do you believe it?*

C2: *I will get better*, she repeats in an even stronger tone.

LMW: You *believe you will get better.*

C2: *That's a fact! I will get better.*

C1: *But uh, some people don't.*

C2: *I know.*

LMW says to the oldest daughter: *And you are, what, sort of unsure whether she'll get better?*

C1: *No, I think she'll get better. It's just we don't know when, and so it may be indefinite. I mean we don't know for sure. We think she'll get better, and we're pretty sure she'll get better, but we don't know for sure. I think that's the major thing.*

C2: *The doctors know that I'll get better. I mean everybody that has this gets better, but they just don't know how long it will take.*

C1: *Exactly, so that's why I said it's indefinite because it may last years, it may last months, it may last weeks.*

This exploration was particularly relevant because of the uncertainty around the temporal aspect of this illness. It was impressive to hear Sarah's confident belief that she indeed would recover from CFS. She just did not know how long it would take. As other family members expressed their uncertainty, this teenager expressed more and more certainty that she would recover from CFS, a very facilitating belief indeed.

Another poignant example of distinguishing beliefs about prognosis occurred with Mark, the young man experiencing MS. The therapeutic conversation quickly moved from one about diagnosis to one of prognosis. More accurately, it moved from the story of suffering at the time of diagnosis to Mark's current suffering about his future.

MARK: *They sent me to an ophthalmologist, and he did a vision range or field on a big cloth thing...*

LMW: *Yes?*

MARK: *And he found I had a blind spot, and he said, "I don't want to ruin your holiday, but either this is something unrelated to anything, just an isolated incident, or that's how MS starts..."*

LMW: *Well, it must have been quite a shock for you to hear this.*

MARK: *Oh yes, I was on a holiday having a good time...*

LMW: *Yes? So that was the first time and then what happened from there?*

MARK: *That would have been February...*

MOTHER: *Yes, February, it was.*

MARK: *And I was diagnosed in December of that year. So, nine months later.*

LMW: *Nine months later. Well, you've been dealt quite a challenge in your life, Mark, haven't you, to cope with MS. I think this is, of course, one of the reasons your mom and dad were interested in coming here* [to FNU] *is because it's quite a challenge for family members too when there's a serious illness in the family. So I'd be curious to know from you, what problems or concerns do you have at the moment? Either for yourself or within the family as a whole? Either with dealing with your illness or dealing with other things?*

MARK: *I've just seen how bad some people get.*

LMW: *Yes.*

MARK: *And there's no way to know if I'm going to get that bad.*

LMW: *Is that a worry for you? Do you worry about how bad your situation is going to become? Is that on your mind?*

MARK: *Not a lot.*

LMW: *Not a lot, but ...*

MARK: *But it's a concern ...*

LMW: *Yes, so one of your concerns is what does your future hold. How do you understand your MS? What has been explained to you about it?*

MARK: *Well, it's a neurological disorder.*

LMW: *Yes, so when you think about your future, what do you think about? What do you see for yourself? Like you said, you're concerned. You've seen what's happened to other people.*

MARK: *I'm not really too worried about the financial end.*

LMW: *Okay ...*

MARK: *Just concerned about how bad it's going to get.*

One nodal point in this segment was when the clinician moved to validate this young man's suffering by stating that he had been "dealt quite a challenge in [his] life." In our clinical experience, the deliberate and open acknowledgment of suffering frequently opens the door for the disclosure of other fears or worries not previously expressed.

The clinician also embedded the idea that the parents were impacted by this illness experience. Then a couple of questions were asked that refined the son's present concerns by making distinctions between self and family and between dealing with illness and dealing with other things. Offering this opportunity for refinement of his concerns, on the heels of validating the tremendous challenge he has been given in life, moves the son to respond, "I've just seen how bad some people get."

For the first time, he now expresses concern about his prognosis. This disclosure reveals that his present illness suffering is more about the future (prognosis) than about the past (diagnosis). In our clinical experience, we have learned that clients are more concerned or troubled by their diagnosis when their beliefs about diagnosis differ from those of health professionals or other family members. When there is no disagreement about the diagnosis, clients tend to focus on their prognosis; that is, on how their futures will develop.

Beliefs have a tremendous effect on the optimism and hope that individuals experience about their illness. Hope is different from expectations, wishes, and desires. The existence of hope can be ascertained by asking family members their beliefs about their future with the illness. To be able to focus on the future in the face of a chronic or life-threatening illness enables families to experience the healing phenomenon of hope. Some of the most challenging clinical work with families arises when there are divergent beliefs about the future among family members. If a mother believes that her 16-year-old child with leukemia will die soon, conflict will arise when the father brings home university catalogs based on his belief that the child will live and go to college.

Hope is also different from "the will to live", which may be experienced as satisfying or unsatisfying. At a Japanese health center, "meaningful life therapy" assists cancer patients to continue in a satisfying life, even in the face of horrendous illness.

The place of beliefs about hope and optimism in the illness experience has generally not been addressed by the dominant medical system. This is perhaps one explanation of the increasing appeal of alternative or complementary healing approaches. Many persons suffering with illness experience these approaches as more positive than the conventional medical approach because complementary healing approaches do not shy away from some of the big questions surrounding illness: Why has this sickness happened to me? Why do people get sick despite living well? Why do some people die "before their time?" These kinds of questions about suffering inevitably open the door to spirituality as the meaning of suffering is queried and postulated (Wright, 2005).

Useful Questions to Distinguish Beliefs about Prognosis

- What do you believe the future holds for you [with this illness]?

- What do family members anticipate the future of this illness will look like?
- Are they hopeful or pessimistic about the outcome of the illness?
- What have health care professionals told you about the prognosis?
- Is there agreement or disagreement between family members about the prognosis?"

Micromove: Beliefs about Religion/Spirituality

The influence of family members' religious and spiritual beliefs on their illness experience has previously been one of the most neglected areas in family work. Our clinical experiences with families have taught us that the experience of suffering becomes transposed to one of spirituality as family members try to make meaning out of their suffering and distress (Wright, 2005, 2008). When health care providers explore family members' religious and spiritual beliefs, they are often concerned about the issue of religious pluralism. To understand how family members offer compassion and what efforts are made to soften suffering, it is useful to explore religious and spiritual beliefs. Cattich and Knudson-Martin (2009) conceptualized spirituality as a relational process and found that spiritual beliefs, couple communication, and problem solving were intertwined in how couples managed diabetes.

The domains of religion and spirituality provide many rich and useful ideas about beliefs. It is important and helpful to make a distinction between religion, which is extrinsic, and spirituality, which is intrinsic. Spirituality is whatever or whoever gives *ultimate* meaning, purpose, and connection in one's life that invites particular ways of being in the world in relation to oneself, others, and the universe (Wright, 2005). Religion is the affiliation or membership in a particular faith community who share a set of beliefs, rituals, morals, and sometimes a health code centered on a defined or transcendent power, most frequently referred to as God.

It has been our clinical experience that persons and families with illness cope better if there is an absence of spiritual suffering or distress. Spiritual suffering is usually the inability to invest life with meaning, purpose, and connection. To find meaning in all major events that arise in our lives seems to be a basic human need. Meaning can be framed within the context of spiritual or religious beliefs or through adherence to a particular ideological viewpoint, be it philosophical, psychological, or political. By being clear about our view of life and possessing facilitating beliefs about life, we are less threatened by unexpected or unusual experiences.

The challenge of health care providers in working with family members who are experiencing spiritual suffering is to avoid falling into the trap of offering ready answers. They are there to listen, accept, and be curious. In so doing, one hopes that family members will discover their own meanings for illness and reasons for believing what they do about their illness.

It is further hoped that the beliefs they adopt will assist them to soften their spiritual suffering. Unfortunately, there are religious healers who attribute setbacks to the lack of spiritual purity of the patient or the impulses of God's will. This belief is often used as an explanation for failures to heal or respond to treatment. Some practitioners in the field of holistic health, with its emphasis on mental control over physical states and the importance of mind-body-spirit integration, have offered similar explanations for failures.

Congruence between spiritual and/or religious beliefs and one's behavior results in a general sense of wellbeing and wholeness, whereas a lack of congruence frequently results in guilt or shame. One delightful exception to this correlation is seen in the story of a 90-year-old woman experiencing difficulty remembering past events and enjoying the game of bingo for the first time in her life. Her granddaughter relates that her grandmother does not remember that she does not believe in gambling.

Illness begs answers to the big questions in life, and frequently spiritual or religious beliefs offer meaningful and comforting answers as well as being an integral part of the healing process. Are health care providers prepared to aid family members in their search for the answers to the big questions? If health care providers are to be helpful, we must acknowledge that suffering and, often, the senselessness of it are ultimately spiritual issues.

For a more in depth reading of the connection between beliefs, suffering, and spirituality, known as the Trinity Model, we refer you to Lorraine Wright's book *Spirituality, Suffering, and Illness: Ideas for*

Healing published by F.A. Davis in 2005.

One clinical family we were privileged to assist consisted of a common-law couple and their 8-year-old daughter. The mother's presenting concern was her daughter's behavior problems at school and aggressive behavior toward the mother at home. During the first session (mother only present), the mother's belief about the connection between the child's behavior, the mother's recurrent breast cancer, and the recent separation of the parents was revealed. Also, the mother expressed concern about the relationship between the daughter and father after her death. The following dialogue occurred in the third session, with the mother, father, and child present.

LMW: *How much do you think Natasha* [daughter] *understands about death or about dying?*

FATHER: *I think Natasha has a peaceful understanding of that because of the church: reincarnation and perpetuation of the soul.*

MOTHER: *Natasha was born with these ideas.*

LMW asks the mother: *And what are your religious beliefs about death?*

MOTHER: *I don't have religious beliefs. I just have a spiritual philosophy.*

LMW: *Yes, and what is that?*

MOTHER: *I believe that my soul is immortal and no one can touch it except me. I am the only one who can change it. It doesn't stop if my body dies.*

LMW again asks the mother: *And what do you think Natasha's beliefs are?*

MOTHER: *Christian Scientist Sunday School and prayer can heal headaches.*

LMW: *Natasha, can you help me understand what your mom is saying?*

When your mom is sick and if she does die, what do you believe will happen? [long pause] *Can you tell me what you think? It's a pretty tough question. A hard one, isn't it?*

FATHER: [to daughter] *Have you thought about it much?*

NATASHA: *No.*

LMW: *Natasha, do you believe that when people are sick they can make themselves better?*

NATASHA: [nods yes]

LMW: *Do think there are ever times when people get sick and no matter how hard they pray or what they do that they can't get better, that their body can't do what they want and they still might die? Can that happen?*

NATASHA: *Yes.*

Later in the session, the following therapeutic conversation took place:

LMW: *Do you think at this point in time that Natasha is doing quite well with her understanding of your illness and the possibility of your life being shortened?*

MOTHER: *She has a good basic foundation. But there is some denial there because she believes that if I wanted to get well, then I could. But I'm at peace. I don't mind moving on.*

Uncovering the family members' beliefs about death and dying was quite significant. We learned that this young mother was at peace with the possibility that her life would be shortened but that her young daughter believed that if her mother wanted to be well, then she would be. We later discovered that the father's belief was similar to his daughter's and that he was also concerned that the mother had given up and was not trying anymore. Discussing these ideas openly and frankly with the family members proved to be a useful exercise. This young mother sadly did die a few months later, and we had the privilege to work with the father and Natasha again. At that time, Natasha was concerned about keeping her mother's memory alive, and we discussed ways that she was already doing that and other ideas that she might entertain.

Useful Questions to Distinguish Beliefs about Religion/Spirituality

- Are there any religious or spiritual beliefs that have been particularly helpful to you during your illness?
- Are there any religious or spiritual beliefs that have NOT been helpful to you during your illness (or perhaps even increased your suffering)?
- What do your religious or spiritual beliefs suggest about health and health care?
- Are there any religious or spiritual practices that you find helpful to cope with your illness? For example, do you pray about your illness? If so, may I ask what you pray for?

Micromove: Beliefs about the Place of Illness in Lives and Relationships

Integration of illness in our lives and relationships can consist of making a place for illness, living alongside illness, putting illness in its place, and/or overcoming illness. Temporal distinctions are often useful in understanding various approaches to managing the illness experience. In the early phases of illness, particularly at the time of diagnosis, there occurs the need for "making a place for illness."

LMW worked with a 25-year-old woman who was experiencing chronic pain. This client was asked by LMW to monitor her activities for two weeks and rate her levels of pain each day. In the second session, she stated she now realized that she had not made a place for pain in her life—that she had wanted to continue all of her activities without "making a place" for illness.

In another family, a 45-year-old wife and mother was newly diagnosed with MS. Her husband remarked, "It may sound selfish, but I was hoping we could just carry on with our lives while we adjusted to this news. But now I see that MS requires some time and attention; carrying on with our lives means including MS." Both of these examples highlight one of the greatest initial challenges with any illness; that is, making a place for it in our lives. However, the North American phenomenon of busyness and no time for illness makes the inclusion of illness an irritant and an add-on to life rather than an integral part of life.

The place that is made for illness may change over time. For example, the space and place of a newly diagnosed illness in family members' lives will be different from that of an illness diagnosed several years previously. There is also a distinction between "making a place" in a life for illness (as in the case of the early days of diagnosis) versus "living alongside illness" in order to have a life (as occurs with the long haul of chronic illness).

In one family, a woman who was successfully living alongside her illness was invited to write a letter to a young woman experiencing MS who was not yet as successful. The letter gave the recipient hope and encouragement. The older woman expressed that writing the letter was a highly "cathartic" experience for her. She also went on to say, "MS is still here, but it does not dominate our lives and occupies only a small space over in the corner." This woman was successful at living alongside of illness. This idea enables persons outside of the family to acknowledge the family member's progress and competence at living alongside illness or putting illness in its place.

The following therapeutic conversation illustrates how a 13-year-old daughter, Sarah (C2), experiencing Chronic Fatigue Syndrome was successful in taking charge of another illness in her life, diabetes, and how she integrated that illness into her life by putting it in its place. The conversation takes place with Sarah (C2), her older sister (C1), and her parents. This leads to a useful comparison and notion of balance between the two illness experiences. It also enables the clinician to offer a new reflection, a new facilitating belief, that perhaps what she has been able to do is keep "diabetes in its place." This precise choice of words fosters the belief that illness can be in one's life but does not have to be in one's face. It also embeds the idea that success invites success; that is, being successful in coping with one illness (diabetes) may predict success in coping with another (CFS).

LMW: *What else do you do to keep diabetes in its place? To keep diabetes in its place, you take insulin; what other kinds of things do you do?*

C2: *Well, my diet.*

LMW: *Yes, what else do you do?*

C2: *Blood tests.*

LMW: *Blood tests. How often do you have to take those?*

C2: *I'm supposed to do it about four times a day, but I only do it about two.*

C1: *She doesn't do it every day, usually. She usually does it...*

LMW: *So, has your sister been pretty much in charge of her diabetes then?*

C1: *Yes.*

LMW: *You don't have to assist her with the insulin; she's pretty much in charge of all that?*

C1: *Yes, she is. She won't let us draw it up for her.*

LMW: *WOW! We certainly know of families and other patients with whom we've worked where adolescents that have diabetes don't really take very good charge of it. So, that's terrific!*

FATHER: *She's very good.*

LMW: *When did you start taking charge of your diabetes like that?*

C2: *Oh...*

MOTHER: *Almost right after she got it.*

C2: *I got it when I was eight, and I was sort of confused and stuff. I just didn't know how to really deal with it and then I sort of relied on my parents to draw it up* [insulin] *and give it and everything and then...*

C1: *Yes, but that was only for a month.*

C2: *And then after a while I started getting braver and giving it myself.*

LMW: *Well, that's impressive! So you must be pretty impressed with your daughter with the way she's...*

C1: *I know if I had diabetes, I would have, well, I like being independent. I don't think I could rely on somebody else drawing it up and giving it for me. I think my sister is the same way. I think it was the way we were raised. Like not being dependent on others.*

LMW: *Where did you get this sort of leadership and take-charge kind of attitude? Where did that come from?*

FATHER: *It wasn't us.*

C1: *I think that we've just always had it.*

LMW: *Yes, but you said...*

C1: *Upbringing...*

LMW: *Part of your upbringing.*

C1: *Because I remember that my sister and me were always the most mature out of all the kids we hung around with. We always took charge and stuff like that, so I think it's been throughout.*

LMW: [to parents] *Do you agree they obtained this sort of "take charge" approach to things from you folks?*

FATHER: *I think so, in that sense.*

LMW: *So it sounds like you've really been able to put diabetes in its place, but it doesn't sound like you've been able to put Chronic Fatigue Syndrome in its place yet. You're still trying to figure out how to put it in its place?*

This move offers and supports the belief that managing an illness successfully involves "putting the illness in its place." This is an important facilitating belief because it challenges the constraining belief that "managing an illness successfully equals eliminating the illness from one's life." Illness can be *included* in a life. Illness and a good life can coexist. One way of integrating illness into one's life is to "put illness in its place."

An important developmental question in the history of the illness with the adolescent with CFS was, "When did you start taking charge of your diabetes like that?" This question embeds a commendation for this young woman of taking personal responsibility for her illness. The clinician is broadcasting the success in the context of the therapeutic conversation. Other family members validate Sarah's past success at taking personal responsibility for the illness. The concepts of volition and responsibility are then added on and framed as leadership. Careful use of the words suggests to Sarah that she has influence over the diabetes. She and other family members respond quickly to this use of language. There seems to be a fit between the words the clinician uses and the family's experience.

Next, the commendation to Sarah is enlarged to include the parents: Perhaps the daughter obtained this "take charge" kind of approach to illness from her parents. The clinician then makes an important connection: Sarah has been able to put diabetes in its place but, as yet, has not been able to put CFS in its place. This balancing and comparing of illnesses has remarkable leverage in opening space for Sarah to see the possibility of having some influence over the CFS: the uncertain and mysteriously non-temporally bound illness. The embedding of expectations and probabilities of success on the basis of a client's previous success story offers invitations for confidence in putting CFS in its place.

Through the therapeutic conversation, Sarah's experiences and expertise are elevated using the family's former experience and past successes. This embeds hope for the present situation because the adolescent is distinguished as victor, not a victim of illness. Possibilities for future change are opened through the uncovering of past illness experiences.

It is tremendously useful to offer distinctions to families about making a place for illness, living alongside illness, or putting illness in its place. It challenges a common belief in our culture that to have a satisfying life, one cannot experience illness. Instead, the clinician offers the more optimistic idea that illness does not need to consume one's whole life. Persons experiencing illness can make a place for it and can decide how much space the illness is going to occupy in one's life. This belief offers an element of volition in that family members decide what place and space illness will have in their lives. It allows for more acceptance of illness, less blaming for failure to manage the illness, and less blaming of the fact that illness exists or has arisen in the first place.

Useful Questions to Distinguish Beliefs about the Place of Illness in Lives and Relationships

- Are you the kind of person that believes it is best to work towards overcoming your illness or adapting to living alongside your illness?
- Do you believe it is best to give a place for illness in your life or to try and ignore your illness?
- As a family, do you believe that your father's illness has too much status and prominence in your family life? If so, what do you think could be done to reduce the status but still be compassionate to your father?
- If you create a place for illness in your life, do you believe you will have more influence on it, or less?

Conclusion

The macromove of Distinguishing Illness Beliefs involves a purposeful and continued effort on behalf of the clinician to draw forth illness beliefs with curiosity, respectfulness, and appreciation of family members in their experience of illness. This chapter has given a sampling of some of the micromoves used to explore and distinguish illness beliefs, namely, beliefs about illness suffering; diagnosis; etiology; healing and treatment; mastery, control, and influence; prognosis; religion/spirituality; and the place of illness in lives and relationships. Additional questions are also available in the instruments that explore illness beliefs in research and in clinical practice (see Part III, Resource Three).

By drawing forth illness beliefs, the clinician is able to co-assess with family members what beliefs are constraining (that invite suffering) and which are facilitating (that soften suffering) in the management of an illness experience. Of course, there are no correct beliefs for families to hold when experiencing serious illness; only beliefs that are more freeing, useful, and facilitating in the lives and relationships of family members.

References

Cattich, J., & Knudson-Martin, C. (2009). Spirituality and relationship: A holistic analysis of how couples cope with diabetes. *Journal of Marital and Family Therapy, 35*(1), 111-124.

Cousins, N. (1989). *Beliefs become biology* [Videotape]. Victoria, British Columbia, Canada: University of Victoria.

Lindbergh, A.M. (1973). *Hour of gold, hour of lead: Diaries and letters of Anne Morrow Lindbergh, 1929-1932.* New York: Harcourt Brace & World.

Robinson, C.A. (1994). Nursing interventions with families: A demand or an invitation to change? *Journal of Advanced Nursing, 19*, 897-904.

Selvini Palazzoli, M., Boscolo, L., Cecchin, G, & Prata, G. (1980). Hypothesizing, circularity, and neutrality: Three guidelines for the conductor of the session. *Family Process, 19*, 3-12.

Tomm, K. (1988). Interventive interviewing: Part III. Intending to ask lineal, circular, strategic, or reflexive questions. *Family Process, 27*(1), 1-15.

White, M. (1988/1989). Externalizing of the problem and re-authoring of lives and relationships. *Dulwich Centre Newsletter,* 3-21.

Chapter 8: Distinguishing Illness Beliefs

White, M. (2007). *Maps of narrative practice.* New York: W.W. Norton.

White, M., & Epston, D. (1990). *Narrative means to therapeutic ends.* New York: W.W. Norton.

Wright, L.M. (2005). *Spirituality, suffering, and illness: Ideas for healing.* Philadelphia: F.A. Davis.

Wright, L.M. (Producer). (2007). *Spirituality, suffering, and illness: Conversations for healing.* [DVD]. (available from: www.lorrainewright.com)

Wright, L.M. (2008). Softening suffering through spiritual care practices: One possibility for healing families. *Journal of Family Nursing, 14*(4), 394-411.

Wright, L.M., & Leahey, M. (2009). *Nursing and families: A guide to family assessment and intervention.* (5th ed). Philadelphia: F.A. Davis Company.

Wright, L.M., Watson, W.L., Bell, J.M. (1996). *Beliefs: The heart of healing in families and illness.* New York: Basic Books.

CHAPTER NINE
Challenging Constraining Beliefs

"Although the world is full of suffering, it is also
full of the overcoming of it."
—Helen Keller

In the *Illness Beliefs Model*, we conceptualize and offer micromoves/
interventions that target the systemic, recursive, and reciprocal
relationships between the beliefs of the ill individual, family members, the
health care providers, and the larger cultural and societal belief systems
they are nested within. The specific beliefs that we hope to target are those
that limit problem solving and solutions and increase suffering (for more
background information, see Chapters 2, 4, 5, and 6). What can a clinician
offer that will invite reflections in family members and hopefully challenge
their constraining beliefs and nurture healing? Out of a myriad of possible
micromoves/interventions, which ones have we found most useful in our
clinical practice with individuals and families?

In this chapter, we identify and describe several micromoves from our
research and clinical practice that are integral to the *Illness Beliefs Model*.
Challenging constraining beliefs through various micromoves is where
the heart of therapeutic change takes place. Some of these micromoves
evolved through our own clinical practice with individuals and families;
others were derived from the systemic intervention literature and our
own learning at conferences and workshops; while still others arose from

the research we conducted about our practice (Bell & Wright, 2007). Regardless of their origin, the purpose of all of these micromoves is to invite more facilitating beliefs through reflection: i.e., facilitating beliefs of family members *and* facilitating beliefs of the clinician/clinical team (see *Figure 13*). This is not an exhaustive list of the micromoves that we use to challenge constraining beliefs, but these are the ones that best characterize our work with families and that we have found to be the most beneficial to soften suffering.

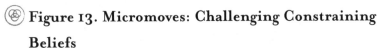 **Figure 13. Micromoves: Challenging Constraining Beliefs**

•**Asking interventive questions**

•**Speaking the unspeakable**

•**Offering alternative beliefs**

•**Using research findings**

•**Offering externalizing conversations**

•**Writing therapeutic letters**

•**Offering commendations**

•**Using reflecting teams**

Micromove: Asking Interventive Questions

We were initiated into the interventive world of questioning through the work of the Milan team (the late Dr. Mara Selvini Palazzoli; the late Dr. Gianfranco Cecchin; Dr. Luigi Boscolo; and Dr. Guiliana Prata). They first offered their ideas to the North American community through workshops in Calgary in the early 1980s (Tomm, 1984a, 1984b). Dr. Lorraine Wright asked Dr. Mara Selvini Palazzoli, one of the original members of the Milan team, "What is the best way to teach nurses to be helpful to families?" Her answer was, "Teach them to ask relationship questions," (M. Selvini

Palazzoli, personal communication, 1985). Since that time, we have drawn on the beneficial and elegant interventive questions (circular, reflexive, relative influence questions, etc.) that have been described, typologized, and illustrated elsewhere (Fleuridas, Nelson, & Rosenthal, 1986; Loos & Bell, 1990; Tomm; 1985, 1987a, 1987b, 1988; Wright, 1989; Wright & Leahey, 2006, 2009).

In the *Illness Beliefs Model,* interventive questions assist us in our therapeutic efforts to "structurally couple" with another person in a therapeutic conversation, create a context for changing beliefs, distinguish current facilitating and constraining beliefs, challenge constraining beliefs, and introduce new facilitating beliefs.

The beliefs of clinicians are embedded in the questions we ask. As the clinician asks questions, family members reflect on their beliefs, and the process of challenging constraining beliefs and/or strengthening facilitating beliefs begins. In our therapeutic conversations, we use three variations on the theme of asking questions:

(1) asking interventive questions that invite a reflection;
(2) inviting family members to externalize internalized questions; and
(3) inviting family members to ask questions.

(1) Asking Interventive Questions that Invite a Reflection

Interventive questions are used in the *Illness Beliefs Model* to open space for reflection. Part of opening space for reflection within family members occurs with the seemingly simple lead-ins to the questions we ask. We have found that it is not just the questions that are important but the lead-ins; they serve as a "drum-roll" for messages and meanings embedded in the questions that follow. These lead-ins introduce the interventive questions and increase the likelihood that the questions (the triggers) that follow the "drum-roll" will be experienced as a perturbation and invite a family member to a reflection. Maturana and Varela's definition of a reflection: "…is the moment when we become aware of that part of ourselves which we cannot see in any other way" (1992, p. 23).

In the following example, LMW uses a lead-in to prepare the family for the move of an unusual and strange question about the benefits of MS: *"I'm going to ask you a question that may seem a bit strange, but*

I've been curious: has there been any good that's come out of having MS [multiple sclerosis]?" The preparation and the "strange question" that follows acknowledges the problematic, troublesome, suffering aspects of the illness that have been previously discussed and, at the same time, offers an alternative view of the experience of the illness.

As in most therapeutic conversations, context is key. It is rarely one question alone that triggers a perturbation, but the timing, spacing, placing, and sequencing of questions—the contextualizing of questions—that perturbs and opens space for new beliefs.

"Lead-ins" and contextualizing of questions are useful, yet we also acknowledge times when the therapeutic conversation "peels back the onion" to distinguish a core belief. In those times, no lead-in is given, and a question is asked that seems to come out of the blue and cuts to a core belief—the belief at the heart of suffering. In the following example, LMW is speaking with Julie. The conversation had co-evolved with Julie describing her husband's violent behavior toward her:

JULIE: *It's not just violence. We don't have to go very far into a fight. It doesn't even have to reach a point where it could accomplish something before Robert tells me to get out, pack my bags, he doesn't need me. And you don't have to have much of a fight for that to happen.*

LMW: *So, are you feeling loved enough in your marriage these days?*

This question took the therapeutic conversation into the heart of the wife's suffering—her belief about not being cared for in her marriage. The conversation culminated in ideas about how to draw forth loving experiences for both husband and wife and how to diminish the anger and violence. The unexpected timing and sequencing of this question were important, as was the use of language. If the clinician had left out the word "enough" and asked instead whether the woman was feeling loved in her marriage these days, this woman may have said, "I know that he loves me" or "I know that he doesn't love me," and the conversation would have ended. The word "enough" seemed to be important in opening space for this woman to reflect on her beliefs in a different way.

In the *Illness Beliefs Model*, we are interested in developing questions that target beliefs and assess the congruence of beliefs at various systems levels. We have developed a series of questions to help clinicians think about possible interventive questions they might ask in a therapeutic conversation. We call this hypothesizing about the connection between illness beliefs and suffering and find the following questions useful to prepare for a session:

- Given the significant events from the last therapeutic conversation and/or literature review, what might be two useful belief hypotheses for this individual/couple/family?
- What individual, family, health care provider, and/or societal beliefs might be identified as constraining or facilitating beliefs in this illness experience?
- How might the intersection of these beliefs perpetuate suffering?
- How might the suffering perpetuate the beliefs?
- Provide circular pattern diagrams specific for each belief hypothesis.

Questions that support or refute the clinician's hypothesis might involve some of these interventive questions:

- Who in your family do you believe is suffering the most?
- Are you a couple who believes you can overcome this major disappointment; or are you a couple who believes this is what marriage is all about?
- Where did you find the courage to stand up to the societal belief that disability is a weakness?
- What is the biggest mistake you have made to convince your husband that your beliefs about his diagnosis are more correct than his beliefs?
- If your physician were here, what changes would she say she has noticed in your beliefs about treatment?
- Do you believe that you have control over how this illness is going to affect your life, or not?
- Where do you believe this idea came from that the best way to help your child heal from his illness was to remove him

permanently from school?

Another form of interventive question is the hypothetical facilitating belief question, developed by our colleague, Dr. Wendy Watson Nelson, that targets a core constraining belief. It embeds a new belief and is an indirect way of challenging a constraining belief. The hypothetical nature of this interventive question invites a sense of playfulness and experimentation with a new way of thinking. The question invites family members in a gentle yet powerful manner to consider an alternative facilitating belief, a belief often diametrically opposed to their current constraining belief.

The question also embeds the suggestion that altered beliefs may give rise to new behaviors. In that process of suspended speculation, we observe changes: changes in affect, behavior, and thinking. As people hypothetically entertain a belief that is an alternative to the core constraining belief, we believe internal changes in their bio-psychosocial-spiritual structure occur. We have found it helpful to ask family members questions such as the following:

- If you were to believe_____, what would be different? (This question opens space for new ideas and offers a non-threatening, reflexive view of the present problem.)
- What would need to be different for you to believe_____?
- What part of you already believes _____?

Temporal distinctions also assist in the offering of the "If you were to believe _____" question. When the conceptual leap that is offered through the new embedded facilitating belief is large, couching the question in small time increments facilitates the perturbation: *If just for the next ten minutes you were to believe _____, what difference would that make (in your suffering, in your marriage, managing your illness, etc.)?*

In a therapeutic conversation with a family, the couple reported feeling overwhelmed by the husband's arthritis and believed they could do nothing to influence the illness, particularly the husband's experience of pain. It was hypothesized that this lack of influence invited the couple to withdraw from each other, which invited conflict. The following hypothetical questions were offered to them: *If you were to believe that you could have 10% more control over the pain, what would be different in your marriage? If you were to believe that you could unite as a couple against the arthritis, what do you think might happen to the pain?* Several weeks later, the couple reported more communication and an increased sense of "team effort" around pain management, in contrast to their previous experience of withdrawal and isolation.

The "If you were to believe…" question is also useful in challenging clinicians' beliefs and inviting hypothesizing in preparation for therapeutic conversations. The clinician might ask him or herself, "If I were to believe that my role is to co-evolve therapeutic conversations that target beliefs, what interventive questions would help me:

- Create a context for changing beliefs?
- Identify constraining beliefs that contribute to illness suffering?
- "Peel back the onion" to distinguish a core illness belief?
- Invite family members to reflection about their beliefs?
- Open space for facilitating beliefs?

Although all of these questions may not always be used in the family session, the thoughtful preparedness and willingness to challenge one's own beliefs may carry the clinician into new ways to soften illness suffering. We believe that the following "If I were to believe _____" questions are important for family clinicians to ask themselves as they continue co-evolving therapeutic moves that are useful to the family:

- If I were to believe that "illness is a family affair" and that each person in this family is experiencing the illness (insert the presenting problem) along with "the patient," what questions would I ask and of whom?
- Whose beliefs would I most want to commence gathering?
- Whose illness suffering would I be most drawn to?
- If I were to believe that acknowledging suffering paves the way for healing, how would I bring forth the suffering in a compassionate and caring manner?
- If I were to believe that all families have strengths, how would I help families to recognize them?

(2) Inviting family members to externalize internalized questions

It is important to ask questions of individuals and families that they usually do not ask themselves, because it may invite reflection and lead to new, facilitating beliefs. However, we also believe that it is important to access the questions that family members *do* ask themselves: *"What are you asking yourself these days?"* What family members ask themselves indicates their current illness beliefs, what emotions will be drawn forth from those beliefs, and ultimately how they will behave and manage their illness. Understanding the questions family members are currently asking themselves in their own internal conversations is one way of distinguishing their current constraining or facilitating beliefs.

To have a family member verbalize their most frequent internal questions usually indicates the most troublesome aspects of the illness and is an important step in understanding their bio-psychosocial-spiritual structures. We have also found that it is within these internalized questions where the greatest suffering lies. We invite clients to externalize (say out loud) their internalized questions through the lead-in: "We all have a lot of internal conversations, conversations with ourselves…"

- what kinds of conversations have you been having with yourself these days?
- what kinds of questions do you ask yourself in a day?
- what do you ask yourself on a bad (good) day?
- when you talk to yourself, what's the most discouraging (encouraging) question you find yourself coming back to?

Internalized questions are usually indicative of an individual or family's deepest suffering. Careful exploration of these internalized questions such as "Why me?", "Why did this tragedy happen to our family?", "What did I do to deserve this illness?" offer clinicians an opportunity to diminish emotional, relational, physical, or spiritual suffering.

Frequently, these internalized questions involve the meaning and purpose of life and invite an exploration about spiritual beliefs (McLeod 2003; McLeod & Wright, 2001, 2008; Wright, 2005, 2007, 2008; 2009). With one family, LMW asked the husband/father: *What questions do you find yourself asking these days?*

He responded immediately: *I ask myself the same questions every day. I ask "would it be cruel to divorce my wife due to her Alzheimer's disease?" "Would this be acceptable to my children, my wife's family, and especially to God?" "Do I have to honor my wedding vow 'in sickness and in health' when it has become unbearable to live like this and not know how many more years she will live?" I feel like my life is on hold and that part of me has died.*

This husband's internal questions were those embedded with great suffering and a moral and spiritual struggle. The clinician explored his core beliefs about what constitutes a good husband when his ill wife cannot recognize him anymore. His desire to leave his wife uncovered his constraining belief that he could not live while still being married to a wife experiencing Alzheimer's. He revealed that he was most worried about God's acceptance. The clinician (LMW) asked a hypothetical facilitating belief to the husband: *If you were to believe that God preferred that you are a loving person to your wife whether married or not, would that make your decision easier or not?*

He became very emotional at that moment and replied: *That's it. I thought I would not be a loving person if I divorced my wife. This question makes me realize that of course I can. If I did leave my wife, I always told myself that I would still visit her regularly and look after her in whatever way that I could.*

Amazingly, this husband chose to stay in his marriage. He explained that he did not feel as trapped once his constraining belief was challenged about the possibility of loving his wife whether married or divorced. Inviting the "internalized" questions enabled the clinician to fully encounter his suffering that was so evident in the questions he was asking himself.

(3) Inviting family members to ask questions

Another way to access family members' beliefs is by inviting them to ask questions of each other or of the clinician or clinical team. For example:

- Are there any questions you wish I had asked you or another family member?
- Is there any question you would like to ask us or another family member?

- If there was just one question you would most like to have answered during our work together, what would that one question be? (This is the "One Question Question" developed by Wright, 1989.)

In the following clinical example with a family experiencing a life shortening illness of breast cancer, the conversation had shifted to the couple's relationship (they were not legally married but had been partners for more than ten years). The team learned that Igor had noticed that his partner Ivana was no longer optimistic about her future. She had accepted that she would die and was now focusing on her relationship with their daughter (Natasha) to teach her all she could in the time she had left. Igor felt guilty that this shift had occurred at a time when Ivana gave up hope of reconciling their relationship (she had previously discovered he was having an affair and had left the partnership). In the middle of the conversation of their beliefs about how two people who cared so deeply for each other had managed to become "bogged down" in their relationship, LMW invited them to ask questions of each other. The focus was on this couple's struggle concerning whether or not they should marry.

LMW: *If you could look ahead in the future, ten years from now, say even if you did pass on, Ivana, do you think it would be useful for Natasha to know that her parents did marry, or would that matter? Will it make a difference for her life?*

IGOR: *I've seen my father and brother get married and divorced. If we did get married, I would be doing it more for Ivana. She's more traditional. A more important lesson for Natasha is love.*

IVANA: *I think for the future what will make a great deal of difference for Natasha is how we deal with this. She'll probably script her life by how we resolve our problems.*

LMW: [5 minutes later] *Are there any last things you want to say to each other or ask each other?*

IGOR: [to Ivana] *Do you feel it is necessary to get back together to give Natasha the right lesson?*

IVANA: *Yes.*

LMW: *Is it essential for Natasha, or is it more essential for you?*

IVANA: *It is important to me, but it's like I want to leave her some essence of my values, so I should live them. If we just split up and he has girlfriends coming in and out of her life, she won't get that. I want to be sure that Natasha and Igor can get along together when I pass on.*

The question that Igor asked Ivana invited a conversation that challenged the belief that they could be helpful to Natasha only if they were married or together as a couple. This helped them to join forces in the common goal of helping Natasha.

In a survey to explore the responses of family members and those of nurses to the "One Question Question," stark differences were revealed (Duhamel, Dupuis, & Wright, in press). Family members were more concerned with the impact of the illness on their lives and relationships and having health care providers appreciate their suffering. Nurses' responses to the "One Question Question" were more focused on how to improve their skills and how to deal with difficult families and/or families in denial or dysfunction. It is our belief that words like "difficult," "denial," and "dysfunction" are used too often with families when nurses should be appreciating and recognizing that these families are likely experiencing intense suffering.

Micromove: Speaking the Unspeakable

Speaking the unspeakable is a powerful therapeutic move used to distinguish beliefs that are central to the problem with which a family is struggling and most often connected to their illness suffering. These core beliefs may be outside a family member's awareness or may be too explosive, frightening, or painful for family members to articulate because they are connected to the beliefs of the family or beliefs of society about what is and what is not appropriate to speak about. Conversations about money, sexuality, death, and family secrets are among the taboo subjects in North American culture. When the clinician breaks the rules and deliberately goes against family or societal beliefs to sensitively raise these issues in a therapeutic conversation to promote healing, the family's constraining belief about their inability to discuss sensitive issues is challenged, and new, facilitating beliefs may arise. Therapeutic change occurs when the belief that is at the heart of the matter is distinguished and examined (for further information see Chapter 5, Beliefs about Change, and Chapter 6, Beliefs about Clinicians).

In Mark's family (the young man experiencing MS), the clinician (LMW) learned that the care-giving parents had not been able to take a holiday together since they began caring for their chronically ill, adult son. In the following dialogue, the clinician explores the parents' belief about what constrains them from taking a break together. After learning that the parents believe they need to ask their son's permission to leave, the clinician uncovers the core belief that constrains them.

LMW: *But you would have to ask your son first, you're saying, to see if he would be okay about that, if he would give his permission to that?*

FATHER: *I wouldn't just bring somebody in and say, "Here, we're going away."*

LMW: *When do you think you would be comfortable asking Mark about that, his permission on that, for the two of you?*

MOTHER: *That's it, you don't know how to…*

FATHER: *…approach him.*

LMW: *Approach him on that?*

FATHER: *Yes.*

MOTHER: *…I don't like to upset him.*

LMW: *Because what would happen if you did?*

MOTHER: *Oh, I just feel that, you know, maybe it's not good* [the father speaks in agreement at the same time], *to be upset with...*

LMW: *So you think it could make his illness worse if you upset him?*

FATHER: *Possibly, yes.*

LMW: *Okay, have you been told that, or is that something...*

MOTHER AND FATHER: *NO!*

FATHER: *No, it's just something that I would think, ah...*

LMW: *Something you believe that, perhaps, it could make his illness worse...*

The clinician speaks the unspeakable when she suggests the parents believe it could make his illness worse if they upset him. By persistent and sensitive probing (What would happen if you did?), the clinician uncovers the fear that constrains the parents from seeking respite together. The very nature of uncovering the core belief and saying it out loud—that the parents could make their son's illness worse by taking a vacation and upsetting him—invites the couple to examine their belief. Where did the belief come from? What impact does the belief have on them? The process also invites the couple to reconsider the usefulness of the belief. The act of speaking the unspeakable out loud challenges a constraining belief and its clandestine power and fearful grip over families.

Speaking the unspeakable around the issue of violence is a situation frequently encountered in clinical work with families, even with families experiencing serious illness. In the following example with a family, violence was even more unspeakable than usual: The couple had presented with concern about the husband's cardiac illness, not spousal violence. Notice the non-threatening, non-defensive curiosity of the clinician (LMW). At the beginning of the third session, the wife (Julie) shows sadness and discouragement. The clinician is persistent in exploring what the wife is troubled about and uncovers the belief that Julie thinks the clinician is allied more closely with her husband than with herself. As the clinician states a position of advocating for the relationship rather than for either person, Julie seems to feel it is safe to disclose a violent incident that is troubling her:

JULIE: *I was really afraid to say what I said because I know it's going to make him angry. And yet, that's what I see happening. I didn't come in here to say he's a "bad guy" and he did this and he did that, but unless I do some of that, I'm not giving you a clear picture of how I feel either.*

LMW: *Well, I'm trying to understand what would constrain you from getting your anger out.*

JULIE: *Well, first, I don't want to make him mad. I don't want to hurt him,* she says while crying softly.

LMW: *So, what would be wrong with getting him mad? So what? So he gets mad.*

JULIE: *It's really unpleasant when he's mad.*

LMW: *Oh, it's unpleasant. Well, that's different then. So, you're saying if you come in here and tell me some "not nice" stories about your husband, that you don't want him to get mad. But you're saying, it's not just that you don't want him to get mad—he's not nice when he's mad. Is that right? So what's the worst thing he does when he's mad?* There's a long pause.

JULIE: *He loses his, loses control.*

LMW: *He loses control.*

JULIE: *I already told you when I made the first appointment. Things had been really bad . . .*

238

LMW: *Yes.*

JULIE: *And I don't want to give the impression that it happens all the time, but he grabbed me and tried to throw me out of the house. And our kids heard and saw that, it was awful, and I won't ever have it happen again.*

LMW: *And nor should you ...Is this the worst thing about Robert that you want me to know?* [Julie is crying.] *Okay, and is this the balancing that you're trying to help me to understand, that last time you were concerned that I would walk away thinking he's Mister Good Guy when he does not-so-nice-guy things to you?*

Throughout this dialogue, we see the continual persistence and curiosity of the clinician, which uncovered the husband's spousal violence. Notice the particular questions that helped the wife speak the unspeakable: What would constrain you? What would be wrong with getting him mad? What's the worst thing he does when he's mad? Is this the worst thing you want me to know about your husband? This is accompanied by the clinician's clear declaration that violence is not acceptable.

By offering opportunities to speak the unspeakable about violence, the clinician makes the therapeutic conversation safer for women and less threatening for men. Speaking the unspeakable challenges the wife's belief that discussing the violence may have negative consequences for her husband's health. By reducing the grip of this constraining belief, she begins to view her husband as capable of handling conflict.

The "unspeakable" takes as many unique forms as there are families. Over the years of seeing families experiencing difficulties with illness, we have come to appreciate that the unspeakable issues surrounding illness frequently center on death and mortality (Tapp, 1997). This is not surprising. Family members and health care providers alike often enter into "conspiracies of silence" motivated by a belief that withholding conversations about death may serve to protect the ill family member.

Having worked with many families experiencing life-shortening and life-threatening illness, we have learned that it is useful to make a distinction between dying and death. Speaking about the process—the anticipation

239

and knowledge that one's life is being shortened—is very different from trying to have knowledge about the time of death (Wright & Nagy, 1993). Once this secret of time is acknowledged as being undetermined, families are more able to talk about the knowledge of dying and the associated suffering of anticipated loss and grief.

In another therapeutic conversation with a clinical family, various family members reported their grave concern about the health habits of the 55-year-old father, who had experienced a heart attack and cardiac bypass surgery. Their concern was shown through their disapproval and nagging when the father indulged in behaviors such as overeating, not exercising, and smoking. In fact, the 25-year-old son reported that his disapproval had escalated to intense anger and fighting with his father on several occasions. Notice the clinician's (LMW) deft probing for beliefs at the heart of the conflict.

LMW: *Do you think your father knows he can count on you folks to worry?*

SON: *Definitely.*

LMW: *Have you decreased your worry for him?*

SON: *No, but I try to handle it better. I used to bug him and he'd bite back at me. I just care about him. I want him to be around forever. My dad's the strong man...*

LMW: *And your biggest worry is what?*

SON: *I just want him to be around forever.*

LMW: *So your biggest worry is...?*

SON: [crying] *I just want him to treat himself better. I just want him to be around till he's seventy or eighty.*

LMW: *So your biggest worry is that he'll die prematurely?*

SON: *Yes.*

LMW: *That's an awful worry, isn't it?*

SON: *And he's a great person. He has a lot to show still.* All members of the family begin to cry, including the father as the son continues, *I have a lot to learn from him in terms of business and getting my career in line. And I don't want my mom to be by herself; she loves him dearly...I know he can't live forever.*

LMW: *So you get sad about this and discouraged. Does he know you have felt this strongly? Does he know the depth of your worry for him?*

SON: *No.*

FATHER: *No, I knew he cared, but I never knew he worried this much.*

SON: *I want my dad to be there. He's my buddy.*

By inviting the son to speak the unspeakable, the family members' worry became more understood. The son feared his father would die. The opportunity to speak this fear aloud altered the meaning of nagging and fighting and created new understanding and appreciation between family members (Tapp, 2004). The belief that drew forth conversations of accusation and recrimination (see Chapter 2 for a discussion of therapeutic conversations) concerning the father's noncompliance was, "He doesn't care enough about his health or our family." This belief was transformed into a facilitating belief that invited conversations of affirmation and affection: "I love my father and worry about him because I want him to live forever."

Micromove: Offering Alternative Beliefs

The clinician's offering of alternative beliefs can be an extremely useful micromove after a context for change has been created. The alternative beliefs can be about family members' lives, relationships, or illness. Families frequently privilege the voice of health care providers, and if it is used wisely, the professional voice may diminish suffering. We have found that family members most often open space for new ideas or beliefs when the ideas are framed in a manner that makes them inviting. To offer a particular idea to a family, we have found it useful to recount for families that we have embraced and learned this knowledge from our work with other families.

With children, we have found it useful to invite the parent to confirm the new belief that is being offered. The following clinical example illustrates this point. A clinical family presented at our outpatient clinic with the mother's primary concern being her 9-year-old daughter's behavior problems at school and aggressive behavior toward her at home. During the first session with the mother only, the mother revealed her beliefs about the connections between (a) her daughter's (Natasha's) behavior and her own struggle with recurrent breast cancer and (b) Natasha's behavior and the separation of her parents.

Children are frequently burdened by two questions when a parent becomes ill: "Am I to blame?" and "Who will take care of me?" During the second session, the clinician spent the first half hour creating a context for change with Natasha. After exploring what Natasha had been told about her mother's illness, the clinician offered the idea that Natasha might be blaming herself for her mother's illness and invited the mother to challenge that belief:

LMW: *Some kids have told me that when their mom and dad stop living together that they think it is their fault. Do you think that?*

NATASHA: *Yes.*

LMW: *And sometimes kids have told me that when their mom or dad get sick, they think it is their fault. Do you think it is your fault that your mom has got sick?*

NATASHA: *Half and half.*

LMW: *How would it be your fault?*

NATASHA: *With my dad fighting with my mom, it is hard to raise me.*

LMW: *Do you think that caused her cancer?*

NATASHA: *Yes.*

LMW: *So half of you thinks it's your fault? A lot of kids think that. I would really like your mom to tell you what she thinks. Would you like to hear from your mom?*

NATASHA: *Yes.*

MOTHER: *Cancer is nobody's fault. It's a sickness like you catch a cold; you don't blame it on somebody, it's nobody's fault. An illness is like that. And I certainly don't think that you are to blame for me being sick, not even a little bit. You make me feel well. You have helped me to get better every time I'm in the hospital.*

LMW: *Your mom has told you something really important. Do you believe her when she tells you that?*

NATASHA: *Yes, I do.*

MOTHER: *And it's not your fault that your dad and I split up.*

LMW: *Something else I have learned from other kids is that even though Mom and Dad tell them this, they tell me that it helps them to hear about this more than once. Are you like that or is once enough?*

NATASHA: *Sometimes, I like to hear it more than once.*

The clinician then invited the mother to ask Natasha in a couple of days if she wanted to once again hear that she was not to blame for either the mother's illness or the breakdown of her parents' relationship. The clinician offered the idea that family members, particularly children, frequently feel they are to blame for illness or marital breakdown. But the

243

clinician carefully offered this new idea by informing the family that this notion was gleaned in work with other families.

The process of this micromove continued with the clinician inviting the mother into the conversation to offer the alternative belief that her daughter was not to blame for her mother's cancer. Beliefs about etiology have a powerful influence on family members' healing and treatment. It is particularly crucial to offer an alternative belief about how an illness may arise when one family member believes they are to blame for an illness. This latter belief can be far more destructive to family members than the belief that illness just happens or is due to fate or some external influence such as pollution.

Another way we have found useful to offer alternate beliefs in the *Illness Beliefs Model* is through sermonettes and storytelling. Sermonettes and storytelling offer families the clinician's beliefs, most frequently alternative beliefs to those currently held by family members. The offering of sermonettes occurs in our clinical work when we believe there is a need for information that goes to the heart of the matter. Families are invited to open space to information by being offered the option to hear the information. This information is often stated through questions such as, "Would you be interested in a story of another family?" The rationale for asking is to avoid imposing the clinician's view and to create a dialogue rather than a monologue. If the family says no, the information is not given. The idea is to give a choice whereby the client selects what fits and what does not. We have learned that the respectful offering of an option to receive or not receive information is the most effective way to help families open space both to hearing information and to being receptive to it.

The following is an example of offering and giving a sermonette. In this session, the clinician chose to have a therapeutic conversation with the husband (Robert) and wife (Julie) individually. The following transcript illustrates how sermonettes are presented. First, there is the question of whether to offer ideas and the consideration of whether they will be useful.

LMW: *Well, should I offer a couple of more thoughts?*

ROBERT: *Sure.*

LMW: *Or not? We run the risk again of you trying and it may not be that useful. I do appreciate your efforts in doing more housework, which seems to be a big, a really big, area for her. But I have two thoughts for you; whether that makes it better or not I don't know. But they're two things that if you would be willing to try, I have the belief, Robert, that you have the ability to make a very big difference and to influence her happiness. And I'll tell you what really stood out for me. I mentioned it in our pre-session discussion: your compliment to her last time that she does a good job, she was just hungry to hear that from you...*

ROBERT: *Yes, I can see that, 'cause I'm not good at that.*

LMW:*...to know that.*

ROBERT: *It's one of those things that I've never been able to do, and I think it probably stems from my past, the emotional things I never had. I never was hugged. I never had a close relationship with my parents, so it's very difficult. It's always been difficult for me to show that side, that emotional side. I've never been good at it, and it's got to stem back, I think, from how I was brought up. My father told me how stupid I was, that I would never amount to anything, and my mother never paid any attention to me. I grew up in that. I left home at sixteen because there was nothing there, there was no relationship, family relationship. My father was an alcoholic, so I think for me, I've never been able to show emotion.*

LMW: *But you do show emotion in here. So, I don't know what kind of emotion you mean.*

ROBERT: *Well of gratitude, thanks, love.*

LMW: *Oh, okay.*

ROBERT: *Anger, I can show.*

LMW: *Yes.*

ROBERT: *Because that's a defense mechanism in a way, I think.*

LMW: *I think this is the core for your wife. I think she's hungry for that from you. This is why I wanted to meet you individually; I didn't want to be saying these kinds of things in front of your wife because I want her saying at home that you're just doing this because...*

ROBERT: *That's what I'd be afraid of too, all of a sudden she sees this change...*

LMW: *Dr. Wright is saying this to you.*

ROBERT: *Yes.*

LMW: *But, I wanted to point out to you that you do have an incredible influence on her. I believe it is because she is hungry for affirmation and affection from you, a compliment, an affirmation that she's doing a good job at home, that kind of thing. So, I had two things in mind for you. I know it's asking you to do the very thing that you're saying you're not good at. That's a bit paradoxical, isn't it, but I think that's where the greatest assurance can come. I think she needs reassurance from you that she's loved and cared about and appreciated. And I don't think it matters what I say or the kids say, she needs to hear it from you. Just the way she responded to your one idea that you thought she did a good job; she sat up and commented on it. It obviously really stood out and meant a lot to her. So, what [I am] asking is, can you look for more opportunities to do that? Maybe it won't be easy and maybe it won't be like falling off a log, but if you can work at that, to get into the habit of that, I think it would have great payoffs for her. And I think she would feel a lot better, because then she'd know what you think about her and how you feel toward her. But I'm asking you to do the very thing that is the hardest for you.*

ROBERT: *Yes. Well, you know, I mean, it just takes trying to do it.*

LMW: *Yes, and there's many ways to try and do it, eh? Sometimes you* *can learn to do it more by writing a note: "Thanks for doing this" or "I appreciated your efforts on that" or whatever. It's just trying to be more conscious about saying something at least every other day to her, something that will build her up so that she knows that she's cared about by you. Because, we know that in your heart...*

ROBERT: *Yes, you tend to take it for granted in a way because you know what they know and...*

LMW: *And I think your wife is a woman that needs to hear it and really feels good when she does hear it from you. So that was the one idea I had. And I didn't realize I was asking you, till we've now talked a bit more, that I'm asking you to do the very thing that's the most difficult. But you've done a lot of difficult things, haven't you?*

ROBERT: *Yes.*

LMW: *You've overcome a lot of difficult things. I admire you—with the kind of family background you describe—the type of person you've become, how you have matured in spite of your family.*

ROBERT: *I didn't do it alone; I had help along the way from different people.*

LMW: *Yes, and the second thing that I would like you to consider is to apologize for the two incidents of physical abuse. Whether you felt justified, whether you felt...*

ROBERT: *Oh, I never felt justified.*

LMW: *...provoked, but I think it's an area that she needs an apology. And I'm saying that to you as a woman and as your counselor. I think that would also mean a lot to her...So when the time seems right, you know when that would be, what the situation would be, that you could offer her an apology.*

ROBERT: *Okay.*

LMW: *I'm not saying these are cure-alls. But trying to get to some of the real core issues of concern. We can talk about housework and doing this and that...*

ROBERT: *It's not the cause of what's going on.*

LMW: *Exactly. All of that can be worked out when someone knows that they're really loved and cared about. We all can put up with a lot more and tolerate a lot more when we know we're really loved and cared about, and I think she needs that...*

ROBERT: *And I should know that.*

LMW: *...so much from you. She needs, I believe, to hear those words and she needs to hear it from you. So, are you willing to...*

ROBERT: *Yes.*

LMW: *...give it a try? Great. And for the moment, I would put a moratorium on the kinds of things we talked about here today. I don't think rehashing it and going over it again and again is helpful.*

ROBERT: *No.*

LMW: *I think you should, and I'm going to say that to Julie as well, I think you just need to press on from here and say, "That was difficult, it was hard." You both obviously have a lot of hurts and resentments from the past and different ideas and perceptions about them but you need to try and press forward and do some things differently. Except for that one piece of the past, that I think offering her an apology would mean a lot to her.*

ROBERT: *Okay.*

LMW: *Okay, great. Well, I'm going to see Julie now for a few minutes.*

In just four minutes of a therapeutic conversation, the husband transforms from a man telling the clinician he does not know what his wife wants to a man who says he is willing to do the hardest thing for him: to offer affirmations to his wife. He also convincingly tells the clinician "It just takes trying to do it." How did this transformation take place? It began by the clinician increasing the husband's curiosity and thereby decreasing his resistance and by the clinician declaring the uncertainty of the usefulness or outcome of her "two thoughts." The first idea is given credence, however, by the clinician providing evidence from a previous session that the wife is experiencing affirmation deprivation. The clinician also challenges the husband's family-of-origin explanation of his belief that the past rules the present and future. He says, "I've never been able to show emotion," but the clinician points out with direct evidence from the session, "but you do show emotion in here" and then invites a distinction about what kinds of emotion he shows.

The clinician acknowledges the husband's difficulty by stating, "I'm asking you to do the very thing that is hardest for you." The client responds to this acknowledgment with a mini-sermonette of his own: "It just takes trying to do it." The receptivity of the husband enables the clinician to offer ideas of how to implement an alternative belief by suggesting that there are many ways he could affirm his wife; she concludes with significant words for this couple experiencing cardiac disease: "We know that [you care about her] in your heart."

A former constraining belief of the husband is countered with a new, alternate belief in hopes that he would not only challenge his belief but open space to a new behavior. Specifically, the husband's belief that the past rules the present was offered back to him as, "You've done a lot of difficult things, overcome a lot of difficult things…in spite of your family." This sermonette also embeds beliefs about relationships: the positive correlation between tolerance and love ("We can all tolerate a lot more when we know we're really loved…"). Finally, this sermonette suggested putting a moratorium on conversations of accusations and recriminations while the couple moves toward conversations of affirmation and affection. Sermonettes can embed useful ideas that can alter or challenge constraining beliefs when approached from an "offering" and "inviting" stance.

Telling stories of oneself or, more frequently, telling stories of other families with whom one has worked changes the conversational flow: The clinician stops asking questions and begins telling stories. This change in the clinician's conversational behavior invites family members into a listening mode. We have found it to be extremely useful for embedding alternative beliefs and validating one family's experience through the telling of a story of another family.

The following is an example of storytelling. Family members were expressing their apprehension about Ritalin being prescribed for the daughter.

LMW: *So are you of the belief now that your daughter's problems are more psychological, biological, or both?*

ROBERT: *Probably both, but we have to do something. I've got reservations as anyone would with drugs. I mean I think most drugs can have both good and bad about them, but the thing with our daughter is, the drugs help her because she has a hard time…it's not a good life, you know what I mean?*

LMW: *Would you be interested in hearing about an adolescent I just saw yesterday who is on Ritalin? Would that be of interest to you?*

ROBERT: *Mmm.*

JULIE: *Especially for him [referring to husband]; I've heard lots of stories…*

LMW: *This is just so timely. I just saw this young person last night. I've been working with her parents, and they like me to see their daughter from time to time individually. So I did last night. I hadn't seen her for probably five or six months. One of the real concerns of the parents is that this young woman had a dreadful history in school all of her life. She'd had just a horrendous school career, failure after failure, poor grades, and she was a very big girl. She had just turned sixteen, but even when she was fourteen and fifteen, she was very large. So socially, she hasn't really fit in.*

So they've had this long history. Well, she came back yesterday. I hardly recognized her.

JULIE: *Yeah?*

LMW: *Because she'd lost weight, because of the Ritalin, and she felt good about herself. But the other thing that was far more fascinating to me was that she was so focused. She was right with me, and I said to her, "There's something different about you. What is it that's so different about you?" And do you know what she said? "I can concentrate now, I can concentrate!"*

ROBERT: *We've heard it put, "that I can hear with one voice now."*

LMW: *Yes. She said, "Now I'm able to focus," and I said, "Well, just talking with me, I notice a difference in you." Well, she was so taken by my comments. I said to her, "I'm so happy for you. This must be just wonderful. That must really do a lot for you," and she said, "Yes."*

JULIE: *See, that's the thing, if it can do that.*

LMW: *If it can do that. So here she's had years and years of history of this, and because I think I was so pleased with how she was doing, and I was so thrilled for her that she said to me, "I can really work on things with my family now." So, I don't know, I mean that's just one example.*

The "Are you of the belief…?" question was followed by a story. The story was meant to open space for the consideration of options about Ritalin. This conversational sequence was followed by the lead-in question, "Would you be interested in hearing…" If the family responds with yes, the conversation is very different than it would be if this question were not asked. The clinician's words, "This may or may not fit for you," shows respect for the family.

The storytelling in this clinical vignette enabled the parents of this young daughter to hear a success story of a young woman who was taking Ritalin. It enabled the clinician to be enthusiastic about the change of another young person, but it also embedded a little cautionary note by offering the idea that this was "just one example." The whole intent of this storytelling is to offer hope to the family that this might be one solution to their daughter's difficulties and thus alter their present constraining belief that the option was not to be considered.

Another of the clinician's beliefs becomes evident from this therapeutic conversation. The belief that "If clinicians are too passionate about change, they can begin imposing their ideas and thus close space to change." By offering the option to hear an idea—"Would you be interested in hearing my idea?"—a domain of requests evolves rather than of demands. If a family member agrees to listen, the resulting perturbation is entirely different in nature because the person is listening differently. There is an underlying assumption of respect that family members can absorb only what their present bio-psychosocial-spiritual structures will allow.

Micromove: Using Research Findings

Given the preeminence of science and technology in our society, knowledge derived from research has been given powerful status. This privileging of research has created novel opportunities in the *Illness Beliefs Model* to use both research findings and the process of research to challenge constraining beliefs.

We have used research findings to draw new distinctions. The clinician must first determine the family members' beliefs about the influence of research by directly asking, "Do you believe in research?" If the family members value research, the clinician may use specific, relevant research reports to challenge constraining beliefs. Efforts are consistently made to have family members open space to the offering of the clinician's ideas. If a family does not "believe in research," the offering of ideas from research will not be a fit and no beliefs will be altered or challenged.

We worked with a family where the parents, Nicole and John, believed they had little influence or control over their younger daughter's uncertain illness of Chronic Fatigue Syndrome. The clinician (LMW) used research findings as a way of challenging this constraining belief. Notice the way that the clinician "drum rolls" the move and heightens the anticipation of the research information when she introduces the idea to the family. The clinician does not impose her ideas through instructive interaction such as:

"Here is what you need to know and how you must behave in the future." She builds up and heightens the need to know, culminating in an offer: "Do you believe in research?" This is similar to other invitations such as, "Would you be interested in my ideas?" or "Is it useful at this time to hear an idea?" Other possibilities include, "Are you in the mood to hear this idea today?" or "Would you like to wait till next week?" We hypothesize that this buildup, or "drum roll," increases family members' curiosity about what will be offered and invites them to open space to the ideas.

The paced introduction of a therapeutic offering is also an intervention for clinicians. It slows clinicians down and tempers their enthusiasm for their own ideas. It keeps clinicians from plunging in prematurely, imposing their ideas, being invested in the rightness of their opinions, or becoming too enthusiastic or passionate about the direction, pace, or outcome of change. (But we are enthusiastic and passionate about the occurrence of change.) If the family agrees to listen to the idea, the perturbation may be experienced differently because they have chosen to listen rather than being forced to listen. There is an underlying assumption of respect: that the listeners have a choice about receiving the opinion or information and will take in what fits for them.

LMW: *There are a couple of research studies that were brought to my attention by my students that were so interesting. The researchers were looking at families who were experiencing chronic illness and trying to see how come some families seem to adjust to the chronic illness and seem to live alongside of it or manage and other families don't. I just want to say you match what the research is saying. And what the research is saying is, families that start to feel that they have a sense of confidence and mastery over the illness adjust to the illness better than families that feel like the illness is ruling them. Those families have no sense of mastery or any sort of confidence to live alongside this illness. And all the things you've been telling me today validate that piece of research.*

You're [daughter] saying, "As I'm feeling better, and as I feel like I'm mastering this more, I'm not worrying about it as much and we're adjusting to it." And you're saying, "I'm not as anxious." People are giving you different ideas about what you can do to set the date for the uncertainty about this illness to be over, and you're all coming up with some good ideas about what you could do.

NICOLE: *I agree with that too, because the feeling that I had when she was first sick, we didn't know what it was and then we did know what it was. But then that's what we felt like, this illness was like a blanket that was smothering us all. You know, it was like being claustrophobic; there was no way out.*

LMW: *Sure, it just feels like it's oppressing you and it's ruling you. When you feel like that, you're not having a sense of mastery or confidence. It doesn't mean that you're going to cure your illness necessarily, but at least if you feel like there's some areas that you have some control in what you're doing, the research is saying people seem to be able to live alongside the illness better.*

NICOLE: *Well, I think that's true.*

JOHN: *As long as you don't get too overconfident.*

The family's experience, expertise, and curiosity are elevated when posing the question, "Do you believe in research?" The content of the research findings about mastery is customized to fit exquisitely with the family's constraining belief, "We have no control over the illness." This new distinction is offered in a manner that gently embeds the suggestion that if they were to have more influence over the illness, they would experience more mastery. It is important to note that this move has three stages: opening space by heightening curiosity, embellishing the idea through research findings, and inviting family reactions to the ideas offered. When family members are asked to respond to an idea and verbalize it, the languaging of the idea helps the family to remember it.

Later in the second session, the clinician asks the family to elaborate on the degree to which they believe they can influence the illness. The mother's, Nicole's, response is to acknowledge change: "I think now I can see that we're getting there." This statement is in sharp contrast to her earlier comment about illness smothering the family like a blanket: "There was no way out." The clinician punctuates the shift in beliefs by again referring to the research findings. This time she commends the family by offering, "You are the family that validates the research findings."

Research is again used to draw a new distinction. The implication is that the family is more expert than the research. Julie's experience is another clinical example of using research findings to challenge beliefs. She believed she could trigger another heart attack in her husband Robert if she raised conflictual issues or burdened him with her worries. She kept these concerns to herself, thereby protecting her husband, but increasing her own stress. In a reflecting team discussion, team members used research findings to challenge the wife's belief.

LMW: [to graduate team members specializing in families with cardiac illness] *What ideas does the research have about how to help families get out of this? How protective do spouses have to be around each other?*

TEAM MEMBER 1: *Actually, there isn't a lot out there [in the cardiac research literature] that has concrete solutions for cardiac couples. It is very much a matter of openly discussing concerns and openly discussing feelings about all of the changes that they've been experiencing so they understand where each other is coming from. There is very little in the literature that would substantiate that stress from a marital discussion will aggravate a heart attack.*

LMW: *There's little to substantiate that? Say that again. I think they really need to hear this one.*

TEAM MEMBER 1: *Sure. There's little in the cardiac literature that substantiates that a heart attack will be triggered by marital disagreement. Marital conflict is very common following a heart attack, but it's not something that is seen as a cause of a recurrence of a heart attack.*

TEAM MEMBER 2: *In fact, there is evidence that trying to protect each other is, in fact, much more stressful than having open communication.*

TEAM MEMBER 1: *Yes, that's a good point.*

TEAM MEMBER 2: *And I think that's important for people to know because you're spending all this energy trying to protect each other.*

LMW: *Yes, that's certainly been my experience in working with families where there has been a coronary like this. They get more stressed trying to protect each other than if they could just deal with the issues more frankly. I think, in a very curious kind of way, [this family is] doing that today. They are being very frank with each other today, and they're even being frank with their compliments today. I mean Robert says he thinks these very nice things about Julie, but he doesn't say them. And even today, he's saying them, and she's being very frank about wanting him more involved in family responsibilities.*

The team used research findings to challenge the wife's constraining belief by identifying the lack of evidence for the idea that stress could trigger another heart attack and offering the idea that protecting each other might be more stressful and take more energy than being open with each other. On the basis of this new information, the couple wrestled with the question, "Is stress that is shared doubled, or is stress that is shared halved?" At the fifth and last session, the couple provided evidence for a shift in the constraining belief. The protective pattern they had been using in their marriage had changed. The wife reported that there was "less conflict—I'm not backing off anymore."

Micromove: Offering Externalizing Conversations

When we engage in externalizing conversations, we practice seeing the person as separate from and in a relationship with the problem (Freedman & Combs, 1996). This micromove, used in the *Illness Beliefs Model*, originated from the clinical work of the late Michael White (White, 1988/89, 2007; White & Epston, 1990) who was a brilliant thinker and clinician in the movement known as Narrative Therapy. In our work with families experiencing serious illness, the "problem" is conceptualized as the beliefs that people hold about their illness.

Families, like George and Linda, whose illness narrative begins in Chapter 1 of this book, often experience the presence of illness in their lives as overwhelming and all encompassing. As one family told us,

"Illness is everywhere in our home—it has even sneaked into the closets." Offering externalizing conversations targets family members' beliefs about mastery, control, and influence with the intent to challenge these beliefs if they are constraining.

Linda and George sought help because they felt overwhelmed by the challenges of chronic illness. Linda was diagnosed with numerous chronic illnesses including hypertension, diabetes with neuropathy, cardiac arrhythmia, and depression. One of the most troubling symptoms was her fatigue. Linda was suffering physically because she believed she was a burden financially, emotionally, and physically, and not keeping up her end of the partnership. The couple reported increasing distance and isolation in the relationship and a sense of disconnection. As Linda's illness symptoms and fatigue increased, she reported she felt more like a patient than a wife; George felt more like a nurse than a husband.

When the clinician (JMB) inquired about the couple's beliefs about mastery, control, and influence, we learned that the couple experienced a sense of helplessness and powerlessness in their abilities to have influence over the illness that pervaded their daily lives and relationships. Our team identified this belief as a core constraining belief. When the clinician asked the couple if they had a name for the illness, George immediately called it "The Monster." Linda recalled, "As soon as George said it ['The Monster'], I thought right away—that's it—it came into our lives and it's just overwhelmed us both. It is in our face 24/7."

We learned about this core constraining belief by asking interventive questions known as *relative influence questions* to begin the process of separating their lives and relationships from the problem of illness:

- What degree of influence do you (or your family) have over your illness?
- What degree of influence does your illness have over you (or your family)?
- What degree of influence would you (or your family) prefer to have?
- These questions encourage individuals and families to map the influence of their constraining beliefs about mastery, control, and influence and explore suffering associated with these

beliefs. As family members begin to experiment with ways to have more influence over the symptoms or experiences of illness and perhaps to put illness in its place, relative influence questions continue to be used to bring forth and strengthen new facilitating beliefs about their resourcefulness and competence.

George and Linda displayed remarkable courage to stand up to the monster of chronic illness (for more information see their No Illness and Fatigue Talk [NIFT] letter, 2006). Their creative efforts to contain illness talk strengthened their beliefs about mastery, control, and influence and served to significantly reduce their illness suffering. They began to believe that the monster was just one of "the little thorns of life" as their influence over the illness increased dramatically. Their beliefs about their couple relationship and their connection with each other also shifted as they reported, "Together we can conquer anything."

Micromove: Writing Therapeutic Letters

The micromove of therapeutic letters used in the *Illness Beliefs Model* had its origins in the creative clinical work of David Epston of New Zealand and the late Michael White of Australia (Epston, 1994; White, 1995; White & Epston, 1990). The power of therapeutic letters was first observed in our team's clinical work in the Family Nursing Unit with an estranged mother and daughter (Wright & Watson, 1988). Since then, we, along with graduate students who were members of our clinical team, have written hundreds of therapeutic letters to families. We have received very positive feedback about the healing aspects of these letters (Bell, Moules, & Wright, 2009, Moules, 2009b).

We have found therapeutic letters—in sealed, personally-addressed envelopes—to be a useful medium for carrying into the homes, minds, and hearts such things as:
- Commendations to individual family members and/or to the family as a whole
- Acknowledgement of illness suffering (hearing the "cries of the wounded")
- Questions we would have or could have asked in a session

258

- Words, phrases, and ideas that particularly stood out for us from a session
- Highlights of our work with a family and what we learned from our work with them
- Any particular therapeutic move that we wish to highlight

Therapeutic letters can offer some things that a therapeutic session cannot do, such as invite nonparticipating family members to a session, follow up on "no shows," and help students or supervisors to articulate more clearly their own constraining beliefs about a family (Bell et al., 2009). A therapeutic letter can also do many things that a therapeutic session *can* do. We have used therapeutic letters to create a context for changing beliefs, challenge constraining beliefs, and strengthen facilitating beliefs. At a narrative therapy conference, Michael White asked, "How many sessions is a therapeutic letter worth?" The answers from clinicians in the audience ranged from five to ten! Recent publications by Pyle (2009) and Rodgers (2009) have added to our understanding of unique ways that therapeutic letters strengthen the therapeutic relationship and invite healing.

To understand more about the effect and usefulness of therapeutic letters written to individuals and families seen in the Family Nursing Unit, University of Calgary, Dr. Nancy Moules (2000, 2002, 2003, 2009a, 2009b) conducted a notable qualitative research study—the first of its kind to examine therapeutic letters. She found that therapeutic letters serve as a particularly effective micromove for softening suffering by challenging constraining beliefs. Families in her study reported that they returned to the therapeutic letters they had received and reread them when needed to have a boost of encouragement and/or hope. In particular, she found that acknowledging illness suffering was an important element of the therapeutic letter. Immediately after her research findings were available, we made several changes and refinements to our practice of writing therapeutic letters.

Here is an example of a therapeutic letter written to George and Linda (see Offering Externalizing Conversations, above) to summarize the clinical work that was offered to them over seven sessions in the Family Nursing Unit (reprinted with permission from SAGE Publications: Bell et al., 2009):

Example of a Family Nursing Unit Closing Therapeutic Letter

Dear George and Linda,

Greetings from the Family Nursing Unit! It was a pleasure to meet with you in March for our final session. We wish to highlight what we have learned from you during our work together, as well as what we believe we have been able to offer you in our conversations together.

Linda and George, we appreciate the commitment you have shown to our work together as we explored the experience of illness suffering in your lives. Together you found the strength to enter into some difficult and painful conversations with us about your experience of suffering with both the loss of loved ones and the uncertainty of pain and chronic illness. We have been impressed with the perseverance you have demonstrated in pursuing creative ways to influence the challenges that the presence of chronic illness has brought into your lives and relationships.

What we have learned from you:

1. *Linda, you taught us how women who live with chronic illness and pain face distinct challenges. Learning to live alongside unrelenting illness, fatigue, and pain while trying to maintain your role as a wife creates the unique challenge of finding balance between caring for self while also nurturing your marriage relationship with George. You helped us realize how the invisible and unpredictable nature of chronic illness invites physical pain and emotional isolation from the ones you love most. We have learned that this loss of emotional connection may be harder to bear and invites more suffering than the illness itself.*

2. *George, you offered us a new appreciation of the complexity of being both a family caregiver and a husband in the presence of illness. We learned about the tremendous impact that illness has had on your marriage and how the uncertainty around which role (nurse or husband) you believe you need to offer in*

any given moment can invite confusion, anger, and suffering. George, you have reaffirmed what we have learned in our work with other families: that giving the illness a name and an identity can help a family shift the illness from robbing your lives to viewing it as an external, manageable circumstance.

3. *Together, you have reminded us that remaining connected and aligned as a couple improves and strengthens your ability to defeat the influence of chronic illness. With your careful formulation of the No Illness and Fatigue Talk (NIFT) Day we learned how a couple can use their creativity to negotiate changed patterns of behavior one day per week. Furthermore, you helped us to understand how persisting in changing this one day has the potential to result in changing many beliefs about yourselves and the illness. You skillfully demonstrated to us the breadth and depth of your wisdom surrounding your illness experience by offering an elaborate, beautifully crafted letter about how you both experimented with new ways of behaving and thinking. Linda, your eloquent reading of your and George's letter in our sessions permitted us further understanding of how much suffering you and George have experienced, and how much work you have done together to become masters over the monster of chronic illness in your lives* [for more information about this letter see NIFT Day at: www.janicembell.com].

What we believe we offered you:

1. *In our work together we witnessed and celebrated the tremendous strength you have as a couple. It has been a privilege to observe the special connection of your relationship. In having your relationship witnessed and reverenced, we reminded you of what we believe you already knew: that you are a spiritual couple who has a sacred relationship, worthy of nurturance and nourishment. We wonder in what ways you will continue to nurture your marital relationship as you live alongside of chronic illness.*

2. *We believe that we challenged your beliefs about your abilities to influence and control the space that chronic illness occupies in your lives. We encouraged you to "name" the chronic illness as a way to invite you to view illness as separate from Linda's being and outside of your marriage. You agreed to call it the "monster." In our efforts to support you to find ways to manage the "monster" and keep your marriage strong we encouraged each of you to experiment with ways in which to give your marriage more status than the monster of chronic illness.*

3. *We offered you our belief that you are an empowered couple with the resourcefulness and creativity to navigate challenges that will arise, including the influence of the monster of illness. We offered you the idea that you can use your skills at mastering illness to conquer anything! We spoke with you about how chronic illness robs couples of the most intimate aspects of their marriage and challenged you to rediscover the meaning and place of sexual intimacy in your marital bond. How might you continue to reclaim a life of creativity, strength, and joy?*

George and Linda, it has been delightful to come to know you as individuals and as a couple. You are a family who has shown remarkable strength and courage in the face of illness suffering. It is often difficult for families to transition into living well and living at peace with chronic illness. Your dedication to the work with us at the Family Nursing Unit to soften your illness suffering is inspiring. We want to express what a privilege it has been to work with you, and we wish you the best in your continued success as you live with this difficult illness experience. The insights you have shared with us will undoubtedly enhance our work with other couples and families who are suffering in the midst of chronic illness.

As part of our work together, a research assistant will contact you within six months to learn whether you would be willing to evaluate what was helpful or not-so-helpful in our work together so that we can continue to improve our practice with families.

With warm regards,

Janice M. Bell, RN, PhD, Director, Family Nursing Unit
Amy Marshall, RN, BN, 2nd year Master of Nursing Student
Marianne Boucher, RN, BN, 1st year Master of Nursing Student
and other members of the clinical team

Micromove: Offering Commendations

The offering of commendations is a central micromove that characterizes the *Illness Beliefs Model*. Fabie Duhamel (1994) examined the clinical practice provided at the Family Nursing Unit, University of Calgary, to families experiencing hypertension. Her analysis of the clinical work brought to our awareness our practice of commenting on family strengths. Lorraine Wright chose the word "commendation" to name the clinical move in which the clinician draws forth and highlights family strengths and resources. We now offer commendations to every individual and family in every therapeutic conversation, both during the interview and at the end-of-session summary of our impressions, ideas, and recommendations. We prefer emphasizing strengths and competencies rather than deficits, dysfunction, and deficiencies in family members (Bell, 1995).

Our clinical observations and research of families' reactions to the immediate and long-term positive effects of commendations indicate that they are an extremely powerful micromove for challenging constraining beliefs (Bohn, Wright, & Moules, 2003; Houger Limacher, 2003, 2008; Hougher Limacher & Wright, 2003, 2006; McLeod & Wright, 2008; Moules, 2002).

Wright and Leahey (2009, p. 150) have defined commendations as "observations of patterns of behavior that occur across time (i.e., 'Your family members are very loyal to one another') whereas a compliment is usually an observational comment on a one-time event (i.e., 'You were very praising of your son today')." Commendations are often connected to the family's illness narrative.

The deliberate drawing forth and elaborating on family strengths and resources has a profound impact on families. Family members frequently respond to the perturbation in a dramatic, affective manner. They voice confirmation that they feel heard or understood (sometimes for the first time in years), or they become tearful as they describe how validated the commendation makes them feel. Often families coping with health problems have not been commended for their strengths or made aware of them (Bohn et al., 2003; Hougher Limacher & Wright, 2003, 2006; McElheran & Harper-Jaques, 1994; Robinson & Wright, 1995).

Through our consistent use of commendations over many years, we have noted that when we commend a family about a particular strength or a resourceful behavior they are showing, they seem to be more open to ideas offered by the clinician. We believe that commendations increase structural coupling between the family members and the clinician and invite the family to open space to new ideas. They are, in essence, conversations of affirmation and affection between the clinician or clinical team and the family and thereby open possibilities for healing.

There are many forms of commendations. In the following clinical example, the clinician (LMW) capitalizes on an opportunity within the session to commend the client (Connie) in a comparative way, pointing out how wise she is in comparison to "society." A distinction is drawn between society's beliefs about therapy and the client's wisdom.

LMW: *What do you tell yourself about coming for counseling?*

CONNIE: *Well, I thought about it quite a while. I need some help and I want to get it.*

LMW: *Well, I admire you, because we still unfortunately have the idea in our society that going for help is embarrassing or shameful. Yet, I look at it quite differently. I prefer to think that it's a wanting to get past the problem—you've exhausted your own resources, you've tried things on your own. You've tried them and, yes, some things have helped somewhat, but it seems like you want to get past the problem. You want to get further with it.*

CONNIE: *And if I don't, I'm going to end up somewhere, I don't know,* *'cause I can't take it anymore.*

A commendation that summarizes and highlights the family's story is another form of commendation. This type recognizes more than a single idea. It is a sustained pattern of commendations, an elaborate reflection on the family's story, which confirms for the family that they have been heard and understood. In the first session, the clinician (LMW) offers an end-of-session commendation to the parents who were caregivers to their adult son experiencing multiple sclerosis (MS).

LMW: *First of all, I want to tell you that my team and I are just incredibly impressed with the two of you as a couple and as a mother and father. I think you've gone above and beyond what most parents do for their children. You've had an unusual circumstance enter your family. Most families do not have to have this challenge of coping with having a son with MS. It has been an incredible challenge your family has been hit with. You have really risen to the occasion. We're just very impressed by you. For whatever reasons, one of your lots in life and your missions in life seems to be the role of caring for people and taking care of people. How do you do that—how do you keep your own health through that and your own sanity through all the pressures...?*

FATHER: *Struggle along.*

LMW: *Yes, it's something we want to talk to you about. We've been very impressed with your dedication and devotion to your son. We've certainly worked with lots of families where there have been health problems, but you're the first family that I've met where the parents have left their home to come and care for their child. More often my experience has been that it's the child who goes back home to care for the parents. Or if the child is not well, then they usually go back to where they grew up or something to make it a bit easier. But you're quite remarkable; to give up your home, your family, your friends, and your social life, your activities and all of that, to come here to care for your son is just quite remarkable. This is the first I've ever heard of this. I've usually seen it the other way.*

MOTHER: *Well, he's your child, you brought him into the world.*

LMW: *Oh sure, I'm just saying, it's the first I've heard. You're a very unique couple, you're to be admired. You've just gone above and beyond as parents and sacrificed. You know, if he had gone back home and you were caring for him there, I would have said that was a tremendous sacrifice.*

FATHER: *At least you'd have all your friends...*

LMW: *You'd have your friends, your family. I would have been commending you for that and say it's a tremendous thing you've done to have your son come home and to care for him and look after him as best you can. You would have to make a lot of sacrifices and adjustments, but you'd be around, like you say, you'd be around your family, your friends, and maybe get some relief once in a while. However, here you're pretty much on your own, because I don't know how many people you [know] here. Not really anybody.*

MOTHER: *No we don't, not really too many.*

LMW: *So now it seems like even your health is being sacrificed somewhat. The tension is perhaps having some effect on that—not being able to have breaks together. We were wondering if your body isn't trying to tell you something. Perhaps maybe, we don't know, we're just guessing here—is it even going a bit too far if it's coming to the point of sacrificing your health, because if your health is affected, then how will you be able to care for your son?*

MOTHER: *Well, I just pray every night that we keep up.*

FATHER: *Me, too.*

LMW: *Yes, well, we can hope your prayers are answered in the positive vein, but I guess the question we as a team have is, "How far are you willing to go to continue to make these sacrifices? Is there any limit to the sacrifices you would make for your son?"*

The elaborate commendation not only summarizes the family's story but distinguishes many family strengths. The embellished nature of the commendation paves the way for the clinician to pose a reflexive question that challenges the couple's beliefs about care-giving: "Is there any limit to the sacrifices you would make for your son?"

Commendations that highlight and acknowledge strengths that are outside the family members' awareness have extra potency and therapeutic value. This form of commendation challenges constraining beliefs by drawing forth a new identity or belief about the family or about their situation.

Houger Limacher (2003, 2008) has contributed significantly to our knowledge by conducting the first research project that examined the micromove of commendations as practiced by our clinical team at the Family Nursing Unit, University of Calgary. She interviewed family members who had received commendations and clinicians who had offered commendations in a therapeutic conversation. She found that commendations brought forth "goodness" in therapeutic conversations that invited healing (Houger Limacher & Wright, 2003, 2006). This bringing forth of goodness is a relational phenomenon in the context of the clinician/patient/family relationship. Commendations have the power to create and bring forth "goodness", or what we refer to as bringing forth "a particular kind of person" who possesses a "particular way of being in the world." A "particular kind of person" and a way of being in clinical practice are represented by a person "who looks for strengths amid suffering, hope amid despair, and meaning amid confusion" (Wright, 2005, p. 209).

Micromove: Using Reflecting Teams

A reflecting team is a powerful therapeutic medium for offering a variety of ideas from which family members may select. Team members behind a one-way mirror observe the conversation between the clinician and family members and then reverse vantage points. The team comes into the interview room, and the clinician and family members go behind the mirror to listen to the reflections of their conversations about the clinician-family conversations. Subsequently, viewing angles are shifted once again, and the clinician and family return to the room to hear the family's reflections on the team's reflections. In this way, reflections on reflections and dialogues about dialogues continue. Andersen's (1987, 1991) approach to dialogues about dialogues has flattened the family hierarchy, facilitated multiple levels of reflections, and made a tremendous contribution to clinical work with families.

In our clinical practice, we have found variations on the traditional format to be a powerful invitation to a reflection. As clinical supervisors and educators, we have experienced that inviting graduate students to participate in a reflecting team is one of the best ways to invite systemic, non-blaming, nonjudgmental conversations of "what is happening in the family" and avoid the "wicked witch of linear thinking."

Although there is no one right way to participate in a reflecting team, there are certain behaviors of team members that are more useful to the meaningfulness of reflecting teams. Some of the suggestions we offer to initiate a new team member include the following:

- Offer commendations to family members or to the family as a whole that are based on evidence from the family session or from research or professional or personal experiences.
- Acknowledge individual and family suffering.
- Validate one family member's position (I can understand that point of view because…). Other team members will validate others' positions.
- Offer alternative views and beliefs about family members' lives, relationships, and experiences of illness.
- Offer personal experience that is triggered by the family's stories and beliefs.
- Offer ideas from research or literature review.
- Offer alternative views concerning questions family members have posed to the team.
- Offer answers to the question, "What will you never forget about this family?"

Consistently, family members and clinicians report their appreciation of the multiple perspectives, beliefs, and recommendations of the reflecting team and the opportunities this micromove offers for challenging constraining beliefs.

Conclusion

This chapter on challenging constraining beliefs has offered the micromoves that are most salient to the *Illness Beliefs Model* at this time. It is through the offering of these micromoves that the clinician is nudging, shifting, moving, and challenging those constraining beliefs that are impeding healing. With each new encounter with an individual and/or family, we believe that new, serendipitous, spontaneous learning occurs. Through this learning, we continue to learn which micromoves are the most successful to lessen the intensity of the suffering through the challenging of constraining beliefs. In the next chapter, we will offer ideas of how to strengthen the facilitating beliefs that are more helpful in nurturing healing.

References

Andersen, T. (1987). The reflecting team: Dialogue and meta-dialogue in clinical work. *Family Process, 26*(4), 415-428.

Andersen, T. (Ed.). (1991). The reflecting team: Dialogues and dialogues about the dialogues. New York: W.W. Norton.

Bell, J.M. (1995). The dysfunction of "dysfunctional" [Editorial]. *Journal of Family Nursing, 1*(3), 235-237.

Bell, J.M., Moules, N.J., & Wright, L.M. (2009). Therapeutic letters and the Family Nursing Unit: A legacy of advanced nursing practice. *Journal of Family Nursing, 15*(1), 6-30.

Bell, J.M., & Wright, L.M. (2007). La recherché sur la pratique des soins infirmiers a la famille [Research on family interventions]. In F. Duhamel (Ed.), *La sante et la famille: Une approche systemique en soins infirmiers* [Families and health: A systemic approach in nursing care] (2nd ed.). Montreal, Quebec, Canada: Gaetan Morin editeur, Cheneliere Education. (An English version of this book chapter is available from DSpace at the University of Calgary Library: https://dspace.ucalgary.ca/handle/1880/44060.)

Bohn, U., Wright, L.M., & Moules, N.J. (2003). A family systems nursing interview following a myocardial infarction: The power of commendations. *Journal of Family Nursing*, 9(2), 151-165.

Duhamel, F. (1994). A family systems approach: Three families with a hypertensive family member. *Family Systems Medicine, 12*, 391-404.

Duhamel, F., Dupuis, F., & Wright, L.M. (in press). Families' and nurses' responses to the "One Question Question": Reflections for clinical practice, education, and research in family nursing. *Journal of Family Nursing*.

Epston, D. (1994). Extending the conversation. *Family Therapy Networker, 18*(6), 31-37, 62-63.

Fleuridas, C., Nelson, T.S., & Rosenthal, D.M. (1986). The evolution of circular questions: Training family therapists. *Journal of Marital and Family Therapy, 12*, 113-127.

Freedman, J., & Combs, G. (1996). *Narrative therapy: The social construction of preferred realities*. New York: W.W. Norton.

Houger Limacher, L. (2003). *Commendations: The healing potential of one family systems nursing intervention.* Unpublished doctoral thesis. University of Calgary, Alberta, Canada.

Houger Limacher, L. (2008). Locating relationships at the heart of commending practices. *Journal of Systemic Therapies, 27*(4), 90-105.

Houger Limacher, L., & Wright, L.M. (2003). Commendations: Listening to the silent side of a family intervention. *Journal of Family Nursing*, 9(2), 130-135.

Houger Limacher, L., & Wright, L.M. (2006). Exploring the therapeutic family intervention of commendations: Insights from research. *Journal of Family Nursing, 12*, 307-331.

Loos, F., & Bell, J.M. (1990). Circular questions: A family interviewing strategy. *Dimensions in Critical Care Nursing, 9*(1), 46-53.

McElheran, N.G., & Harper-Jaques, S.R. (1994). Commendations: A resource intervention for clinical practice. *Clinical Nurse Specialist, 8*(1), 7-10, 15.

McLeod, D.L. (2003). *Opening space for the spiritual: Therapeutic conversations with families living with serious illness.* Unpublished doctoral thesis, University of Calgary, Alberta, Canada.

McLeod, D., & Wright, L.M. (2001). Conversations of spirituality: Spirituality in family systems nursing – making the case with four clinical vignettes. *Journal of Family Nursing, 7*(4), 391-415.

McLeod, D.L., & Wright, L.M. (2008). Living the as-yet unanswered: Spiritual care practices in Family Systems Nursing. *Journal of Family Nursing, 14*(1), 118-141.

Moules, N.J. (2000). *Nursing on paper: The art and mystery of therapeutic letters in clinical work with families experiencing illness.* Unpublished doctoral thesis, University of Calgary, Alberta, Canada.

Moules, N.J. (2002). Nursing on paper: Therapeutic letters in nursing practice. *Nursing Inquiry, 9*(2), 104-113.

Moules, N.J. (2003). Therapy on paper: Therapeutic letters and the tone of relationship. *Journal of Systemic Therapies*, 22(1), 33-49.

Moules, N.J. (2009a). The past and future of therapeutic letters: Family suffering and healing words. *Journal of Family Nursing, 15*(1), 102-111.

Moules, N.J. (2009b). Therapeutic letters in nursing: Examining the character and influence of the written word in clinical work with families experiencing illness. *Journal of Family Nursing, 15*(1), 31-49.

NIFT Letter. (2006). Written by George and Linda Jensen. Available at: www.janicembell.com

Pyle, N. (2009). Therapeutic letters as relationally responsive practice. *Journal of Family Nursing, 15*(1), 65-82.

Robinson, C.A. (1994). *Women, families, chronic illness and nursing interventions: From burden to balance.* Unpublished doctoral dissertation, University of Calgary, Alberta, Canada.

Robinson, C.A., & Wright, L.M. (1995). Family nursing interventions: What families say makes a difference. *Journal of Family Nursing, 1*(3), 327-345.

Rodgers, N. (2009). Therapeutic letters: A challenge to conventional notions of boundary. *Journal of Family Nursing, 15*(1), 50-64.

Tapp, D.M. (1997). *Exploring therapeutic conversations between nurses and families experiencing ischemic heart disease.* Unpublished doctoral dissertation, University of Calgary, Alberta, Canada.

Tapp, D.M. (2004). Dilemmas of family support during cardiac recovery: Nagging as a gesture of support. *Western Journal of Nursing Research, 26*(5), 561-580.

Tomm, K. (1984a). One perspective on the Milan systemic approach: Part 1. Overview of development, theory and practice. *Journal of Marital and Family Therapy, 10,* 113-125.

Tomm, K. (1984b). One perspective on the Milan systemic approach: Part 2. Description of session format, interviewing style and interventions. *Journal of Marital and Family Therapy, 10,* 253-271.

Tomm, K. (1985). Circular interviewing: A multifaceted clinical tool. In D. Campbell & R. Draper (Eds.), *Application of systemic family therapy: The Milan approach* (pp. 33-45). London: Grune Stratton.

Tomm, K. (1987a). Interventive interviewing: Part I. Strategizing as a fourth guideline for the therapist. *Family Process, 26*(1), 3-13.

Tomm, K. (1987b). Interventive interviewing: Part II. Reflexive questioning as a means to enable self-healing. *Family Process, 26(6),* 167-183.

Tomm, K. (1988). Interventive interviewing: Part III. Intending to ask lineal, circular, strategic, or reflexive questions? *Family Process, 27*(1), 1-15.

Tomm, K. (1989). Externalizing the problem and internalizing personal agency. *Journal of Strategic and Systemic Therapies, 8*(1), 54-59.

White, M. (1988/1989). Externalizing of the problem and re-authoring of lives and relationships. *Dulwich Centre Newsletter,* pp. 3-21.

White, M. (2007). *Maps of narrative practice.* New York: W.W. Norton.

White, M. (1995). Therapeutic documents revisited. In M. White (Ed.), *Re-authoring lives: Interviews and essays.* Adelaide, Australia: Dulwich Centre Publications.

White, M., & Epston, D. (1990). *Narrative means to therapeutic ends.* New York: W.W. Norton.

Wright, L.M. (1989). When clients ask questions: Enriching the therapeutic conversation. *The Family Therapy Networker, 13*(6), 15-16.

Wright, L.M. (2009). Spirituality, suffering, and beliefs: The soul of healing with families. In F. Walsh (Ed.), *Spiritual resources in family therapy* (2nd ed., pp. 65-80). New York: Guilford. (Previous edition: 1999).

Wright, L.M. (2005). *Spirituality, suffering, and illness: Ideas for healing.* Philadelphia: F.A. Davis.

Wright, L.M. (Producer). (2007). *Spirituality, suffering, and illness: Conversations for healing.* [DVD]. (available from: www.lorrainewright.com)

Wright, L.M. (2008). Softening suffering through spiritual care practices: One possibility for healing families. *Journal of Family Nursing, 14(*4), 394-411.

Wright, L.M., & Leahey, M. (Producers). (2006). *How to use questions in family interviewing.* [DVD]. (available from www.FamilyNursingResources.com)

Wright, L.M., & Leahey, M. (2009). *Nurses and families: A guide to family assessment and intervention* (4th ed.). Philadelphia: F.A. Davis.

Wright, L.M., & Nagy, J. (1993). Death: The most troublesome family secret of all. In E. Imber Black (Ed.), *Secrets in families and family therapy* (pp. 121-137). New York: W.W. Norton.

Wright, L.M., & Watson, W.L. (1988). Systemic family therapy and family development. In C.J. Falicov (Ed.), *Family transitions: Continuity and change over the life cycle* (pp. 407-430). New York: Guilford.

CHAPTER TEN
Strengthening Facilitating Beliefs

"Healing may not be so much about getting better, as about letting go of everything that isn't you—all of the expectations, all of the beliefs—and becoming who you are."
—Rachel Naomi Remen

The intent of each and every macromove, as well as the micromoves within the *Illness Beliefs Model*, is to offer healing for illness suffering. Just as suffering may be physical, emotional, relational, spiritual, and/or all four (Wright, 2005), we conceptualize healing to be a process of change in the beliefs held by individuals, families, health care providers, larger systems, and/or culture and society. Offering interventions that will perturb beliefs at the systems level that offers the greatest leverage for change is the desired outcome of the therapeutic conversation. The healing may also be physical, emotional, relational, spiritual, or all four.

Guided by the ideas of structural determinism (Maturana & Varela, 1992), we remain humbled and acutely aware that while we, as clinicians or family members, may desire therapeutic change and healing, we cannot be invested in the direction or pace of the change that leads to healing (for more elaboration of these ideas see Chapter 5, Beliefs about Therapeutic Change and Chapter 6, Beliefs about Clinicians).

But how does a clinician sustain the changes that have evolved?

What micromoves will assist individuals and families to continue on their path of healing? This chapter describes our own learning process of noticing, observing, and distinguishing change as well as the most useful macromoves for strengthening the change and the accompanying facilitating beliefs.

Within the literature that advocates a family systems perspective for clinical practice with families experiencing serious illness, the focus has largely been on *outcome research*, which asks the question, "Are we helpful to families?" (Kazak, 2002; Law, Crane, & Berge, 2003; Sexton, Ridley, & Kleiner, 2004). This is an important question that has been examined by several integrative reviews about the effectiveness of family interventions in health care (Campbell, 2003; Campbell & Patterson, 1995; Gilliss & Davis, 1993; Martire, Lustig, Schulz, Miller, & Helgeson, 2004).

What began as a need to demonstrate efficacy and justify involving families in health care has evolved into asking research questions about the change process itself. The focus has broadened from, "*Does* the intervention work?" to "*How does* the intervention work?" and "*How do* we make sense of therapeutic change?" (Bell & Wright, 2007; Heatherington, Friedlander, & Greenberg, 2005; Pinsof & Wynne; 2000). These are exactly the kinds of questions our team (Drs. Janice Bell, Lorraine Wright, and Wendy Watson Nelson) found ourselves asking in the early 1990s when we designed an innovative research project to examine therapeutic change in our clinical practice with families. Our interest in this kind of unique *process research* used a qualitative approach called hermeneutic inquiry (Benner, 1994; Dreyfus, 1991; Heidegger 1927/1962) and resulted in the publication of our first book about the *Illness Beliefs Model* (Wright, Watson, & Bell, 1996). The unit of data collection and analysis in this research was "change segments" defined as segments of the therapeutic conversation salient to the process of therapeutic change that we observed in the selected families, with therapeutic change corroborated by the family themselves through outcome data. Across the five families we chose for this research who showed observable therapeutic change, we examined nineteen therapeutic conversations and harvested ninety-two change segments for our research analysis.

What is most fascinating and relevant to the discussion about the macromove of "Strengthening Facilitating Beliefs" in this chapter, is that as a clinical team we were largely unaware of the interventions we were using to distinguish therapeutic change in our practice with families. We knew that change happened in families, we were thrilled when change happened, and we talked with families about change when they noticed and reported it; but we did not have a language to describe the insightful, and somewhat invisible, work we were actually doing to ask about change, observe for change, be curious about change, and even mine for change in our therapeutic conversations. When we began our research analysis of the change segments described above, we were often amazed at how curious we were as clinicians and as a clinical team about therapeutic change and how, when we sensed change in the therapeutic process, we held it up, examined it, got excited about it, and made a big deal of it! This research allowed us to bring forth in language the specific and carefully elaborated micromoves we offer here about how to strengthen facilitating beliefs.

It is therefore no surprise when we say with conviction that we believe change needs to be distinguished to become a reality. If change is not distinguished, noticed, observed, and languaged by a person, it is not present for that individual. To distinguish therapeutic change is to bring change forth: to bring change forward from its background, to "see" change, to determine what change has occurred, and to uncover the facilitating beliefs that we believe are foundational to the change.

Persistent Scrutiny of Changed Beliefs

This fourth macromove of the *Illness Beliefs Model* focuses on strengthening facilitating beliefs whenever they arise in the therapeutic conversation. Facilitating beliefs open possibilities for change and growth, thereby softening illness suffering. Facilitating beliefs may be distinguished within the first few minutes of an initial therapeutic conversation with an individual or family, or after many hours of intensive effort directed at carefully creating a context for changing beliefs, distinguishing a core illness belief that is the heart of the suffering, and challenging this constraining belief. For the purposes of the discussion in this chapter, we will focus on micromoves that the clinician may use to strengthen facilitating beliefs that usually arise *after* a core constraining illness belief has been challenged, altered, or modified through the therapeutic conversation(s).

Distinguishing therapeutic change involves therapeutic moves that watch for, identify, and strengthen facilitating beliefs. Listen for the shift from constraining beliefs to facilitating beliefs in the following clinical vignettes that have been used as exemplars throughout this book.

Initially, the parents of the 34-year-old man experiencing multiple sclerosis (Mark) embraced the constraining belief that "good parents caring for their son cannot take a holiday." But through the course of the clinical sessions, they challenged this belief with the heart-wrenching question of how to ask their son for some respite. However, when they finally did go away for a short holiday, the rewards were substantial.

"I did not know how I could say this to him," the mother explained to us after returning from their first holiday in years: "Can we go away somewhere together?" To anyone else, this may have seemed an easy question for a parent to ask of their child. For this particular family, it was a question that brought about guilt and heartache for the parents, to the point they were burning out completely because they felt they couldn't ask it. "But it was just wonderful," she said smiling widely. "It has changed our life completely."

In another family, the mother of a daughter experiencing Chronic Fatigue Syndrome expressed her new facilitating belief this way: "I now realize there are always solutions if we can just keep talking." Her previous constraining belief had been, "We are sick and tired of being tired and sick. There is nothing more we can do."

Another profound facilitating belief arises from Julie, the wife of a man who had experienced a heart attack: "Things are going better. There's not the conflict; I am not backing off anymore. I don't believe I have to protect him. I believe he can take it." Her core constraining belief had previously been, "If I upset my husband, he'll get angry and have another heart attack." She had been hiding her true self and therefore her own health was at risk from her self-silencing.

And in yet another family, the 13-year-old experiencing Chronic Fatigue Syndrome, Sarah, offered this confident comment in our final session with the family: "I can control my illness. It doesn't control me." This was a dramatic shift from her previous constraining belief of, "My illness controls me. I am a victim of Chronic Fatigue."

In order to watch for changed beliefs that are connected to therapeutic change and thus a softening of suffering, the clinician needs to stay as alert and curious about facilitating beliefs as possible. As the conversations progress, he or she will become sensitized to listen for and watch intently for constraining beliefs. Staying alert to changed beliefs requires the clinician's persistence. Beliefs that are foundational to the *Illness Beliefs Model* about the connection between therapeutic change and new facilitating beliefs include:

- Change is always happening, both in our internal structures and in our environment (Maturana & Varela, 1992).
- Individuals and families are frequently unaware of the changes they are making.
- Individuals and families may sometimes, if invited, notice change in their behaviors or affect but are frequently unaware about changes in their beliefs.
- Therapeutic change consists of a change from a core constraining belief that invites suffering to a facilitating belief that softens suffering.
- Through talking about and reflecting about changed beliefs, therapeutic change is drawn forth as a reality; that is, therapeutic change is distinguished.
- Through the distinguishing of changed beliefs, change is solidified.
- Strengthening the facilitating belief by talking about it and examining it makes it more likely that therapeutic change will be sustained and maintained.

These clinician beliefs invite wonderment, awe, and an insatiable curiosity with respect to being vigilant for facilitating beliefs. The clinician anticipates change but it must be distinguished to be real for the clinician as well as the family and connected to a change in beliefs. Every possible aspect about change is rolled over, described, explored, amplified, and magnified to make it real, to know that it truly has happened, that it exists. Often when families have been oppressed with an illness or loss for a long time, it is not readily evident to them that change has occurred and almost always not within their awareness that they have changed their beliefs.

It is not just one aspect of the therapeutic change that makes it stand out; it is the composite of the distinctions that makes it real. The persistent scrutiny for change and the micromoves needed to connect therapeutic change to changed beliefs is an ethical obligation of the skilled clinician who uses the (see *Figure 14*).

Figure 14. Micromoves: Strengthening Facilitating Beliefs

- **Seeing change**
- **Exploring change**
- **Inviting observations of others about change**
- **Exploring effects of change**
- **Inviting explanations of change**
- **Targeting new facilitating beliefs**
- **Celebrating change**
- **Publishing change**

Micromove: Seeing Change

What do you see? Maturana and Varela (1992) remind us that we are all observers, constantly observing ourselves and others. What we are structurally able to see influences our relationships with others. In turn, our relationships with others influence our structure and thus what we are able to see. Influenced by these ideas, the clinician asks directly about what family members are observing: What have you noticed about yourself, your family, your relationship, etc. since the last time we met? How have you experienced our conversation today? Are you noticing anything different about the way you were thinking or feeling at the start of our work together compared to the way you are thinking or feeling now?

In some families, members spontaneously offer what they see. One example occurred with Julie and Robert, the couple suffering with marital conflict in the context of the husband's heart attack. When the clinician asked about what had happened since the previous session, Julie offered the following: "I see [my husband] making efforts…I see him stopping short when he would have said something and thinking about things."

She was able to distinguish her husband's efforts. His changes were noticeable to, and noticed by, her. His new behavior was a difference that made a difference to her and emerged out of the background of "no change" for her. For this woman, her husband's changes were real!

In the following example in which the youngest daughter, Sarah (C2), had been experiencing Chronic Fatigue Syndrome, the clinician (LMW) follows up on a conversation about "putting uncertainty in its place." The mother spontaneously comments, "I *feel* that she is making some progress." Notice how readily the mother, father and eldest sister (C1) respond when the clinician asks what they are *seeing*:

LMW: *What do you* see?

MOTHER: *I* see *her up for longer periods. I* see *her able to interact. Like if a friend comes over, she may be tired, but she'll stick with her friend for a long time and she may fall into bed after that.*

LMW: *So for longer periods? Socializing longer?* [The clinician is trying to focus the conversation on the actual changes that have taken place.]

FATHER: *I think she bounces back quicker* [he says to the mother]. *Don't you find that?*

MOTHER: *Yes. And it doesn't take her as long.*

LMW: [Turning her attention to Sarah] *Wow! Do you notice that yourself? Are you up for longer periods, socializing longer?*

C2: [She nods.] *I was going to try to go to school today because I was feeling not bad for a while. But this morning I got up and I just knew, no way, I couldn't.*

C1: *Her attention is coming back too. She has a longer attention span.*

MOTHER: *Because her attention is coming back, she can read for longer periods, but her memory is getting worse.*

C2: *I'll read a book then forget about it.*

LMW: *But your memory is—you don't remember sometimes just what you've read?*

C2: *No.*

LMW: *Wow, this is a lot. So, what else?*

The clinician discovers what changes various family members are selecting out: what changes they are able to "see" and what changes they are each able to distinguish. In this process the clinician learns that the changes family members are *seeing* range from positive changes of Sarah socializing longer, bouncing back quicker, and attending school longer to a negative change in the daughter's memory. The clinician expresses her own amazement at the amount of change that the family members are able to see after only one session, and in a "true," ever-curious therapeutic style, she inquires about what else they are seeing these days.

In our clinical work, we are as amazed and curious about therapeutic change as we are about challenges and suffering. At a conference with the late Michael White, we learned about his phrase, "falling off my chair with excitement" when discussing therapeutic change. When we are supervising student clinicians who receive early glimpses of change from families, we often phone into the interview room and tell the student, "Fall off your chair!"—a shorthand way of inviting more excitement, animation, enthusiasm, and curiosity about the change that is being reported. Other words and phrases like "Wow," "That's incredible," "Really?" "Tell me more" are ways of operationalizing this micromove of seeing change, which, in turn, hopefully invites even more scrutiny and observation of change.

Michael White also taught us about the value of "audible note-taking" as another response to reports of seeing therapeutic change. Writing something down in our culture usually means that it is important. We try to take careful notes of the specific changes that are reported and make lists of these changes as a way to demonstrate that the changes the family are seeing are vitally important and fascinating to the clinician as well (for more ideas, see *Celebrating Change* later in this chapter).

Micromove: Exploring Change

Change is not linear, nor is the exploration of change. The systems theory axiom that "a change in one part of the system affects other parts of the system" implies that when therapeutic change is being distinguished, it needs to be explored in different areas of the system and from different points of view. To distinguish change, the exploration of change is thorough, systemic, and nonlinear. No turn in the loop of change is left unexplored.

In the following change segment, the clinician (LMW) distinguishes change by exploring change from the husband's point of view, exploring the wife's view of the husband's view, and exploring the wife's view. Change becomes real as the clinician turns the change that is being described over and over, looking at it from various angles and points of view.

LMW: *Well, tell me, how are Robert and Julie doing together as a couple? You've told me a lot about the kids and how you're doing individually. How are you doing as a couple?*

JULIE: *What do we really do together?* [She leans heavily on the word "do."] *We're always with kids and family. We don't do a whole lot just as a couple.*

ROBERT: *No, we do it as a...*

JULIE: *We're not fighting.* [Julie continues with the theme of what they are not doing as a couple, which begins change.]

LMW: *Well, okay.* [The clinician is trying to bring the conversation back.] *Maybe I don't mean doing activities together.*

ROBERT: *I've become more comfortable.*

283

LMW: *Let me ask you this question then in a different way. . . How are you getting on together?*

ROBERT: [enthusiastically] *I'm happy. I'm comfortable. I'm in love. I'm in admiration.*

LMW: [looking carefully at the expression on Julie's face] *She's looking at you like...*

ROBERT: *I like the relationship. . .*

LMW: *Julie's looking at you like . . .*

ROBERT: [continuing] *. . .that we have.*

LMW: *But Julie looked kind of quizzical when you said admiration.* [The clinician explores the explanation for the wife's quizzical look, discovering that this is the first time the wife has heard that her husband is "happy, comfortable, in love, in admiration."]

LMW: [drawing forth the wife's experience] *And what about for you, Julie? How are you? How do you feel things are going for you in your marriage?*

From a variety of angles and with an undaunted stance, the clinician explores change, never assuming that one family member's experience is the same as another's, always curious about the impact of one person's description of change on another.

In the therapeutic conversations with George and Linda, who initially reported being oppressed by "The Monster" of chronic illness 100% of the time in their lives and in their marriage relationship, the clinician (JMB) challenged the couple's constraining beliefs about mastery, control, and influence by asking a series of relative influence questions. As the couple began experimenting with ways to have more influence over the chronic illness, they returned to the third session feeling discouraged that they had not made much progress. As they talked about their experiment with the NIFT Day (2006), many changes were uncovered and explored. Scaling questions were again helpful to explore the change by using a 0-10 point scale or percentage of influence. What percentage of influence did the monster of illness have over them now as compared to before? What percentage of influence did the couple believe they had over the monster now compared to before?

This exploration of change was very useful to the couple because it helped them see change in concrete terms. Realizing that their ability to influence the monster of illness had increased from 0% to 30% because of their efforts, gave them a language to explore their changed beliefs and to define themselves as a competent and resourceful team with the potential to have even more influence in the future. As our clinical team shared with them in a between session therapeutic letter:

> We were struck with the magnitude of the changes you have made and we wondered if part of the reason you hadn't fully realized the full impact of these changes yourselves was related to the deceptiveness of the monster. We believe that it is important to notice each and every act of protest as you develop an anti-monster plan for your lives. We hope that as you continue to refine the NIFT day, you will spend time reviewing the changes that you have noticed in each other and in yourselves at the end of these experimental anti-monster days—even if the changes seem small.

Micromove: Inviting Observations of Others about Change

"Everything said is said by an observer to another observer," (Maturana, 1978, p. 31). If everything said is said by an observer, our interest becomes, "Who is the observer noticing change and what are they saying about the change?" An "observer-perspective question" (Tomm, 1988) about therapeutic change becomes any question that draws forth any person's perspective about change, including the person observing him or herself, because all are observers.

Operating from a systemic stance, the perspective of multiple observers is useful in the previous example in which family members were experiencing the Chronic Fatigue of the daughter, Sarah. Each offered his or her perspective on changes observed. Directly or indirectly, we inquire about such aspects as (a) others' perspectives on changes "seen," (b) others' explanations of how changes have occurred, and (c) others' perspectives of the effects of change. Examples of observer perspective questions about change include:

- What changes, if any, are you noticing in your daughter?
- What change in your sister do you think has caught your mother's attention?
- What is it about the change your wife made that allowed you to notice it?
- Who else is noticing the change you are making?
- If your father were here, what would he say has contributed to this change?
- What would your sister need to see or experience that would convince her that you have changed?

One woman (Connie) was challenging her beliefs about herself and experiencing a decrease in her anxiety. The clinician (LMW) invites the client to notice others' noticing of her changes.

LMW: *Well, I'm wondering if anybody else noticed this change in you?*

CONNIE: [firmly] *No.*

LMW: *Nobody's noticed. You don't think that they did? Were you pretty good at masking your anxiety?*

CONNIE: *Yes.*

LMW: [noticing a shift in Connie's demeanor] *So your friends, your husband, your kids wouldn't have picked up on this?*

CONNIE: *Oh, I think my husband knows. I'm not so crabby all the time; you could put it that way.*

LMW: *Ah. So, that's one difference. If he were here, he may not comment on the anxiety, but he would notice that difference in you?*

CONNIE: *Yes.*

LMW: *Not as crabby? Anything else that your friends and family would notice about you?*

Here, the client's view of her changes is shored up when the clinician solicits the client's view of others' views of her changes. When the client initially says no one has noticed, the clinician explores the hypothesis that no one has noticed the dramatic changes because the client was so good at masking her problem. The question embeds a commendation about the amount of change: The client would have to be "pretty good at masking the anxiety" for others not to notice now the change in her anxiety.

Following this question, the clinician gives the client another opportunity to view others' viewing of her. This time her view has shifted, and she is able to notice that her husband would notice less crabbiness. This willingness to open space to others' observations of change (particularly if those observations are offered from people who matter) may provide information to the family system that will encourage even more change in family members and sustain the change that is occurring.

Micromove: Exploring Effects of Change

When changes have happened, one way to strengthen and solidify them within the *Illness Beliefs Model* is to explore the effects of the changes on various family members. Exploration and reflection are involved in this process. The couple who presented with respite issues concerning managing their son, Mark's, multiple sclerosis (MS) held the following constraining beliefs:

- Good parents of a son with MS sacrifice all they have, including their own health, for the well-being of their son.
- Good parents of a son with MS need to do all the nursing care themselves.
- Good parents of a son with MS can never take a holiday,

especially without their son's permission.

While masterful therapeutic moves were involved in identifying and challenging the constraining beliefs, equally important to the work with this family were the therapeutic moves to draw forth and strengthen the facilitating beliefs. The last two sessions were focused solely on strengthening facilitating beliefs: drawing forth and affirming facilitating beliefs and the corresponding affective and behavioral changes. During the course of four sessions, the issues of family members shifted from worry about the son's trips to the bathroom and the parents' fear of his tripping and falling down in their absence, to the parents' making plans for respite: their vacation trip to Las Vegas.

In following up on an assignment, the clinician (LMW) heard the report from Mark that he'd made phone calls securing information about nursing services available for himself, which would allow respite for his care-giving parents and a change for him in being cared for by someone other than his parents. The son could receive respite from his parents' care giving just as the parents could receive respite. LMW's efforts to draw forth and affirm facilitating beliefs involved pursuing the effect of this new information ("new" on many levels) on family members.

One seemingly small but important aspect of exploring the effects of change is sequencing. To whom do you address the first question? To affirm the facilitating belief that Mark can manage his illness, the clinician initially addresses questions to him, asking his opinion first, a move that is not minor but is saturated with meaningful messages. By addressing questions initially to Mark, the clinician supports his newly claimed leadership position in the family. Mark comes to the foreground, de-ranking the debilitating illness to the background. These changes serve as possible perturbations for other family members and their relationships.

The following clinical vignette demonstrates sequencing while exploring the effects of change. Mark has just told the clinician of his accessing the life-liberating information regarding nursing care services available to him.

LMW: *Congratulations! That's wonderful. I'm really pleased to hear that. What do you think this information has done for your parents? Do you* *think it's done anything for them?* [By directing these questions to Mark, the clinician invites him to a reflection about the impact of the change on his parents.]

MARK: *Well...it's taken a load off their shoulders, I would think. They want to go...*

LMW: *Knowing that they have that option now and knowing that you're supportive of it. Remember last time we met, you really were very clear about that, that you're very supportive of them having a holiday. And now knowing how they could arrange it.*

MARK: *Yes.*

LMW: [to his parents] *Is that so? Has it given you...*

PARENTS: *Yes. It's a big relief...*

MARK: *Having that registered nurse or whatever... They know I'll be in good hands.*

LMW: [to his parents] *Yes. So, is Mark accurate when he says it's taken some pressure off?*

PARENTS: [agreeing] *Oh, it sure has...*

LMW: *Knowing you've got that option now, being able to...*

PARENTS: *Yes.*

LMW: [Turning to Mark and checking the information in another way by bringing up the formerly forbidden topic of travel] *When do you think they're going to take off?*

MARK: *I think they...*

MOTHER: [firmly] *October.*

MARK: ...*said October.* [Mark finishes, confirming his parents' plans.]

LMW: *Ah, so you are planning. Great!*

The clinician then invites the parents into a conversation about the holiday they might take, allowing them to create a new belief about themselves right in the session. The new belief is about themselves as a traveling couple instead of as permanent, full-time 'nurses.' The clinician then asks, "What do you think this information has done for your son? Do you think it's made any difference for him?" The clinician provides the son an opportunity to give his reflection on his parents' reflections. In this manner, the son has had the first and last word, and the belief that the son can take leadership and manage his illness is gently solidified and strengthened. It was a poignant moment in the clinical work.

Micromove: Inviting Explanations of Change

Persistently seeking the explanation for how change has come to be is another way to distinguish change and make it real:
- What made you aware of this new behavior/affect?
- How do you explain that you have been able to make this important change?
- How have you accomplished this remarkable change?
- How were you open to having your previous belief challenged?

As family members are invited to offer explanations about their changes, they are concurrently invited to a reflection about the change and hopefully begin to have new beliefs about themselves and their illness. Both the change and the family members' efforts become more real. Our belief is that if change can be explained, it is more likely to be maintained.

Micromove: Targeting New Facilitating Beliefs

Facilitating beliefs are those that open the possibility for a greater variety of solutions and new and empowering ideas about one's self, relationships, and abilities. Facilitating beliefs soften illness suffering.

How does one invite individuals and families to reflect on and articulate their new beliefs so that further refinement and solidification of change can happen? When a change is observed by an individual, family members, or the clinician, it is useful to target and explore the facilitating beliefs that are connected to the change.

- What have you come to believe about yourself [your spouse, your marriage, life] through our work together?
- What else have you come to believe?
- What questions/statements do you find you saying to yourself these days?
- What do you think your ability to make this change says about you?
- What new beliefs fit with the change that you are noticing?

The therapeutic conversation that unfolds to distinguish the facilitating belief provides an opportunity for family members to see themselves and other family members differently, in a new light, and become more aware of the shift that has occurred in their beliefs. As new facilitating beliefs are brought forth, illness suffering is softened.

Micromove: Celebrating Change

When change has occurred, change needs to be drawn forth, languaged, commended, even celebrated. How does one invite an individual or family to celebrate change? How can a clinician provide opportunities for conversations of commendation and celebration? The following are some of the ways that we have found useful and fun in our clinical work with individuals and families:

- Use celebratory language: wow, really, incredible, fantastic, terrific!
- Refocus back to the celebration of change.
- Repeat the client's words.
- Concretize change by audible note taking.
- Elevate, specify, and celebrate client effort, giving credit to the client for the change and specifying client behavior that

led to the change through persistent inquiry.

- Do not allow diminishing of client effort.
- Offer commendations that distinguish individual and family strengths and resourcefulness to make significant change.
- Offer comparative commendations: commendations pointing out, for example, how wise or courageous the client is in comparison to others in the situation.
- Offer commendations that highlight what the individual/family has taught you that you will remember when you work with other families.
- Encourage individual and family rituals to celebrate the change.

In the *Illness Beliefs Model*, we make conscious efforts to celebrate change. The following segment of the fourth and final session with a family who were experiencing difficulties with the younger daughter's Chronic Fatigue Syndrome, is a typical example of our efforts. Listen as the accolades abound and sincere commendations are offered with enthusiasm to solidify the changes. None of the celebration can be feigned. The clinician must believe at a deep "cellular-soulular" level that she is witnessing change. When the clinician believes in the celebratory worthiness of the change, corresponding palpable emotion and therapeutic cheerleading behavior will be present. Change is magnified through therapeutic inquiries—what did your family say?—and by pursuing the client's internal conversations: How did you make the decision to go each day like that? What did you say to yourself while doing this? What does this tell you about your ability to control the disease?

Following is a segment of therapeutic celebration from the consultation with the 13-year-old youngest daughter, Sarah (C2), who experienced Chronic Fatigue Syndrome:

LMW: *And anything else new since I've seen you last, before we talk about your assignment?*

C2: [quietly] *The week I saw you, what day was that?*

LMW: *That was the twenty-sixth of May.*

C2: *Yeah, well, I think I didn't go to school that week, but then the next week and the week after and the next week and the next week I went for about the whole week.* [It is interesting that the daughter who has been immobilized by Chronic Fatigue has been going so regularly to school that she now doesn't think she went to school that first week. School is such a part of her repertoire of behaviors, she cannot remember when it started to be so.]

LMW: *Did you?*

C2: *Yeah, in the mornings.*

LMW: *Wow! Congratulations! That's fantastic! Let me get this down. So, not the week I saw you, but the next week and the week after... You went in the mornings? Dynamite!* [The clinician emphasizes the importance of this change by audibly taking notes. This underlines the importance to the girl of what she's accomplished—it's so important that it must be written down. Distinguishing what is important is important. Family members then feel valued for their comments.]

C2: *And there was a dance* [she picks up the excitement of the clinician]. *I really wanted to go, right? So I asked the counselor and everything and the principal and they said, "Yes, that would be okay." So I went, and then I was really tired for the next week.*

LMW: *So you went to the dance. Well, I can imagine after not being out dancing for a while, that you would be tired. Did you actually get up and dance?*

C2: *Not really. I just sort of hung out.*

LMW: *Hung out, yes. Just hung out and visited with your friends. Well, that's incredible! That's really terrific! What did your family say?* [At this point, the clinician shifts to enlarge the celebration, exploring the client's view on others' views of her accomplishment. She explores responses of family members by broadening the audience of change. They were happy with it.] *And how did you make the decision to go each day like that, because we talked about, um…*[the clinician embeds volition by strengthening the client's belief about herself. Note the wonderful response of the client, who now, from a position of strength, interrupts the clinician.]

C2: [with immense joy] *Me controlling the disease instead of the disease controlling me!* [The fact that the client chose to interrupt the clinician is rich evidence of significant, meaningful change. It shows the client's understanding of the change and clearly brings forth the new facilitative belief.]

LMW: *We talked about pacing it, maybe every other day. How did you figure out that you could handle it every morning?* [Again, the clinician is embedding and inviting the client to a reflection.]

C2: *Well, I just, I don't know, I was feeling good. Like I was feeling better than I was, so I thought that I could add to it.* [The client's structure is being perturbed. Perhaps this "trying-to-sort-it-out, confused" languaging is an indicator of the beginnings of a structural change, a change in beliefs.]

LMW: *Well, that is just fantastic! That's a real accomplishment! What did you say to yourself when you were doing this?*

C2: *Oh, I thought, well, I just wanted to get back to school…*

LMW: *Yes, I know.*

C2: *I was tired a little bit, but I was better than I was, I think.*

LMW: *Well, I'm sure you would be a little bit, but that's just a tremendous accomplishment* [the clinician reinforces]. *So what does this say [to you] about your ability to control this disease a little more instead of it always ruling you? What does this tell you?*

In these few minutes within a therapeutic conversation, change has been distinguished through celebration, and the possibilities for more change have been opened.

Micromove: Publishing Change

Sometimes strengthening facilitating beliefs involves publication of change. We first encountered this micromove through the clinical work of White and Epston (1990) and have since expanded these ideas with many families. Publishing change involves (a) exploring the desirability of publicity (e.g., would you like anybody else to know of your success?) and (b) elevating clients' experiences of success and expertise by connecting the experience to the clinician's future work with families. This is done in a manner that recaps the client's whole story, validating, amplifying, and solidifying the changes and strengthening the new facilitating beliefs. The clinician might ask:

- What advice would you give to health care professionals who care for families with your health concern?
- What advice would you suggest I give to another person/family who is suffering with a similar illness/challenge?
- Would you be interested in writing a letter about the changes you've noticed in your beliefs and behavior and how you accomplished this so that I could share your experience with other families who are dealing with similar issues?

We have had many families over the years that have been very interested and willing to write us a letter about the changes that they have experienced. George and Linda were very interested in telling others about the dramatic shift in their beliefs about mastery, control, and influence as they experimented with living alongside chronic illness. Our team suggested that perhaps they could write a letter briefly describing their illness story and emphasizing how they had been successful and what they specifically did to reduce the influence of "the monster" of illness in their lives and marital relationship. We were very impressed by their altruism as they developed their No Illness and Fatigue Talk (NIFT) Letter

(2006) and read it aloud in our therapeutic conversation. They encouraged our clinic to distribute it as widely as possible to health care providers and other families. Another family with whom we worked co-authored a journal publication with our team which highlighted what we had learned together about healing following the death of their adolescent son (Levac et al., 1988).

Publishing change by putting it on paper is to have the changes documented through text rather than through spoken words. Recording changes in the form of written words concretizes the changes for the family members. The written word can be read, reread, and shared with others and thus published over and over again. We routinely send a closing therapeutic letter to every family with whom we are privileged to work. In the closing letter we specifically highlight what we have learned from the family and what we believe we offered the family (for more information about therapeutic letters, see Chapter 9).

The closing letter that follows was written to a family who had recently experienced the tragic deaths of two members of their family. The young son/brother was killed in an accident and the father/husband died a year later following a myocardial infarction while the family was vacationing together. (Reprinted with permission from SAGE Publications: Bell, Moules, & Wright, 2009.)

Example of a Family Nursing Unit Closing Therapeutic Letter

Dear Connie, Samantha, and Jeremy:

Greetings from the Family Nursing Unit. As part of completing our clinical work with families, we send a closing letter as a summary and record of our time spent together. From February 24 to April 14 we had an opportunity to meet with you on three occasions.

We would like to share what we learned from your family and what we believe we offered to you in these sessions. We were very touched and privileged with your sharing of the tragic experience of losing William and Aaron [husband/father and son/brother], and your continuing journey in finding your own ways to live with your losses.

What we learned from your family:

296

1. *You shared with us your powerful story of experiencing two traumatic and unexpected losses in your family [through the deaths of William and Aaron]. We heard that living with loss and grief has been the most challenging and difficult journey you have endured as individuals and as a family. You have taught us about strength and courage in the face of loss and grief. Although we believe that families have amazing resilience and resources in difficult situations, you demonstrated an exceptional capacity to rise to this challenge and emerge with courage and sensitivity.*

2. *We have been impressed with your ability to remain a very close family, one that supports and respects each other and one that has been able to share so openly about deeply painful issues. In choosing to remain united and committed to one another, we learned again of the power that families have when they work together. The team witnessed an extension of this commitment when you openly expressed your hopefulness and optimism for an "untainted" future. You taught us that even amidst sorrow, pain, and grief there can be joy, as you shared the changes and blessings in your family that evolved as a result of William and Aaron's deaths.*

3. *We learned that you are a very spiritual family and your strong spiritual beliefs invited the team into the privilege of experiencing William and Aaron's spirit in our sessions. Your belief that God loves you unconditionally and has a reason and purpose for this loss seems to have helped you make sense of this experience. You reminded us how one's strong spiritual beliefs and faith in God is sustaining and can diminish suffering and contribute to healing.*

What we believe we offered you:

1. *Our team offered you our observation of your closeness as a family and we witnessed the concern you have not only for*

your individual well-being but the well-being of your family. We offered our perceptions that some family members seem to have been able to say goodbye to parts of the relationship with William and Aaron more easily, and other members have had an easier experience with saying hello. The team offered our belief that grief is both about saying goodbye and saying hello and we wondered if there could be a way that you could teach and share your abilities with each other. We also offered you our belief that we are most hopeful for your family because of your strength and commitment to one another.

2. *Our team has been very impressed with your insight into your experience. We suggested our belief that you are a family who accepts where each person is with respect to coping and experiencing loss, yet seems able to gently offer individual thoughts and beliefs to help with one another's healing.*

3. *Your family has shown us that it is not only acceptable to be sad but that it is acceptable to be mad at God and we appreciated your belief: "God can handle it". Because of your strong spiritual beliefs, your lack of bitterness, and your ability to continue discovering the many ways you are blessed, you have opened yourselves to the possibility of finding happiness and living a rich life alongside your loss and grief. We suggested that your ability to feel joy, express laughter, embrace hope, and discover a sense of meaning in this experience will serve you well as your continue healing and move forward on your journey.*

We would like to repeat that, as a result of meeting your family, we believe we will be different with and have more to offer other families who are journeying with their own experiences of loss and grief. We thank you for this immense gift and blessing.

We would like to remind you that you will be contacted in about six months time to be invited to participate in a follow-up study, intended to improve our clinical practice with families.

With warm regards,

Nancy L. Moules, RN, MN, Doctoral student
Lorraine M. Wright, RN, PhD, Director, Family Nursing Unit

This closing therapeutic letter is an example of publishing change, that not only observes and celebrates the changes that the family has made, but also serves to highlight and strengthen the facilitating beliefs that have evolved through the therapeutic process. By bringing therapeutic change to life through a written document like a letter we increase the possibility of sustaining the influence of facilitating beliefs in family members' lives which leads to healing.

Whether a closing letter is part of the termination ritual or not, health care providers need to part from their clients in a manner that leaves persons with hope and confidence in their new and rediscovered strengths, resources, and abilities to manage their health and relationships (Wright & Leahey, 2009). Strengthening facilitating beliefs through the micromoves of the *Illness Beliefs Model* offered above can be incorporated into the process of terminating with individuals and families. Madsen (2007) refers to this part of the therapeutic process as a "consolidation interview." The consolidation or termination process may actually occur over more than one session, but the significance of this process is that particular kinds of questions are asked—questions that review the clinical work the family and clinician have done together in the past and also the work that the family is seeking to accomplish on its own in the future. Questions that process the therapeutic relationship and offer what the clinician has learned may also be useful at termination (e.g., What did I do or say that was most helpful in our work together?; What did I do or say that was least helpful?; What feedback do you have for me so that I can improve in my work with families? Here's what I have learned most from your family...). This kind of termination process is a way to reduce feelings of anxiety, fear, or loss on the part of the clinician, an individual/family, or both, and hopefully assists in maintaining and sustaining the changes that have begun.

Conclusion

Distinguishing change, bringing it forth through language, and connecting these changes to new facilitating beliefs is the careful, rewarding, and joyful work of the *Illness Beliefs Model* that strengthens and sustains therapeutic change and healing. In this chapter, clinicians and family members alike are invited to be vigilant in their observations of changed beliefs that soften suffering. By strengthening, encouraging, and sustaining new or modified facilitating beliefs, we believe change is honored and healing continues and grows. As new facilitating beliefs are embraced, behaviors and emotions are also altered and new interactions in our relationships become possible. The ripple effect of changing our beliefs is so profound within each person that it can affect our very biology and so wide ranging to affect our relationships with others and illness.

We close this chapter by asking you the reader to reflect on a belief of yours that has been challenged about families, illness, clinicians, or about therapeutic change itself? What difference has this new belief made in your life and your relationships? How were you open to having your limiting belief challenged? What contributed to this shift in your beliefs? How are you or will you be different in your clinical practice, in your relationships, or perhaps in managing an illness because of the new facilitating beliefs you have embraced? As Maturana and Davila (n.d.) remind us:

> The reflection, as a proper doing of the human manner of living, is also an act that is performed in a particular emotional ambience that is the total acceptance of the legitimacy of the circumstances that he or she lives. The reflection happens as an act that the person abandons its attachment to what he or she knows and is able to contemplate his or her present without prejudice, demands or expectations. The emotion that makes reflection possible is love, since love is the domain of relational behavior through which oneself and the other one arise as a legitimate other in coexistence with oneself.

Across all of the macromoves of the *Illness Beliefs Model*, the clinician drifts towards objectivity-in-parenthesis, inviting facilitating beliefs that will encourage particular kinds of practices in our therapeutic conversations that include among others, affirmation, affection, and forgiveness that will soften illness suffering and heal relationships. Above all, we hope that the *Illness Beliefs Model* will invite you as a clinician, and as a family member to become a particular kind of person. Maturana and Varela (1992, p. 246) remind us, love lets us *see* the other person and open up for him room for existence beside us." We hope the ideas of the Illness *Beliefs Model* will serve as a template for love and compassion to flourish in relationships between clinicians and families and between family members. "Charity suffereth long, and is kind; charity envieth not; charity vaunteth not itself, is not puffed up...And now abideth faith, hope, charity, these three; but the greatest of these is charity." (1 Corinthians 13).

References

Bell, J.M., Moules, N.J., & Wright, L.M. (2009). Therapeutic letters and the Family Nursing Unit: A legacy of advanced nursing practice. *Journal of Family Nursing, 15*(1), 6-30.

Bell, J.M., & Wright, L.M. (2007). La recherche sur la pratique des soins infirmiers à la famille [Research on family interventions]. In F. Duhamel (Ed.), *La santé et la famille: Une approche systémique en soins infirmiers* [Families and health: A systemic approach in nursing care] (2nd ed. pp. 87-105). Montreal, Quebec, Canada: Gaëtan Morin editeur, Chenelière Éducation. (An English version of this book chapter available for public access on DSpace at the University of Calgary Library: https://dspace.ucalgary.ca/handle/1880/44060)

Benner, P. (1994). The tradition and skill of interpretive phenomenology in studying health, illness, and caring practices. In *Interpretive heurmenology: Embodiment, caring, and ethics in health and illness* (pp. 99-127). Thousand Oaks, CA: Sage.

Campbell, T.L. (2003). The effectiveness of family interventions for physical disorders. *Journal of Marital and Family Therapy, 29*(2), 263-281.

Campbell, T.L., & Patterson, J.M. (1995). The effectiveness of family interventions in the treatment of physical illness. *Journal of Marital and Family Therapy, 21*(4), 545-583.

Dreyfus, H.L. (1991). *Being-in-the-world: A commentary on Heidegger's Being and Time, Division I.* Cambridge, MA: MIT Press.

Gilliss, C.L., & Davis, L.L. (1993). Does family intervention make a difference? An integrative review and meta-analysis. In S.L. Feetham, S.B. Meister, J.M. Bell, & C.L. Gilliss (Eds.), *The nursing of families. Theory/research/ education/practice* (pp. 259-265). Newbury Park, CA: SAGE.

Heatherington, L., Friedlander, M.L., & Greenberg, L. (2005). Change process research in couple and family therapy: Methodological challenges and opportunities. *Journal of Family Psychology, 19*(1), 18-27.

Heidegger, M. (1962). *Being and time* (J. Macquarrie & E. Robinson, Trans.). New York: Seabury Press. (Original work published 1927).

Kazak, A.E. (2002). Challenges in family health intervention research. *Families, Systems, & Health, 20*(1), 51-59.

Law, D.D., Crane, D.R., & Berge, J.M. (2003). The influence of individual, marital and family therapy on high utilizers of health care. *Journal of Marital and Family Therapy, 29*(3), 353-363.

Madsen, W. (2007). Working within traditional structures to support a collaborative clinical practice. *The International Journal of Narrative Therapy and Community Work, 2,* 51-61.

Martire, L.M., Lustig, A.M., Schulz, R., Miller, G. E., & Helgeson, V. S. (2004). Is it beneficial to involve a family member? A meta-analysis of psychosocial interventions for chronic illness. *Health Psychology, 23*(6), 599-611.

Maturana, H.R. (1978). Biology of language: The epistemology of reality. In C. A. Miller & E. Lennenberg (Eds.), *Psychology and biology of language and thought: Essays in honor of Eric Lennenberg* (pp. 27-63). New York: Academic Press.

Maturana, H.R., & Varela, F.J. (1992). *The tree of knowledge: The biological roots of human understanding* (rev. ed.). Boston: Shambhala.

Maturana, H.R., & Davilla, X.Y. (n.d.). *Matriztica Institute. International English reflective circles in cultural-biology.* Retrieved March 22, 2009, from: http://www.matriztica.org

NIFT Letter. (2006). Written by George and Linda Jensen. Available at: www.janicembell.com

Pinsof, W.M., & Wynne, L.C. (2000). Toward progress research: Closing the gap between family therapy practice and research. *Journal of Marital and Family Therapy, 26,* 1-8.

Seikkula, J., & Trimble, D. (2005). Healing elements of therapeutic conversation: Dialogue as an embodiment of love. *Family Process, 44*(4), 461-475.

Sexton, T. L., Ridley, C. R., & Kleiner, A. J. (2004). Beyond common factors: Multilevel-process models of therapeutic change in marriage and family therapy. *Journal of Marital & Family Therapy, 30*(2), 131-149.

Tomm, K. (1988). Interventive interviewing: Part III. Intending to ask lineal, circular, strategic, or reflexive questions? *Family Process, 27*(1), 1-15.

Wright, L.M. (2005). *Spirituality, suffering, and illness: Ideas for healing.* Philadelphia: F.A. Davis.

Wright, L.M., & Leahey, M. (2009). *Nursing and families: A guide to family assessment and intervention.* (5th ed.). Philadelphia: F.A. Davis Company.

Wright, L.M., Watson, W.L., & Bell, J.M. (1996). *Beliefs: The heart of healing in families and illness.* New York: Basic Books.

CHAPTER ELEVEN
Grief and Families:
Applying the Illness Beliefs Model to Bereavement

by Dr. Nancy J. Moules

"...this gentleness we learn from what we can't heal"
—Bronwen Wallace

*A*mi *was 3 years old when she was diagnosed with Acute Lymphocytic Leukemia and 6 years old when she died. In between those three short and yet, long years, she and her family lived with the "Damocles Sword" of feasting and fear. After multiple remissions and relapses, Ami was given a bone marrow transplant which was, in theory, successful in eradicating any cancer cells in her blood. Unfortunately, however, the intensity of treatments required to hold her leukemia at bay and to eventually prepare her for her bone marrow transplant took a toll on her young, fragile body. In spite of her strong will, the love of her family, and the dedication of the health care team, Ami died of a cerebral hemorrhage as a result of low platelets.*

I was present with Ami and her family when she died, gave her eulogy at the funeral, and continued to be a part of the continuing love and connection that her family felt for her in spite of her physical absence in their lives. Several weeks after her funeral, I received a call from a family member concerned that Ami's mother, Karen, was not "coping" and "not letting go" as evidenced through her behaviors of maintaining her daughter's room in situ and her "refusal' to be apart from her daughter's ashes. Karen's husband and two small sons were worried along with other members of her large extended family that this behavior was not healthy and that Karen might even be mentally ill.

In response to this family member's concern, I met with Karen, a strong, determined, and charismatic woman, and spoke with her about her family's concern about her choice to carry Ami's urn with her at all times. I asked Karen if she knew why her family was concerned about her. Her response was: "They think I need to let go and move on, that my carrying her ashes is crazy." I asked her how she answered that concern in her own mind and she responded: "There is nothing wrong with me. I had this little girl for only six years and I know she is dead. But I also know that I am not ready to let go of the last physical piece I have of her."

I asked her when she might know when she was ready and she said that she did not know but she would recognize it when it came. She trusted her own knowledge and timing. I applauded Karen's courage in standing up to others' prescriptions of how she was to manage her grief and, instead, to trust in her own instincts.

Two weeks later, I received an invitation for a private family burial of Ami's ashes. I asked Karen how she knew that the time was right and she said that her father had dreamed that Ami wanted to go in a hot air balloon with other children and that she (Karen) was stopping her. At the burial, when some purple (Ami's favorite color) balloons broke away from the tree to which they were tied and floated down towards the ocean, Karen, at my side, with grace, confidence, and connection, said: "There she goes."

Grief is arguably one of the most universal of human experiences and, with few exceptions, powerfully touches family members' lives. The death of a loved one is ultimately inevitable and how families learn to live with the grief that accompanies such a loss is profoundly influenced by the beliefs that are held, embodied, and played out in thoughts, emotions, behaviors, and relationships. Through our program of research around grief and families, and through our clinical work with bereaved families informed by *the Illness Belief Model*, we have come to see that the role of beliefs in the grief experience is at once the source of either suffering or comfort, and also the portal through which healing therapeutic conversations can enter.

Arriving at Commonly Held Beliefs about Grief

Grief, a fundamental part of our human condition, has prompted the call to understand, define, predict, and ultimately eradicate it. Within this call, there has been a distinct evolution of thinking of grief as a process of energy withdrawal involved in the psychic process of releasing and transferring energy and an association between unsuccessful mourning and melancholia; to grief as a disease or pathology with predictable trajectories; to grief as a process involving stages and expectations; to grief as requiring models of clinical practice that involves tasks and accomplishments in the work of letting go.

Shifts in understanding have opened the notion that grief is not something so easily defined or predicted, but rather is an unavoidable life experience that is not anticipated, in spite of any preparation; does not follow a temporal and limited sequence; and ultimately does not result in recovery, resolution, or successful elimination. Rather, it is more currently being regarded as a normal reaction to an event of loss, a response that becomes a part of living and relationships in unique, mutable, lifelong, and life-changing ways (Attig, 1996; Klass, Silverman, & Nickman, 1996; Moules, 1998; Moules & Amundson, 1997; Moules, Simonson, Prins, Angus, & Bell, 2004; Moules, Simonson, Fleiszer, Prins, & Glasgow, 2007; Neimeyer, 2001a, 2001b; Worden, 2000). Ultimately, grief does not result in a "recovery" as seen as a return to the familiar, but in an incorporation of the loss into living forward, and an ongoing connection with the deceased that allows one to continue to move ahead in living (Klass et al., 1996; Moules et al., 2004, 2007; White, 1989).

In spite of these shifts in our understandings, however, we have been left a pervasive legacy that finds its place in everyday experience of grief and loss. We are burdened with the idea that there is a right way to "do" grief, that this right way is measured by the absence of grief feelings, and that ultimately, to stray from these prescribed trajectories implants a stamp of failure, if not pathology, that takes shape in lives and relationships (Moules et al., 2004).

Beliefs that May Show Up in Grief

Clinical practice using the *Illness Beliefs Model* and research (Moules et al., 2004, 2007) have allowed us to examine the types of beliefs that seem to arise in grief experiences. Some of these beliefs center on grief itself and the nature of grief, while others are related to the activities that occur in grief. Other beliefs that surface in grief seem to fall more in the domain of the particularities and complexities of the relationship with the deceased and the events preceding the loss.

Beliefs about Staying Connected

The legacy left to us that viewed grief as a process of energy withdrawal and the work of disconnection with the deceased often creates a belief in the bereaved that they ought to work on "getting over" their loss and learn how to say goodbye to their loved ones. There is a part of grief that absolutely involves a departure, a physical absence, a loss, and ending to a relationship as it once was. We have learned, however, that while simultaneously letting go of the deceased, the bereaved also find ways to remain connected, to redefine their relationship with the deceased. Michael White (1989) first described this as a process of "saying hullo again" in learning to "re-member" the deceased, to call the deceased back into membership in lives and relationships. The nature of this membership, of course, is changed, though often not the character of it. Silverman and Klass (1996) used the language of "continuing bonds" and staying connected by internalizing and incorporating aspects of the lost person such that a physical presence is no longer necessary for the relationship to exist. One family member seen in the Family Nursing Unit stated this realization eloquently: "When my grandmother died, I thought I would lose her, but I didn't—I become more like her every day, so I did not lose her at all."

Another family member expressed her fear that she was losing her memories of her son. The work of staying connected and "re-membering" is also the work of nurturing memories. The beliefs about saying goodbye and letting go are perpetuated and sustained through popular literature, culture, and even some of our therapeutic practices. Experiences of grief, however, contradict these culturally sanctioned beliefs and in the contradiction, many people find themselves subscribing to a sense of personal failure, incompetence, and sometimes even pathology when they believe that their continued experience of feeling connected and in relationship is wrong.

Beliefs about the Time-limited, Sequential Nature of Grief

Over 100 years of theory, literature, and clinical practice has somehow created a culture of beliefs that grief is a process with a trajectory that is limited and that successful achievement of this enormous process is measured by an absence of grief. Our clinical work and research has led us to a different belief that grief is a lifelong and life-changing experience marked by shifts in intensity over time but not measured as successful by the evidence of its absence (Moules, 1998; Moules, Thirsk, & Bell, 2006; Moules et al., 2004, 2007). The contradiction of bereavement experiences suggests this: Grief remains, not with the same intensity of deep, unrelenting sorrow but with aspects of memory, joy, love, connection, celebration and, yes, even pain. As one family member expressed: "We need steps to get on with life, not over him...we're never going to get over his death; we don't want to." Another family member from our research project stated, "I wish that people understood that it wasn't a short-term process, and that it is a lifelong change." A third member pointedly reminded us that:

How long does it last? I hate that question. But if you really, really insist, I would say if after two years you're still where you are now, then you need to be concerned. But the real answer is never...it's not going to be like this forever, but it's not going to go away either.

Stage model theories of grief are pervasive in the literature and such models may be damaging. They involve a movement through predictable reactions to loss that has left an imprint that there is a correct sequencing of actions and affect that, if followed correctly, result in the resolution of grief or, in other words, its ending, and in the "recovery" of the bereaved. The contradictions of experiences of the bereaved again defy these ideas as the bereaved speak of the nature of "recovery" as an impossibility. Life, as it was known before the death of the loved one, cannot be recovered,

Beliefs and Illness: A Model for Healing

and although aspects of it can be reclaimed, there is no absolute recovery. Rather, we are moved into a lifelong process of constructing meaning, re-authoring narratives, and relearning the world, our relationships, and often even our identities (Attig, 1996; Klass et al., 1996; Moules, 2009; Moules et al., 2007; Neimeyer, 2001b; White, 1989).

Stage model theories perpetuate the belief of a "right" and "wrong" or a normal way, or at least parameters to experiences and expressions of grief. As a result, some people believe they are not grieving enough or some too much; some move into a protectiveness in shielding their own grief from other family members; some view seeking support as a weakness; some believe that all family members should suffer the same amount at the same time; some believe that grief emotions should be controlled and managed (Moules, 1998).

Beliefs about Events Connected to the Loss

In the very normal process of reliving, recalling, and reflection that occurs after the death of a loved one, many family members struggle with beliefs around their relationship, their roles, and their responsibilities. These beliefs often arise as beliefs about something they could have done differently in life that may have prevented the death or the nature of the death, around things said or left unsaid prior to the death, about unresolved conflicts, or around concerns about how the dying member may have suffered. At times, these beliefs take the shape of guilt and often this guilt remains unspoken and in its unexpressed containment can become toxic and unrelenting (Moules & Amundson, 1997).

Beliefs about Identity

In our research (Moules et al., 2007; Moules & Simonson, 2009), a well-seasoned grief counselor identified that there are three "red flags" that he is vigilant in watching for in his clients who present around grief experiences. These markers are bereaved people who present with guilt that is so overwhelming that it dominates and obscures other emotions of grief, with unrelenting anger that takes on an embitterment or resentment that casts other aspects of grief into the shadows, and finally when the person who has died was so significant to the identity of the bereaved that there is a feeling of complete loss of self. If the bereaved person believes that they have no identity in the absence of the deceased family member, then this constraining belief can block all of the courage, wisdom, and adventure required of the bereaved, where one enters into an engagement with the loss that is strong enough to sustain it.

Applying the Illness Beliefs Model to Grief

The work that occurs with the bereaved involves an excavation of the beliefs that may be creating, fuelling, or exacerbating the suffering that is already inherent in grief. In the uncovering of such beliefs guided by the *Illness Beliefs Model* and the gentle and directed challenging of them, lies the possibility of healing conversations.

Macromove: Creating a Context for Changing Beliefs

The relationship that takes root in initial conversations with families experiencing grief is foundational to the healing possibilities of suffering in grief; the relationship is, in fact, the first portal to healing. Within the skills and process of engaging, removing obstacles to engagement, and creating a context where healing can occur, the clinician must, first and foremost, be open to hearing suffering. "To enter the world of one who is grieving, we must choose to listen to the pain behind the words" (Gibbons, 1993, p. 599). The death of a loved one is often embodied in many narratives—narratives of lives lived; of illness, anticipated or sudden; of death; of other losses; of complicated relationships; of joys, regrets, remorse, and guilt; and of continued love in presence and in absence. The context for healing in grief work is solidly rooted in this engagement with families as they begin to realize that their suffering is heard, honored, and acknowledged. In grief work, recognizing suffering is a means of remembering and joining families in their need to remember and "re-member" (White, 1989); it is about tending to the woundedness and rawness that lies in loss (Moules et al., 2007).

Macromove: Distinguishing Beliefs

The beliefs that can arise in grief are, as described earlier, as varied as there are family members. Some are connected to cultural discourse, some to circumstances, some to gender, and some to experience. The *Illness Beliefs Model* offers a roadmap through beliefs related to suffering;

diagnosis; etiology; healing and treatment; mastery, control, and influence; prognosis, religion/spirituality, etc., and all of these areas can be unpacked around grief experiences. In the face of many beliefs that may either constrain or create more suffering for families in grief or that may facilitate healing, it is often in discussions of spiritual beliefs where conversations of therapeutic healing are located (Moules et al., 2007). The work of grief is often about making sense of it, searching for meaning and understanding. "The core of work with the bereaved is spiritual in nature because the core of grief is a spiritual experience. It is an experience of making meaning, doubting meaning, or questioning the purpose of lives lived, living, and lost" (Moules et al., 2007, p. 127).

Another belief that often finds its way into therapeutic conversation is the notion of "grief work" as simply letting go or saying goodbye. Karen's family shared this belief and thought that Karen's behavior was an indication that she was not successfully navigating letting Ami "go." In the uncovering of this belief with families, the clinician might recognize the opportunity to gently offer challenge and an invitation to consider grief as a process of connection rather than just separation.

All of the beliefs aforementioned may emerge in this macromove of exploration and distinguishing beliefs. The clinician's attunement to beliefs that commonly tether themselves to grief experiences requires a discernment of which of these beliefs are comforting, sustaining, facilitating, and connecting and which might be adding to the woundedness that lies in grief.

Macromove: Challenging Constraining Beliefs

The challenging of beliefs that contribute to suffering in grief happens in many ways. The challenge is embedded in commendations that recognize families' strengths in the face of immense pain, resilience at times of most wanting to abandon faith and belief, and in the offering of hope in a family's ability to navigate the pain of grief and renegotiate a life that continues in the absence of a loved one's physical presence. The challenge is embedded in thoughtful comments, observations, new ideas, and suggestions offered by reflecting teams and in the ways that therapeutic letters extend and expand the clinical conversation. The challenge lies in skillfully crafted questions that invite reflection and ultimately offer the possibility of new beliefs that might better serve the family. It lies in sermonettes and reflecting comments of the clinician. In all of these carefully considered micromoves, the beliefs of the clinician subtly, tentatively, and sometimes boldly emerge.

Micromove: Offering Alternative Beliefs

Through our clinical work with families and research, we are convinced that one limiting belief in particular must be challenged: the socially sanctioned, constraining belief that grief work only involves the process of saying goodbye. The offering of a "professional" belief that staying connected is also the work of grief seems to have the potential for initial relief and, then, the development of a sustaining sense of peace in the recognition that to feel connected is not only "normal" and "okay" but healthy. For example, in one therapeutic conversation, the clinician offered her belief that grief work is not just about saying goodbye but finding ways to stay connected to the deceased in such a way that there is comfort and relationship; there is re-membering. After this offering of the clinician's belief, a family member offered her insight that, prior to this, she may not have been open to admitting that she did still feel connected. Instead, she might have been conscripted into a conspiracy of silence and hiding, only admitting to herself that she felt connected and had found private ways to allow the connection. With the offering of our belief, she felt the courage and confidence to express her own belief, which the team saw as facilitating. The family member insightfully offered us this comment:

> When you lose somebody, it's almost like you're building a house and when somebody dies, all the top gets taken off but the foundation is still there...So we still have this foundation but we have to build it up again and in that foundation are my dad and brother – still there. They're still there. And they're so much engrained in who we are but all of the physical manifestations of them are gone.

Micromove: Speaking the Unspeakable

Another micromove that seems to be almost a therapeutic obligation in grief work is that of taking the lead in inviting families to speak the unspeakable around many aspects of their loss experience. It is here where the clinician moves into conversations of guilt, remorse, responsibility, fears, normalcy, and sometimes contradictory responses such as the mixture of loss and relief after periods of long suffering in illness. These poignant, fragile yet robust conversations involve courage on the part of the family and the clinician; tenacity, timing, and discernment on the part of the clinician; and ultimately faith that talking is healing. It is often in these conversations that the family is able to shift from beliefs of self-blame to beliefs and actions of forgiveness (of self and others) and of atonement.

Macromove: Strengthening Facilitating Beliefs

The realization of family members that they are doing "okay," that their experiences of the continuing presence of grief is normal; that the continuing sense of connection to their deceased loved one is exactly what is supposed to happen; that guilt is something that needs to sometimes be considered but cannot be allowed to consume; that grief is evidence of having loved well; that suffering, sadness, joy, memory, and celebration can live simultaneously; that there is hope for the future; that they are not alone; and that they are entitled to all their feelings, behaviors, and thoughts *is* therapeutic change and a shift from constraining to facilitating beliefs. In the words of one mother who had lost her 18-year-old son and her husband within one year, change for her meant, "I feel more at peace." She attributed this change to having had the opportunity to be heard, to have witness to her pain, to be challenged around her sense of responsibility, and to "not be alone here having to hold it all together," but rather having had the clinician move into this role, allowing her the luxury and pain of her grief and the expression of her guilt. She also reported that what was offered to her was hope—hope from the clinical team, the clinician, from her family members, and from her heart that there would be joy, there would be laughter, and there would be "good times to come." There *is* hope in grief—hope in the belief in our human capacity to suffer, sorrow, heal, celebrate, and love.

Conclusion

The work of healing in grief is the work of courage and love. It embodies a "character of connection to the living and the dead, a lifelong work that is borne by the bereaved who carry the inherent capacity to heal through love, and clinicians willing and skilled to join in behind" (Moules et al., 2007, p. 139). The *Illness Beliefs Model* offers a therapeutic template, relationship, and possibility for healing that lies in the power of skilled, thoughtful, mindful, and present therapeutic conversations.

Therapeutic conversations are privileged conversations that occur in many contexts, but often are present in nursing. They lie somewhere in intent and outcome, but mostly in outcome. Conversations happen or they do not. We do not get to predict how ideas will be taken up, how questions will be reflected upon, and how conversations will linger. However, we do get to offer our best intentions, our most thoughtful questions, our empirically guided interventions to hopefully create a space where something of value—of nursing, of therapy, and healing—will take root. As witnesses to suffering, nurses are already in the position of listening to and offering presence, experience, and language that may invite healing and diminish or even ameliorate, suffering. This goal is not new in nursing, but rather a cornerstone of nursing itself. The intervention of language in nursing has often been relegated to other professions and disciplines, but the Greek root of *therapeia*, "to nurse," remains firmly tethered to our words and encounters with those in suffering.

References

Attig, T. (1996). *How we grieve: Relearning the world.* New York: Oxford University Press.

Gibbons, M.B. (1993). Listening to the lived experience of loss. *Pediatric Nursing, 19*(6), 597-599.

Klass, D., Silverman, P. R., & Nickman, S. L. (Eds.). (1996). *Continuing bonds: New understandings of grief.* Philadelphia: Taylor & Francis.

Moules, N. J. (1998). Legitimizing grief: Challenging beliefs that constrain. *Journal of Family Nursing, 4*(2), 142-166.

Moules, N.J. (2009). A parent's worst nightmare: Grief, families, and the death of a child. *Relational Child and Youth Care Practice, 21*(4), 63-69.

Moules, N. J., & Amundson, J. K. (1997). Grief: An invitation to inertia. A narrative approach to working with grief. *Journal of Family Nursing, 3*(4), 378-393.

Moules, N.J., & Simonson, K. (2009). Following in behind: An interview with the Reverend Bob Glasgow on his practice with grief work. *Illness, Crisis, & Loss, 17*(1), 51-69.

Moules, N.J., Simonson, K., Fleiszer, A., Prins, M., & Glasgow, B. (2007). The soul of sorrow work: Grief and therapeutic interventions with families. *Journal of Family Nursing, 13*(1), 117-141.

Moules, N. J., Simonson, K., Prins, M., Angus, P., & Bell, J. M. (2004). Making room for grief: Walking backwards and living forward. *Nursing Inquiry, 11*(2), 99-107.

Moules, N.J., Thirsk, L.M., & Bell, J.M. (2006). A Christmas without memories: Beliefs about grief and mothering–A clinical case analysis. *Journal of Family Nursing, 12*(4), 426-441.

Neimeyer, R.A. (Ed.). (2001a). *Meaning reconstruction and the experience of loss.* Washington, DC: American Psychological Association.

Neimeyer, R.A. (2001b). Reauthoring life narrative: Grief therapy as meaning reconstruction. *Israel Journal of Psychiatry and Related Sciences, 38*(3–4), 171–83.

Silverman, P.R., & Klass, D. (1996). Introduction: What's the problem? In D. Klass, P.R. Silverman, & S.L. Nickman (Eds.), *Continuing bonds: New understandings of grief* (pp. 45–58). Philadelphia: Taylor & Francis.

White, M. (1989). Saying hullo again: The incorporation of the lost relationship in the resolution of grief. In M. White (Ed.), *Selected papers* (pp. 29-36). Adelaide, Australia: Dulwich Centre.

Worden, J. W. (2000). Towards an appropriate death. In T. A. Rando (Ed.), *Clinical dimensions of anticipatory mourning: Theory and practice in working with the dying, their loved ones, and their caregivers* (Vol. 13, pp. 267-277). Champaign, IL: Research Press.

Contributor Information: Nancy J. Moules, RN, PhD, Associate
Professor, Faculty of Nursing, University of Calgary, 2500
University Ave N.W., Calgary, Alberta, Canada T2N 1N4

Email: njmoules@ucalgary.ca

PART III

ADDITIONAL RESOURCES ABOUT THE

ILLNESS BELIEFS MODEL

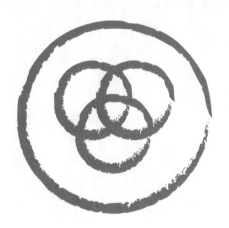

Resource One

Publications by Dr. Lorraine M. Wright and/or Dr. Janice M. Bell and other Faculty and Graduates associated with the Family Nursing Unit

Updated April, 2009. For more recent updates see:
www.janicembell.com or www.lorrainewright.com

This collection of publications and media productions was created by faculty and graduates associated with the Family Nursing Unit, University of Calgary (1982-2007). *The legacy of this family-focused clinical scholarship continues to grow.*

Dr. Lorraine M. Wright (Director 1982-2002); Dr. Wendy L. Watson Nelson (1982-1992); Dr. Janice M. Bell (1986-2002; Director 2002-2007); Dr. Nancy J. Moules (2000-2007)

Many of the publications listed in this bibliography are available for free public access on DSpace at the University of Calgary Library: https://dspace.ucalgary.ca/handle/1880/44060

EDUCATIONAL VIDEOTAPES/DVD

Wright, L.M. (Producer). (2007). *Spirituality, suffering, and illness: Conversations for healing* [DVD]. (Available from: www.lorrainewright.com)

Wright, L.M. & Leahey, M. (Producers). (2006). *How to use questions in family interviewing* [DVD]. (Available from: www.FamilyNursingResources.com)

Wright, L.M., & Leahey, M. (Producers). (2003). *How to intervene with families with health concerns* [DVD]. (Available from: www.FamilyNursingResources.com)

Wright, L.M., & Leahey, M. (Producers). (2002). *Family nursing interviewing skills: how to engage, assess, intervene, and terminate* [DVD]. (Available from www.FamilyNursingResources.com)

Wright, L.M., & Leahey, M. (Producers). (2001). *Calgary Family Assessment Model: How to apply in clinical practice* [DVD]. (Available from www.familyNursingResources.com)

Wright, L.M., & Leahey, M. (Producers). (2000). *How to do a 15 minute (or less) interview* [DVD]. (Available from www. FamilyNursingResources.com)

Maturana, H.R. (1998). *Biology of cognition and biology of love* [Videotapes of a workshop presented at the Faculty of Nursing, University of Calgary in 1998]. (Available from www.janicembell. com)

Maturana, H.R. (1988). *Telephone conversation: The Calgary/Chile coupling* [Phone conversation with Dr. Lorraine Wright and graduate students]. (Transcript available from www.lorrainewright.com)

No longer in circulation:

Watson, W.L. (Producer). (1989a). *Families and psychosocial problems* [Videotape].

Watson, W.L. (Producer). (1989b). *Family systems interventions* [Videotape].

Watson, W.L. (Producer). (1988a). *A family with chronic illness: A "tough" family copes well* [Videotape].

Watson, W.L. (Producer). (1988b). *Aging families and Alzheimer's disease* [Videotape].

Watson, W.L. (Producer). (1988c). *Fundamentals of family systems nursing* [Videotape].

PUBLICATIONS

BOOKS

Wright, L.M., & Bell, J.M. (2009). *Beliefs and illness: A model for healing.* Calgary, Alberta, Canada: 4th Floor Press, Inc.

Wright, L.M., & Leahey, M. (2009). *Nurses and families: A guide to family assessment and intervention* (5th ed.). Philadelphia: F.A. Davis. (previous editions: 1st ed. 1984; 2nd ed. 1994; 3rd ed. 2000; 4th ed., 2005).

Wright, L.M. (2005). *Spirituality, suffering, and illness: Ideas for healing.* Philadelphia: F.A. Davis.

Wright, L.M., Watson, W.L., & Bell, J.M. (1996). *Beliefs: The heart of healing in families and illness.* New York: Basic Books.

Feetham, S.L., Meister, S.B., Bell, J.M., & Gilliss, C.L. (Eds.). (1993). *The nursing of families: Theory/research/education/practice.* Newbury Park, CA: Sage. (selected papers from the Second International Family Nursing Conference.)

Bell, J.M., Watson, W.L., & Wright, L.M. (Eds.). (1990). *The cutting edge of family nursing.* Calgary, Alberta, Canada: Family Nursing Unit Publications. (selected papers from the First International Family Nursing Conference.)

Leahey, M., & Wright, L.M. (Eds.). (1987). *Families & life-threatening illness.* Springhouse, PA: Springhouse.

Leahey, M., & Wright, L.M. (Eds.). (1987). *Families & psychosocial problems.* Springhouse, PA: Springhouse.

Wright, L.M., & Leahey, M. (Eds.). (1987). *Families & chronic illness.* Springhouse, PA: Springhouse.

PROCEEDINGS

Bell, J.M., Wright, L.M., Leahey, M., Watson, W.L., & Chenger, P.L. (Eds.). (1988). *Proceedings of the [First] International Family Nursing Conference.* Calgary, Alberta, Canada: University of Calgary.

CHAPTERS IN BOOKS
2000-Present

Wright, L.M. (2009). Spirituality, suffering, and beliefs: The soul of

323

healing with families. In F. Walsh (Ed.), *Spiritual resources in family therapy* (2nd ed., pp. 65-80). New York: Guilford. (First edition 1999)

Bell, J.M., & Wright, L.M. (2007). La recherche sur la pratique des soins infirmiers à la famille [Research on family interventions]. In F. Duhamel (Ed.), *La santé et la famille: Une approche systémique en soins infirmiers* [Families and health: A systemic approach in nursing care] (2nd ed., pp. 87-105). Montreal, Quebec, Canada: Gaëtan Morin editeur, Chenelière Éducation. [in French] (An English version of this book chapter available for public access on DSpace at the University of Calgary Library: https://dspace.ucalgary.ca/handle/1880/44060)

Moules, N.J. (2006). A whispered story. In C. Sorrell Dinkins & J. Merkle Sorrell (Eds.), *Listening to the whispers: Re-thinking ethics in health care* (pp. 7-9). Madison, WI: University of Wisconsin Press.

Wright, L.M., Leahey, M., & Perry, A.G. (2005). Family nursing. In J.C. Ross-Kerr & M.J. Wood (Eds.), *Canadian fundamentals of nursing* (pp. 295-314). Toronto, Ontario, Canada: Elsevier Mosby.

Raffin Bouchal, S., & Moules, N. (2003). Loss, grieving and death. In S. Raffin Bouchal & S. Hirst (Eds.), *Fundamentals of Canadian nursing: Concepts, process and practice* (pp. 1340-1364). Toronto, Ontario, Canada: Pearson Education.

Levac, A.M.C., Wright, L.M., & Leahey, M. (2002). Children and families: Models for assessment and intervention. In J.A. Fox (Ed.), *Primary health care of infants, children, and adolescents* (2nd ed., pp. 10-19). St Louis: Mosby.

Wright, L.M. (2000). What's love got to do with it? Conversations that heal. In W.L. Watson (Ed.), *The arms of His love* (pp. 148-157). Salt Lake City, UT: Brookcraft.

1990-1999

Wright, L.M. (1997). Multiple sclerosis, beliefs and families: Professional and personal stories of suffering and strength. In S. McDaniel, J. Hepworth, & W.J. Doherty (Eds.), *The shared experience of illness: Stories of patients, families, and their therapists* (pp. 263-273). New York: Basic Books.

Bell, J.M., & Wright, L.M. (1995). L'avenir de la recherche en soins infirmiers de la famille: Les interventions. [Family nursing intervention research] In F. Duhamel (Dir.), *La Santé et la famille: Une approche systémique en soins infirmiers* {Families and health: A systematic approach in nursing care (pp. 87-99)]. Montreal: Gaëtan Morin Éditeur [in French]

Wright, L.M., & Levac, A.M. (1993). The non-existence of non-compliant families: The influence of Humberto Maturana. In S.L. Feetham, S.B. Meister, J.M. Bell, & C.L. Gilliss (Eds.), *The nursing of families: Theory/research/education/practice* (pp.111-117). Newbury Park, CA: Sage (reprinted with permission).

Wright, L.M., & Nagy, J. (1993). Death: The most troublesome family secret of all. In E. Imber Black (Ed.), *Secrets in families and family therapy* (pp. 121-137). New York: W.W. Norton.

Watson, W.L. (1992). Family therapy. In G.M. Bulechek & J.C. McCloskey (Eds.), *Nursing interventions: Essential nursing treatments* (2nd ed., pp. 379-391). Philadelphia: W.B. Saunders.

Wright, L.M., Watson, W.L., & Bell, J.M. (1990). The Family Nursing Unit: A unique integration of research, education and clinical practice. In J.M. Bell, W.L. Watson, & L.M. Wright (Eds.), *The cutting edge of family nursing* (pp. 95-112). Calgary, Alberta, Canada: Family Nursing Unit Publications.

1980-1989

Wright, L.M., & Leahey, M. (1988). Nursing and family therapy training. In H.A. Liddle, D.C. Breunlin, & R.C. Schwartz (Eds.), *Handbook of family therapy training and supervision* (pp. 278-289). New York: Guilford.

Wright, L.M., & Watson, W.L. (1988). Systemic family therapy and family development. In C.J. Falicov (Ed.), *Family transitions: Continuity and change over the life cycle* (pp. 407-430). New York: Guilford.

Bell, J.M. (1987). Assessing marital responses to the threat of breast cancer. In M. Leahey & L.M. Wright (Eds.), *Families & life-threatening illness* (pp. 129-142). Springhouse, PA: Springhouse.

Leahey, M., & Wright, L.M. (1987). Families and chronic illness: Assumptions, assessment and intervention. In L.M. Wright & M. Leahey (Eds.), *Families & chronic illness* (pp. 55-76). Springhouse, PA: Springhouse.

Watson, W.L. (1987). Intervening with aging families and Alzheimer's disease. In L.M. Wright & M. Leahey (Eds.), *Families & chronic illness* (pp. 381-404). Springhouse, PA: Springhouse.

Wright, L.M., & Leahey, M. (1987). Families and life-threatening illness: Assumptions, assessment and intervention. In M. Leahey & L. Wright (Eds.), *Families & life-threatening illness* (pp. 45-58). Springhouse, PA: Springhouse.

Wright, L.M., & Leahey, M. (1987). Families and psychosocial problems: Assumptions, assessment and intervention. In M. Leahey & L. Wright (Eds.), *Families & psychosocial problems* (pp. 17-34). Springhouse, PA: Springhouse.

Watson, W.L., & Wright, L.M. (1984). The elderly and their families: An interactional view. In J.C. Hansen & E. Imber Coppersmith (Eds.), *Families with a handicapped member* (pp. 75-78). Rockville, MD: Family Therapy Collections, Aspen Systems.

Wright, L.M., & Watson, W.L. (1982). What's in a name: Redefining family therapy. In A. Gurman (Ed.), *Questions and answers in the practice of family therapy* (Vol. 2, pp. 27-30). New York: Brunner/ Mazel.

Tomm, K.M., & Wright, L.M. (1982). Multilevel training and supervision in an outpatient service program. In R. Whiffen & J. Byng-Hall (Eds.), *Family therapy supervision: Descriptions of teaching practices* (pp. 211-227). London, England: Academic Press.

Wright, L.M., & Bell, J. (1981). Nurses, families and illness: A new combination. In D. Freeman & B. Trute (Eds.), *Treating families with special needs* (pp. 199-205). Ottawa, Ontario, Canada: The Canadian Association of Social Workers.

ARTICLES

2005-PRESENT

Duhamel, F., Dupuis, F., & Wright, L.M. (in press). Families' and nurses' responses to the "One Question Question": Reflections for clinical practice, education, and research in family nursing. *Journal of Family Nursing*.

Moules, N.J., MacLeod, M., Thirsk, L.M., & Hanlon, N. (in press). "and then you'll see her in the grocery store": The working relationships of public health nurses and high priority families in northern communities. *Journal of Pediatric Nursing.*

Moules, N.J. (2009). A parent's worst nightmare: Grief, families, and the death of a child. *Journal of Relational Child and Youth Care Practice, 21*(4), 63-69.

Moules, N.J., & Simonson, K. (2009). Following in behind: An interview with the Reverend Bob Glasgow on his practice with grief work. *Illness, Crisis, & Loss, 17*(1), 51-69.

Bell, J.M., Moules, N.J., & Wright, L.M. (2009). Therapeutic letters and the Family Nursing Unit: A legacy of advanced nursing practice. *Journal of Family Nursing, 15*(1), 6-30.

Moules, N.J. (2009). The past and future of therapeutic letters: Family suffering and healing words. *Journal of Family Nursing, 15*(1), 102-111.

Moules, N.J. (2009). Therapeutic letters in nursing: Examining the character and influence of the written word in clinical work with families experiencing illness. *Journal of Family Nursing, 15*(1), 31-49.

Wright, L.M. (2008). Softening suffering through spiritual care practices: One possibility for healing families. *Journal of Family Nursing, 14*(4), 394-411.

Bell, J.M. (2008). Highlights of the 8th International Family Nursing Conference, Bangkok, Thailand, June 4-7, 2008 [Editorial]. *Journal of Family Nursing, 14*(4), 391-393.

Bell. J.M. (2008). The Family Nursing Unit, University of Calgary: Reflections on 25 years of clinical scholarship (1982-2007) and closure announcement [Editorial]. *Journal of Family Nursing, 14*(3), 275-288.

Flowers, K., St. John, W., & Bell, J.M. (2008). The role of the clinical laboratory in teaching and learning family nursing skills. *Journal of Family Nursing, 14*(2), 242-267.

Bell, J.M. (2008). Distinguished Contribution to Family Nursing Research Award (2007): Catherine L. Gilliss, DNSc, RN, FAAN. *Journal of*

Family Nursing, 14(2), 157-161.

Bell, J.M. (2008). Distinguished Contribution to Family Nursing Research Award (2007): Suzanne L. Feetham, PhD, RN, FAAN. *Journal of Family Nursing, 14*(2), 147-150.

Bell, J.M. (2008). Distinguished Contribution to Family Nursing Research Award (2007): The research team of Kathleen A. Knafl, Janet A. Deatrick, and Agatha Gallo. *Journal of Family Nursing, 14*(2), 151-156.

McLeod, D.L., & Wright, L.M. (2008). Living the as-yet unanswered: Spiritual care practices in Family Systems Nursing. *Journal of Family Nursing, 14*(1), 118-141.

Bell, J.M., Moules, N.J., & Wright, L.M. (2008). Closure of the Family Nursing Unit brings reflection from colleagues, students. *University of Calgary, Faculty of Nursing, Faculty Links.* Summer, 7.

Bell, J.M., Moules, N.J., & Wright, L.M. (2007). Closure of the Family Nursing Unit (1982-2007), University of Calgary. *University of Calgary, Faculty of Nursing, Faculty Links.* Winter, 8-9.

Bell, J.M. (2007). Innovative Contribution to Family Nursing Award 2007: Recognizing Family Nursing leaders in Thailand. *Journal of Family Nursing, 13*(4), 503-508.

Bell, J.M. (2007). Distinguished Contribution to Family Nursing Award: Dr. Marilyn Friedman [Editorial]. *Journal of Family Nursing, 13*(3), 287-289.

Bell, J.M. (2007). Distinguished Contribution to Family Nursing Award: Dr. Perri J. Bomar [Editorial]. *Journal of Family Nursing, 13*(3), 290-292.

Bell, J.M. (2007). The Family Nursing Unit (FNU) Marks 25th Anniversary. *University of Calgary, Faculty of Nursing, Faculty Links.* Summer, 9-12.

Bell, J.M. (2007). Family Nursing Network. Remembering Dr. Chieko Sugishita. *Journal of Family Nursing 13*(2), 278-280.

Moules, N.J., Simonson, K., Fleiszer, A.R., Prins, M., & Glasgow, B. (2007). The soul of sorrow work: Grief and therapeutic interventions with families. *Journal of Family Nursing, 13*(1), 117-141.

Bell, J.M. (2007). Distinguished Contribution to Family Nursing Award: Dr. Lorraine M. Wright [Editorial]. *Journal of Family Nursing, 13*(1), 3-8.

Limacher, L.H., & Wright, L.M. (2006). Exploring the therapeutic family intervention of commendations: Insights from research. *Journal of Family Nursing, 12*, 307-331.

Wright, L.M. (2006). Facilitating healing in illness: Practical therapeutic techniques for diabetes educators. *The Diabetes Communicator, Jan/ Feb*, 8.

Moules, N.J., Thirsk, L.M., & Bell, J.M. (2006). A Christmas without memories: Beliefs about grief and mothering—A clinical case analysis. *Journal of Family Nursing, 12*(4), 426-441.

Moules, N.J. (2006). A cautionary tale about stories [Guest Editorial]. *Journal of Family Nursing, 12*(3), 231-233.

Wright, L. M. (2005). Family Nursing: Challenges and opportunities-- Marriage: It matters in sickness and in health. *Journal of Family Nursing, 11*(4), 344-349.

Bell, J.M., & Moules, N.J. (2005). Profiles in family nursing leadership: Innovative contributors [Editorial]. *Journal of Family Nursing, 11*(4), 313-323.

Bell, J.M. (2005). Profiles in family nursing leadership: Honoring the authors of family nursing textbooks [Editorial]. *Journal of Family Nursing, 11*(3), 191-194.

Bell, J.M., & Kobayashi, N. (2005). Profiles in family nursing leadership: Dr. Chieko Sugishita [Editorial]. *Journal of Family Nursing, 11*(2), 87-89.

Wright, L.M., & Leahey, M. (2005). The three most common errors in family nursing: How to avoid or side-step. *Journal of Family Nursing, 11*(2), 90-101.

Bell, J.M. (2005). 10th Anniversary of the Journal of Family Nursing [Editorial]. *Journal of Family Nursing, 11*(1), 1-2.

Robinson, D.W., Carroll, J, S., & Watson, W. L. (2005). Shared experience building around the family crucible of cancer. *Families, Systems, &*

Health, 23(2), 131- 147.

2000-2004

Bell, J.M. (2004). Foreword. In P. Bomar (Ed.), *Promoting health in families: Applying family research and theories in nursing practice* (3rd ed.). Philadelphia: Saunders.

Wright, L.M., & Leahey, M. (2004). How to conclude or terminate with families. *Journal of Family Nursing,* 10(3), 379-401.

Rallison, L. & Moules. N.J. (2004). The unspeakable nature of pediatric palliative care: Unveiling many cloaks. *Journal of Family Nursing, 10*(3), 287-301.

Bell, J.M., Moules, N.J., Simonson, K., & Fraser, J. (2004). Marriage and illness: Therapeutic conversations with couples who are suffering. *Vision 2004: What is the future of marriage?* (pp. 47-52). Minneapolis, MN: National Council on Family Relations.

Moules, N.J., Simonson, K., Prins, M., Angus, P., & Bell, J.M. (2004). Making room for grief: Walking backward and living forward. *Nursing Inquiry, 11*(2), 99-107.

Wright, L. M., & Bell, J. M. (2004). Retrospective — Nurses, families, and illness: A new combination [Editorial]. *Journal of Family Nursing, 10*(1), 3-11.

Bell, J.M. (2003). Clinical scholarship in family nursing [Editorial]. *Journal of Family Nursing*, 9(2), 127-129.

Houger Limacher, L., & Wright, L.M. (2003). Commendations: Listening to the silent side of a family intervention. *Journal of Family Nursing*, 9(2), 130-135.

Bohn, U., Wright, L.M., & Moules, N.J. (2003). A family systems nursing interview following a myocardial infarction: The power of commendations. *Journal of Family Nursing*, 9(2), 151-165.

Moules, N.J. (2003). Therapy on paper: Therapeutic letters and the tone of relationship. *Journal of Systemic Therapies*, 22(1), 33-49.

Moules, N.J., & Tapp, D.M. (2003). Family nursing labs: Shifts, changes, and innovations. *Journal of Family Nursing,* 9(1), 101-117.

Cobb, N., Larson, J., & Watson, W. L. (2003). Development of the attitudes about romance and mate selection scale. *Family Relations, 52,* 222 -231.

Moules, N.J. (2002). Hermeneutic inquiry: Paying heed to history and Hermes. *International Journal of Qualitative Methods, 1*(3), Article 1. Retrieved September 2002 from http://www.ualberta.ca/~ijqm/

Moules, N.J. (2002). Nursing on paper: Therapeutic letters in nursing practice. *Nursing Inquiry, 9*(2), 104-113.

Bell, J.M. (2002). 20th Anniversary of the Family Nursing Unit [Editorial]. *Journal of Family Nursing, 8*(3), 175-177.

McLeod, D., & Wright, L.M. (2001). Conversations of spirituality: Spirituality in family systems nursing—making the case with four clinical vignettes. *Journal of Family Nursing, 7*(4), 391-415.

Wright, L.M. (2001). Suffering and family nursing intervention research: A healing combination. *Japanese Journal of Family Nursing, 6*(2), 133-140. [in Japanese]

Watson, W. L. (2001). Ethical roots of marital therapy. *Journal of the Association of Mormon Counselors and Psychotherapists: 25th Anniversary Edition, 25*(1), 64 - 75.

Bell, J.M., Swan, N.K.W., Taillon, C., McGovern, G., & Dorn, J. (2001). Learning to nurse the family [Editorial]. *Journal of Family Nursing, 7*(2), 117-126.

Bell, J.M. (2000). Reflections on the 5th International Family Nursing Conference, Chicago [Editorial]. *Journal of Family Nursing, 6*(4), 317-319.

Bell, J.M. (2000). Editor's choice: Selected bibliography on research with families. *Journal of Family Nursing, 6*(4), 400-404.

Bell, J.M. (2000). Encouraging nurses and families to think interactionally: Revisiting the usefulness of the circular pattern diagram [Editorial]. *Journal of Family Nursing, 6*(3), 203-209.

Bell, J.M. (2000). Transforming your conference presentation into a publishable article [Editorial]. *Journal of Family Nursing, 6*(2), 99-102.

Moules, N.J. (2000). Postmodernism and the sacred: Reclaiming connection in our greater-than-human worlds. *Journal of Marital and Family Therapy, 2*(1), 241-253.

Moules, N.J. (2000). Funerals, families, and family nursing: Lessons of love and practice [Guest Editorial]. *Journal of Family Nursing, 6*(1), 3-7.

1990-1999

Bell, J.M. (1999). Calgary Family Nursing Model: Practical and research tasks in family nursing. *Japanese Journal of Research in Family Nursing, 5*(1), 26-33. [in Japanese]

Bell, J.M. (1999). Therapeutic failure: Exploring uncharted territory in family nursing [Editorial]. *Journal of Family Nursing, 5*(4), 371-373.

Wright, L.M., & Leahey, M. (1999). Maximizing time, minimizing suffering: The 15-minute (or less) family interview. *Journal of Family Nursing, 5*(3), 259-273.

Bell, J.M. (1999). Family nursing in Japan: A firsthand glimpse. *Journal of Family Nursing 5*(2), 236-238.

Moules, N.J. (1999). Suffering together: Whose words were they? [Guest Editorial]. *Journal of Family Nursing, 5*(3), 251-258.

Bell, J.M. (1998). The professional meeting: Revenue generation versus meaningful dialogue [Editorial]. *Journal of Family Nursing, 4*(4), 347-379.

Bell, J.M. (1998). Editor's choice: Selected bibliography on family nursing theory. *Journal of Family Nursing, 4*(3), 334-336.

Bell, J.M. (1998). Rx for certainty in clinical work with families: Insatiable curiosity [Editorial]. *Journal of Family Nursing, 4*(2), 123-126.

Bell, J.M. (1998). Postcard from Valdivia [Editorial]. *Journal of Family Nursing, 4*(1), 3-7.

Levac, A.M., McLean, S., Wright, L.M., Bell, J.M., "Ann", & "Fred". (1998). A "Reader's Theatre" intervention to managing grief: Post-therapy reflections by a family and a clinical team. *Journal of Marital and Family Therapy, 24*(1), 81-94.

Moules, N.J. (1998). Legitimizing grief: Challenging beliefs that constrain. *Journal of Family Nursing, 4*(2), 138-162.

Bell, J.M. (1997). Illness stories and family nursing [Editorial]. *Journal of Family Nursing, 3*(4), 315-317.

Tapp, D.M., Moules, N., Bell, J.M., & Wright, L.M. (1997). Family skills labs: Facilitating the development of family nursing skills in the undergraduate curriculum. *Journal of Family Nursing, 3*(3), 247-266.

Bell, J.M. (1997). Levels in undergraduate family nursing education [Editorial]. *Journal of Family Nursing, 3*(3), 227-229.

Bell, J.M. (1997). Year 3: A state of the union address [Editorial]. *Journal of Family Nursing, 3*(2), 115-119.

Moules, N.J., & Amundson, J.K. (1997). Grief—An invitation to inertia: A narrative approach to working with grief. *Journal of Family Nursing, 3*(4), 378-393.

Moules, N.J., & Streitberger, S. (1997). Stories of suffering, stories of strength: Narrative influences in family nursing. *Journal of Family Nursing, 3*(4), 365-377.

Wright, L.M. (1997). Beliefs, illness, and healing: A dynamic threesome. *AFTA Newsletter,* Summer (68), 15-18.

Wright, L.M. (1997). Suffering and spirituality: The soul of clinical work with families [Guest Editorial]. *Journal of Family Nursing, 3*(1), 3-14.

Wright, L.M., & Bell, J.M. (1997). Beliefs, families and illness: The evolution of a clinical practice approach. *AARN Newsletter, 53*(1), 11-12.

Bell, J.M. (1996). Signal events in family nursing [Editorial]. *Journal of Family Nursing, 2*(4), 347-349.

Bell, J.M. (1996). Advanced practice in family nursing: One view [Editorial]. *Journal of Family Nursing, 2*(3), 244-247.

Gale, J., Chenail, R.J., Watson, W.L., Wright, L.M., & Bell, J.M. (1996). Research and practice: A reflexive and recursive relationship. Three narratives and five voices. *Marriage and Family Review, 24*(3/4),

275-295. [Special issue: Methods and Methodologies of Qualitative Family Research.]

Tapp, D.M., & Wright, L.M. (1996). Live supervision and family systems nursing: Post-modern influences and dilemmas. *Journal of Psychiatric and Mental Health Nursing, 3*(4), 225-233.

Watson, W.L. (1995) [Review of the books *A whack on the side of the head: How to unlock your mind for innovation; A kick in the seat of the pants: Using your explorer, artist, judge and warrior to be more creative*]. *Journal of Family Nursing, 1*(4), 431-434.

Robinson, C.A., & Wright, L.M. (1995). Family nursing interventions: What families say makes a difference. *Journal of Family Nursing, 1*(3), 327-345.

Wright, L.M., Bell, J.M., Watson, W.L., & Tapp, D. (1995). The influence of the beliefs of nurses: A clinical example of a post-myocardial-infarction couple. *Journal of Family Nursing, 1*(3), 238-256.

Bell, J.M. (1995). Avoiding isomorphism: A call for a different view [Editorial]. *Journal of Family Nursing, 1*(1), 5-7.

Bell, J.M. (1995). What is "family"? Perturbations and possibilities [Editorial]. *Journal of Family Nursing, 1*(2), 131-133.

Bell, J.M. (1995). The dysfunction of "dysfunctional" [Editorial]. *Journal of Family Nursing, 1*(3), 235-237.

Bell, J.M. (1995). Wanted: Family nursing interventions [Editorial]. *Journal of Family Nursing, 1*(4), 355-358.

Duhamel, F., Watson, W.L., & Wright, L.M. (1994). A family systems approach to hypertension. *Canadian Journal of Cardiovascular Nursing, 5*(4), 14-24.

Wright, L.M., & Leahey, M. (1994). Calgary Family Intervention Model: One-way to think about change. *Journal of Marital and Family Therapy, 20*(4), 381-395.

Wright, L.M. (1994). Live supervision: Developing therapeutic competence in family systems nursing. *Journal of Nursing Education, 33*(7), 325-327.

Wright, L.M., & Bell, J.M. (1994). The future of family nursing research: Interventions, interventions, interventions. *The Japanese Journal of Nursing Research, 27*(2-3), 4-15. [in Japanese]

Robinson, C.A., Wright, L.M., & Watson, W.L. (1994). A nontraditional approach to family violence. *Archives of Psychiatric Nursing, 8*(1), 30-37.

Watson, W.L., & Lee, D. (1993). Is there life after suicide?: The systemic belief approach for "survivors" of suicide. *Archives of Psychiatric Nursing, 7*(1), 37-43.

Bell, J.M., Wright, L.M., & Watson, W.L. (1992). The medical map is not the territory; or, "Medical Family Therapy?"—Watch your language! *Family Systems Medicine, 10*(1), 35-39.

Watson, W.L., Bell, J.M., & Wright, L.M. (1992). Osteophytes and marital fights: A single case clinical research report of chronic pain. *Family Systems Medicine, 10*(4), 423-435.

Wright, L.M., & Levac, A.M. (1992). The non-existence of non-compliant families: The influence of Humberto Maturana. *Journal of Advanced Nursing, 17*, 913-917.

Wright, L.M., & Simpson, P. (1991). A systemic belief approach to epileptic seizures: A case of being spellbound. *Contemporary Family Therapy: An International Journal, 13*(2), 165-180.

Wright, L.M., Luckhurst, P., & Amundson, J. (1990). Family therapy supervision as counter-induction. *Journal of Family Psychotherapy, 1*(3), 65-74.

Bell, J.M., & Wright, L.M. (1990). Flaws in family nursing education. *The Canadian Nurse, 86*(6), 28-30.

Loos, F., & Bell, J.M. (1990). Circular questions: A family interviewing strategy. *Dimensions in Critical Care Nursing, 9*(1), 46-53.

Watson, W.L., & Bell, J.M. (1990). Who are we? Low self-esteem and marital identity. *Journal of Psychosocial Nursing, 28*(4), 15-20.

Watson, W.L., & Nanchoff-Glatt, M. (1990). A family systems nursing approach to premenstrual syndrome. *Clinical Nurse Specialist, 4*, 3-9.

Wright, L.M. (1990). One way to deal with the perils of polytherapy: A contract for marital privacy. *Australian and New Zealand Family Therapy Journal, 11*(3), 179-181.

Wright, L.M. (1990). Research as a family therapy intervention technique. *Contemporary Family Therapy: An International Journal, 12*(6), 477-484.

Wright, L.M., & Leahey, M. (1990). Trends in the nursing of families. *Journal of Advanced Nursing, 15*, 148-154.

1980-1989

Wright, L.M. (1989). Decisions of competence and preference: An intervention for couples in conflict. *American Psychiatric Nurses Association Newsletter, 1*(3), 3.

Wright, L.M. (1989). When clients ask questions: Enriching the therapeutic conversation. *Family Therapy Networker, 13*(6), 15-16.

Wright, L.M., & Bell, J.M. (1989). A survey of family nursing education in Canadian Universities. *Canadian Journal of Nursing Research, 21*, 59-74.

Wright, L.M., & Park Dorsay, J. (1989). A case of Marilynitis or a Marilyn Monroe infection. Adelaide, Australia: *Dulwich Centre Newsletter*, 7-9.

Wright, L.M., Bell, J.M., & Rock, B.L. (1989). Smoking behavior and spouses: A case report. *Family Systems Medicine, 7*(2), 158-171.

Bell, J.M. (1988). Graduate student acquisition of family systems nursing skills. *Family Health News*, 1.

Wright, L.M. (1986). An analysis of live supervision "phone-ins" in family therapy. *Journal of Marital and Family Therapy, 12*, 187-190.

Wright, L.M., Miller, D., & Nelson, K. L. (1985). Treatment of a non-drinking family member in an alcoholic family system by a family nursing team. *Family Systems Medicine, 3*(3), 291-300.

Wright, L.M., Watson, W.L., & Duhamel, F. (1985). The Family Nursing Unit: Clinical preparation at the Masters' level. *The Canadian Nurse, 81*, 26-29.

Wright, L.M., Watson, W.L., & Duhamel, F. (1985). Une formation clinique en centre familial au niveau de la maitrise [The Family Nursing Unit: Clinical preparation at the master's level]. *L'Infirmiere Canadienne [The Canadian Nurse], 10*, 31-32. [in French]

Leahey, M., & Wright, L.M. (1985). Intervening with families with chronic illness. *Family Systems Medicine, 3*, 60-69.

Wright, L.M., & Leahey, M. (1985). Families with chronic illness: Three intervention approaches. *Continuing Care Coordinator, March*, 35-36.

Wright, L.M., & Imber Coppersmith, E. (1983). Supervision of supervision: How to be "meta" to a metaposition. *Journal of Strategic and Systemic Therapies, 2*, 40-50.

Wright, L.M., Hall, J., O'Connor, M., Perry, R., & Murphy, R. (1982). The power of loyalties: One family's developmental struggle during the launching years. *The Journal of Strategic and Systemic Therapies, 1*, 57-70.

Watson, W.L. (1981, January). A family systems perspective of aging. *Alberta Association on Family Relations Newsletter,* 7-9.

Wright, L.M., & Leahey, M. (1980, July). Discrepancies abound. *American Association for Marriage and Family Therapy Newsletter.*

Wright, L.M., & Leahey, M. (1980, August). Clinical training of marriage and family therapists in Alberta. *Alberta Association on Family Relations Newsletter.*

1975-1979

Tomm, K.M., & Wright, L.M. (1979). Training in family therapy: Perceptual, conceptual and executive skills. *Family Process, 18*(3), 227-250.

Wright, L.M. (1975). A symbolic tree: Loneliness is the root; Delusions are the leaves. *Journal of Psychiatric Nursing & Mental Health Services, 13*(3), 30-35.

DISSERTATIONS

PhD Graduates Specializing in Family Systems Nursing, University of Calgary

Thirsk, L.M. (2009). *Understanding the nature of nursing practices and interventions with grieving families.* Unpublished doctoral thesis, University of Calgary, Alberta, Canada. (Supervisor: Dr. Nancy J. Moules)

Houger Limacher, L. (2003). *Commendations: The healing potential of one family systems nursing intervention.* Unpublished doctoral thesis, University of Calgary, Alberta, Canada. (Supervisor: Dr. Lorraine M. Wright)

McLeod, D.L. (2003). *Opening space for the spiritual: Therapeutic conversations with families living with serious illness.* Unpublished doctoral thesis, University of Calgary, Alberta, Canada. (Supervisor: Dr. Lorraine M. Wright)

Moules, N.J. (2000). *Nursing on paper: The art and mystery of therapeutic letters in clinical work with families experiencing illness.* Unpublished doctoral thesis, University of Calgary, Alberta, Canada. (Supervisor: Dr. Janice M. Bell)

Tapp, D.M. (1997). *Exploring therapeutic conversations between nurses and families experiencing ischemic heart disease.* Unpublished doctoral dissertation, University of Calgary, Alberta, Canada. (Supervisor: Dr. Janice M. Bell)

Robinson, C.A. (1994). *Women, families, chronic illness and nursing interventions: From burden to balance.* Unpublished doctoral dissertation, University of Calgary, Alberta, Canada. (Supervisor: Dr. Lorraine M. Wright)

ADDITIONAL PUBLICATIONS RELATED TO FAMILY-FOCUSED PRACTICE AND RESEARCH

These publications have been written by former graduate students of the University of Calgary who completed one or more clinical practicums at the Family Nursing Unit. This list includes publications that we're aware of at this time, but may not be fully inclusive of all published contributions.

Boyd, M.A., & Houger Limacher, L. (2008). Family assessment and intervention. In W. Austin & M.A. Boyd (Eds.), *Psychiatric care for Canadian practice* (pp. 270-286). Philadelphia: Lippincott Williams & Wilkins.

Bottorff, J. L., Robinson, C. A., Sullivan, K. M., & Smith, M. L. (in press). Lung cancer patient approaches to continued family smoking. *Oncology Nursing Forum.* [These findings were selected to be featured in the *ONS Connect* In-Service Education series for oncology nurses - Becze, E. (in press) Patients with lung cancer encourage family members to stop smoking, *ONS Connect.*]

Campagna, L., & Duhamel, F. (2000). Les croyances : Élément–clef dans une approche systémique familiale de Calgary [Beliefs, a key element in the Calgary Family Assessment Model]. *Sciences pastorales, 19(*2), 119-134. [in French]

Ceri, P.M., Davidson, K.M., DeWitt, P.A., & Slauenwhite, C.A. (1995). Review of the book [The changing family life cycle: A framework for family therapists]. *Journal of Family Nursing, 1*(2), 219-232.

De Young, L, Webster, A.M., Tweedell, D., & Park Dorsay, J. (1994). Family systems nursing to the rescue. *Registered Nurse, June/July*, 31-32.

Dorsay, J.P., Premji, S., Lendrum, B.L., & Royle, J. (1995). Research. Family systems nursing education. *Canadian Nurse, 91*(9), 21.

Duhamel, F. (1994). A family systems approach: Three families with a hypertensive member. *Family Systems Medicine, 12*(4), 391-404.

Duhamel, F. (1995). The practice of family nursing care: Still a challenge! *Canadian Journal of Nursing Research, 27*(1), 7-11.

Beliefs and Illness: A Model for Healing

Duhamel, F. (Dir). (1995). *La santé et la famille: Une approche systémique en soins infirmiers* [Families and health: A systemic approach in nursing care]. Montreal, Quebec, Canada: Gaëtan Morin editeur. [in French]

Duhamel, F. (Dir.). (2007). *La santé et la famille: Une approche systémique en soins infirmiers* [Families and health: A systemic approach in nursing care] (2nd ed.). Montréal, Quebec, Canada; Gaétan Morin éditeur. Chenelière Éducation. [in French]

Duhamel F. (2007). L'analyse du système familial dans des contextes de santé et de maladie [Family analysis in the context of health and illness]. In F. Duhamel (Ed.), *La santé et la famille: Une approche systémique en soins infirmiers* [Families and health: A systemic approach in nursing care] (2nd ed., pp. 39-61). Montréal, Quebec, Canada: Gaëtan Morin éditeur. Chenelière Éducation. [in French]

Duhamel F. (2007). Les interventions systémiques familiales auprès de la famille [Family nursing intervention]. In F. Duhamel (Ed.), *La santé et la famille: Une approche systémique en soins infirmiers* [Families and health: A systemic approach in nursing care] (2nd ed., pp. 63-86). Montréal, Quebec, Canada: Gaëtan Morin éditeur. Chenelière Éducation. [in French]

Duhamel F. (2007). Questions et réponses sur la mise en application des soins infirmiers à la famille [Questions and answers regarding the implementation of family nursing]. In F. Duhamel (Ed.), *La santé et la famille: Une approche systémique en soins infirmiers* [Families and health: A systemic approach in nursing care] (2nd ed., pp. 229-241). Montréal, Quebec, Canada: Gaëtan Morin éditeur, Chenelière Éducation. [in French]

Duhamel, F., & Dupuis, F. (2003). Families in palliative care: Exploring family and health–care professionals' beliefs. *International Journal of Palliative Nursing, 9*(3), 113-119.

Duhamel, F., & Dupuis, F. (2004). Guaranteed returns: Investing in conversations with families of cancer patients. *Clinical Journal of Oncology Nursing, 8*(1), 68-71.

Duhamel, F., & Talbot, L. (2004). A constructivist evaluation of family interventions in cardiovascular nursing practice. *Journal of Family Nursing, 10*(1), 12-32.

Dupuis, F., & Duhamel, F. (2002). Le décès d'un enfant dans la famille:

Intégrer une dimension spirituelle aux interventions familiales [The death of a child in the family: Integrating a spiritual dimension in family interventions"]. *Sciences pastorales, 21*(2), 245-262. [in French]

Fast Braun, V., Hyndman, K., & Foster, C. (in press). Family nursing for undergraduate nursing students: The Brandon University Family Case Model approach. *Journal of Family Nursing.*

Forchuk, C., & Park Dorsay, J. (1995). Hildegard Peplau meets family systems nursing: Innovation in theory-based practice. *Journal of Advanced Nursing, 21*, 110-115.

Friedman, M.M., & Levac, A.M. (1997). The family nursing process. In M.M. Friedman (Ed.), *Family nursing: Research, theory and practice* (4th ed., pp. 49-72). Stamford, CT: Appleton & Lange.

Goudreau, J., & Duhamel, F. (2003). Interventions in perinatal family care: A participatory study. *Families, Systems, & Health, 21*(2), 165-180.

Goudreau J., & Duhamel, F. (2005). La famille : Lorsque des proches participent à la consultation médicale [When the family participates in the medical consultation]. In C. Richard, & M.T. Lussier (Eds.), *La communication professionnelle en santé* [Professionnal communication in health] (pp. 483-502). Montreal, Quebec, Canada: Éditions du renouveau pédagogique (ERPI). (Ce livre a reçu le « Prix Prescrire 2005 du livre médical et pharmaceutique) [in French]

Goudreau, J., Duhamel, F., & Ricard, N. (2006). The impact of a Family Systems Nursing educational program on the practice of psychiatric nurses. A pilot study. *Journal of Family Nursing, 12*(3), 292-306.

Harper-Jaques, S., McElheran, N., Slive, A., & Leahey, M. (2008). A comparison of two approaches to the delivery of walk-in single session mental health therapy. *Journal of Systemic Therapies, 27*(4), 40-53.

Harper-Jaques, S., & Masters, A. (1994). Written communication with survivors of sexual abuse: Use of letters in therapy. *Journal of Psychosocial Nursing, 32*(8), 11-16.

Houger Limacher, L. (2008). Locating relationships at the heart of commending practices. *Journal of Systemic Therapies, 27*(4), 90-105.

Keefler, J., Lach, L.M., & Duhamel, F. (2005). A review of current trends, debates and intervention models in family therapy circa 2005.

Beliefs and Illness: A Model for Healing

Intervention, *123*, 6-16.

Kent-Wilkinson, A. (1993). After the crime, before the trial. *The Canadian Nurse, December*, 23-26.

Kent-Wilkinson, A. (1999). Forensic family genogram: An assessment and intervention tool. *Journal of Psychosocial Nursing and Mental Health*, 37(9), 52-56.

Krusky, M. (2002). Women and thinness: The watch on the eve of the feast. Therapy with families experiencing troubled eating. *Journal of Systemic Therapies, 21*(1), 58-76.

Laliberte, S., Bohn, U., Bartlett, K.R., West, C., & Englehart, R. (2002). Remembering September 11th, 2001: Families and family nursing [Guest Editorial]. *Journal of Family Nursing, 8*(1), 3-10.

Lawson, A., McElheran, N., & Slive, A. (1997). Single session walk-in therapy: A model for the 21st century. *Family Therapy News, August, 15*, 25.

Leahey, M., & Harper-Jaques, S. (1996). Family-nurse relationships: Core assumptions and clinical implications. *Journal of Family Nursing, 2*(2), 133-151.

Leahey, M., Harper-Jaques, S., Stout, L., & Levac, A.M. (1995). The impact of a family systems nursing approach: Nurses' perceptions. *The Journal of Continuing Education in Nursing, 26*(5), 219-225.

Leahey, M., Stout, L., & Myrah, I. (1991). Family systems nursing: How do you practice it in an active community hospital? *The Canadian Nurse*, February, 31-33.

Limacher, L. H. (2007). Tribute to Dr. Maureen Leahey offered by Lori Houger Limacher, RN, PhD [Guest Editorial]. *Journal of Family Nursing, 13*(1), 9-12.

Manassis, K., & Levac, A.M. (2004). *Helping your teenager beat depression: A problem-solving approach for families.* Bethesda, MD: Woodbine House.

Marshall, A.J., & Harper-Jaques, S. (2008). Depression and family relationships: Ideas for healing. *Journal of Family Nursing, 14*(1), 56-73.

342

McElheran, N.G., & Harper-Jaques, S.R. (1994). Commendations: A resource intervention for clinical practice. *Clinical Nurse Specialist, 8*(1), 7-10, 15.

McLeod, A.A. (1997). Resisting invitations to depression: A narrative approach to family nursing. *Journal of Family Nursing, 3*(4), 394-406.

Nanchoff-Glatt, M. (1995) [Review of the book *Families, illness and disability: An integrative treatment model*]. *Journal of Family Nursing, 1*(1), 105-107.

Nordgren, J., & Johnson, M.A. (1995). Using experiences of older adults to teach nursing students. *Nurse Educator, 20*(5), 34-38.

Ran M., Xiang, M., Chan, C.L., Leff, J., Simpson, P., Huang, M., Shan, Y., & Li, S. (2003). Effectiveness of psychoeducational intervention for rural Chinese families experiencing schizophrenia: A randomized controlled study. *Social Psychiatry and Psychiatric Epidemiology, 38*(2), 69-75.

Ran, M., Xiang, M., Simpson, P., & Chan, C.L. (2005). *Family based mental health care in rural China*. Hong Kong: Hong Kong University Press.

Robinson, C.A. (1994). Nursing interventions with families: A demand or an invitation to change? *Journal of Advanced Nursing, 19*, 897-904.

Robinson, C.A. (1995). Beyond dichotomies in the nursing of persons and families. *Image, 27*(2), 116-120.

Robinson, C.A. (1995). Unifying distinctions for nursing research with persons and families. *Journal of Family Nursing, 1*(1), 8-29.

Robinson, C.A. (1996). Health care relationships revisited. *Journal of Family Nursing, 2*(2), 152-173.

Robinson, C.A. (1998). Women, families, chronic illness, and nursing interventions: From burden to balance. *Journal of Family Nursing, 4*(3), 271-290.

Robinson, C.A. (2000). Response to 'Establishing and maintaining trust during acute care hospitalizations'. *Scholarly Inquiry for Nursing Practice, 14*(3), 243 - 248.

Robinson, C.A., & Janes, K. (2001). Is my mom going to die? Answering children's questions when a family member has cancer. *Canadian Oncology Nursing Journal, 11*(2), 62 - 66.

Robinson, C.A. (2003). Healing conversations in the face of persistent or recurring cancer. *Canadian Oncology Nursing Journal, 13*(2), 95 - 99.

Robinson, C.A. (2008). Some thoughts on qualitative research with families. In A. Yamazaki (Ed.), *Family Nursing* . Tokyo: Nankodo. [in Japanese]

Robinson, C.A., Pesut, B., Bottorff, J.L., Mowry, A., Broughton, S., & Fyles, G. (2009). Rural palliative care: A comprehensive review. *Journal of Palliative Medicine, 12*(3), 253-258.

Robinson, C.A., Reid, R. C., & Cooke, H. A. (in press). A home away from home: The meaning of home according to families of residents with dementia. *Dementia: The International Journal of Social Research and Practice.*

Shaw, M.C., & Halliday, P.H. (1992). The family, crisis and chronic illness: An evolutionary model. *Journal of Advanced Nursing, 17*, 537-543.

Simpson, P. (2003). Family beliefs about diet and traditional Chinese medicine for Hong Kong women with breast cancer. *Oncology Nursing Society, 30*(5), 834-840.

Simpson, P. (2005). Hong Kong families and breast cancer: Beliefs and adaptation strategies. *Psycho-Oncology, 14*(8), 671-683.

Simpson, P., & Tarrant, M. (2006). Development of the Family Nursing Practice Scale. *Journal of Family Nursing, 12*(4), 413-425.

Simpson, P., Yeung, K. K., Kwan, T. Y., & Wah, W. K. (2006). Family systems nursing. A guide to mental health care in Hong Kong. *Journal of Family Nursing, 12*(3), 276-291.

Slauenwhite, C.A., & Simpson, P. (1998). Patient and family perspectives on early discharge and care of the older adult undergoing fractured hip rehabilitation. *Journal of Orthopaedic Nursing, 17*, 30-36.

Slive, A., McElheran, N., & Lawson, A. (2008). How brief does it get? Walk-in single session therapy. *Journal of Systemic Therapies, 27*(4), 5-22.

Southern, L., Leahey, M., Harper-Jaques, S., McGonigal, K., & Syverson,

(2007). Integrating mental health into urgent care in a community health centre. *Canadian Nurse,* January, 29-34.

Steele, R., Robinson, C.A., Hansen, L., & Widger, K. (in press). Families and palliative/end-of-life. In J. R. Kaakinen, V. Gedaly-Duff, D.Coehlo, & S.M.H. Hanson (Eds.), *Family health care nursing: Theory practice and research* (4th ed.). Philadelphia: F.A.Davis.

Tapp, D. (1993). Family protectiveness: A response to ischemic heart disease. *Canadian Journal of Cardiovascular Nursing, 4*(2), 4-8.

Tapp, D. (1995). Impact of ischemic heart disease: Family nursing research 1984-1993. *Journal of Family Nursing, 1*(1), 79-104.

Tapp, D.M. (2000). Family nursing in the fast lane: Therapeutic conversations that count. *Canadian Nurse, 96*(6), 29-32.

Tapp, D.M. (2000). The ethics of relational stance in family nursing: Resisting the view of "nurse as expert". *Journal of Family Nursing, 6*(1), 69-91.

Tapp, D.M. (2001). Conserving the vitality of suffering: Addressing family constraints to illness conversations. *Nursing Inquiry, 8*(4), 254-263.

Tapp, D.M. (2004). Dilemmas of family support during cardiac recovery: Nagging as a gesture of support. *Western Journal of Nursing Research, 26*(5), 561-580.

Vosburg, D., & Simpson, P. (1993). Linking family theory and practice: A family nursing program. *Image: Journal of Nursing Scholarship, 25*(3), 231-235.

Updated: April 2009

Resource Two
Publications by Colleagues Utilizing the Illness Beliefs
Model in Clinical Practice and Research

Brazil

Angelo, M. (2009). Cultura e cuidado da família. [Culture and family care].
In E. Nakamura, D. Martin, & J.F.Q.dos Santos (Eds.), *Antropologia
para a Enfermagem*. [*Anthropology for nursing*] (pp. 82-99). Barueri,
Brazil: Manole. [in Portuguese]

Bousso, R.S. (1999). *Trying to preserve the integrity of the family unit:
The family living with the experience of having a child in the pediatric
intensive care unit.* Unpublished doctoral thesis, School of Nursing,
University of São Paulo, Brazil. (Supervisor: Dr. Margareth Angelo)
[in Portuguese]

Bousso, R.S. (2006). *Time for crying: The family making sense of the
premature death of their child.* Unpublished thesis, School of Nursing,
University of São Paulo, Brazil. [in Portuguese]

Bousso, R.S. (2008). The family decision-making process concerning
consent for donating their child's organs: A substantive theory. *Texto
& Contexto Enfermagem, 17,* 45-54. [in Portuguese]

Bousso, R.S., & Angelo, M. (2001). Trying to preserve the integrity of the
family unit: The family living with the experience of having a child in
the pediatric intensive care unit. *Revista da Escola de Enfermagem da
USP, 35*(2), 172-179. [in Portuguese]

Bousso, R.S., & Angelo, M. (2003). The family in the intensive care unit:
Living the possibility of losing the child. *Journal of Family Nursing,
9*(1), 30-45.

Coa, T.F., & Pettengill, M.A.M. (2006). Children's autonomy during
therapeutic procedures: Pediatric nurses' beliefs and actions. *Acta
Paul. Enferm.* [online], *19*(4), 433-438. [in Portuguese]

Cunha, M.L.R. (2009). *Uncertainty and sacrifice: The suffering in family's
life invaded by child cancer.* Unpublished doctoral thesis, School of
Nursing, University of São Paulo, Brazil. (Supervisor: Dr. Margareth
Angelo) [in Portuguese]

Beliefs and Illness: A Model for Healing

Damiao, E.B.C., & Angelo, M. (2004). A experiência da família da criança com doença crônica *[The family's experience of childhood chronic illness]*. In: D.M.R. Gualda, & R.B. Bergamasco (Eds.), *Enfermagem, Cultura e o Processo Saúde-Doença*. *[Nursing, culture and illness and health process]* (pp. 119-134). São Paulo, Brazil: Ícone. [in Portuguese]

Garcia, D.M., & Pimenta, C.A.deM., & Cruz, D. deA.L.M.da. (2007). Validation of the survey of pain attitudes - professionals. *Rev. Esc. Enferm. USP* [online], *41*(4), 636-644. [in Portuguese]

Girardon-Perlini, N.M.O. (2009). *Taking care to keep a family's world supported: Agricultural families' experience of facing cancer*. Unpublished doctoral thesis, School of Nursing, University of São Paulo, Brazil. (Supervisor: Dr. Margareth Angelo) [in Portuguese]

Paula, E.S. de, Nascimento, L.C., Rocha, S.M.M. (2009). Religion and spirituality: The experience of families of children with chronic renal failure. *Rev. Bras. Enferm.* [online], 62(1), 100-106. [in Portuguese]

Pauli, M.C., & Bousso, R.S. (2003). Beliefs about humanized care in a pediatric intensive care unit. *Rev. Latino-Am. Enfermagem* [online], *11*(3), 280-286. [in Portuguese]

Pedroso, G.E.R. (2001). *The meaning of family care: Nurses' beliefs.* Unpublished master dissertation, School of Nursing, University of São Paulo, Brazil. (Supervisor: Dr. Regina S. Bousso) [in Portuguese]

Pedroso, G.E.R.P., & Bousso, R.S. (2003). The meaning of family care in the neonatal intensive unit: Nurses' beliefs. *Ciência, Cuidado e Saúde Maringá*, 2(2), 123-129. [in Portuguese]

Rossato-Abede, L.M., & Angelo, M. (2000). Determining beliefs in nursing care for children in pain: The family context. *Fam. Saúde Desenv*, 2(2), 7-18. [in Portuguese]

Rossato-Abede, L.M., & Angelo, M. (2002). Beliefs determining the nurse's intention concerning the presence of parents in neonatal intensive care units. *Rev. Latino-Am. Enfermagem* [online], *10*(1), 48-54. [in Portuguese]

Silveira, A.O. (2005). *Searching security to develop competences: The experience of the family's interaction.* Unpublished master dissertation, School of Nursing, University of São Paulo, Brazil. (Supervisor: Dr. Margareth Angelo) [in Portugese]

Resource Two: Colleagues' Publications

Silveira, A.O., & Angelo, M. (2006). Interaction experiences of families who live with their child's disease and hospitalization. *Rev. Latino-Am. Enfermagem* [online], *14*(6), 893-900. [in Portuguese]

Canada

Bélanger. L. (1999). *Interventions systémiques auprès de familles dont la conjointe est atteinte d'un cancer du sein* [Family systems nursing for families with a wife who has breast cancer]. Unpublished master's clinical project, University of Montreal, Quebec, Canada. (Supervisor: Dr. Fabie Duhamel) [in French]

Campagna, L., & Duhamel, F. (2000). *Les croyances: Élément clef dansune approche systémique familiale de Calgary* [Beliefs: A key element in the Calgary Family Assessment Model]. *Sciences pastorales, 19*(2), 119-134. [in French]

Carapetian, M. (2008). *Transfert des connaissances en nursing familial sur une unité de médecine* [Knowledge transfer and family systems nursing on a medicine unit]. Unpublished master's clinical project, University of Montreal, Quebec, Canada. (Supervisors: Dr. Fabie Duhamel, Lyne St. Louis, and Diane Breault) [in French]

Caron, I. (2007). *Développement d'un outil d'interventions familiales pour des familles dont un membre est atteint d'un AVC* [Development of a nursing tool]. Unpublished master's clinical project, University of Montreal, Quebec, Canada. (Supervisor: Dr. Fabie Duhamel) [in French]

Coulombe, M. (2006). *Mise en application du rôle de l'infirmière pivot en soins palliatifs* [Implementing the role of a family systems nursing specialist in palliative care]. Unpublished master's clinical project, University of Montreal, Quebec, Canada. (Supervisor: Dr. Fabie Duhamel) [in French]

Dallaire, J. (1999). *Interventions systémiques infirmières auprès de familles dont un membre est en attente d'un placement* [Family nursing interventions for families waiting for a placement for their elderly parent]. Unpublished master's clinical project, University of Montreal, Quebec, Canada. (Supervisor: Dr. Fabie Duhamel) [in French]

Duhamel, F. (Ed.). (2007). La santé et la famille. Une approche systémique

349

Beliefs and Illness: A Model for Healing

en soins infirmiers [*Families and health: A systemic approach in nursing care*] (2nd ed.). Montréal, Quebec, Canada: Gaétan Morin, Chenelière Éducation. [in French]

Duhamel, F., & Dupuis, F. (2003) Families in palliative care: Exploring family and health-care professionals' beliefs. *International Journal of Palliative Nursing, 9*(3), 113-119.

Duhamel, F., & Dupuis, F. (2004). Guaranteed returns: Investing in conversations with families of cancer patients. *Clinical Journal of Oncology Nursing, 8*(1), 68-71.

Dupuis, F. (2003). *Évaluation constructiviste d'interventions systémiques auprès de familles dont un membre en récidive de cancer* [Co-constructive evaluation of family systems nursing at a time of cancer relapse]. Unpublished master's thesis, University of Montreal, Quebec, Canada. (Supervisor: Dr. Fabie Duhamel) [in French]

Dupuis, F., & Duhamel, F. (2002). *Le décès d'un enfant dans la famille: intégrer une dimension spirituelle aux interventions familiales* [The death of a child in the family: Integrating a spiritual dimension in family interventions]. *Sciences pastorales, 21*(2), 245-262. [in French]

Friesen, P. (2002). A case study evaluating nursing interventions with a family, with an older adolescent in which one parent is hospitalized for treatment of lymphoma. Unpublished master's thesis, University of Montreal, Quebec, Canada. (Supervisor: Dr. Fabie Duhamel).

Goudreau J., & Duhamel, F. (2005). La famille : Lorsque des proches participent à la consultation médicale [When the family participates in the medical consultation]. In C. Richard & M.T. Lussier (Eds.), *La communication professionnelle en santé* [Professional communication in health] (pp. 483-502). Montreal, Quebec, Canada: Éditions du renouveau pédagogique (ERPI). (Ce livre a reçu le « Prix Prescrire 2005 du livre médical et pharmaceutique) [in French]

Keefler, J., Lach, L.M., & Duhamel, F. (2005). A review of current trends, debates and intervention models in family therapy circa 2005. *Intervention, 123*, 6-16.

Langlois, H. (2003). *Évaluation d'interventions systémiques auprès de couples lors de l'annonce de diagnostic d'un cancer du poumon* [Co-constructive evaluation of family systems nursing at the time of diagnosis of lung cancer]. Unpublished master's thesis, University of Montreal, Quebec, Canada. (Supervisor: Dr. Fabie Duhamel) [in

French]

Lepac, L. (2007). *Développement et évaluation d'interventions familiales dans un contexte de soins critiques* [Development and evaluation of family nursing interventions in a context of critical care]. Unpublished master's clinical project, University of Montreal, Quebec, Canada. (Supervisors: Dr. Fabie Duhamel and Lyne St. Louis) [in French]

Louissaint, S. (2004). *Évaluation d'interventions systémiques auprès de couples à la naissance d'un enfant premature* [Co-constructive evaluation of family systems nursing in a perinatal clinical context]. Unpublished master's thesis, University of Montreal, Quebec, Canada. (Supervisor: Dr. Fabie Duhamel) [in French]

Ménard, H. (2007). *Développement et évaluation d'interventions familiales dans un contexte de soins intensifs* [Development and evaluation of family systems nursing interventions in an intensive care unit]. Unpublished master's thesis, University of Montreal, Quebec, Canada. (Supervisor: Dr. Fabie Duhamel) [in French]

Noiseux, S. (1999). *Élaboration et évaluation constructiviste d'une intervention infirmière auprès de familles ayant un enfant en préparation à une greffe de moelle osseuse* [Co-constructive evaluation of family systems nursing on a bone marrow transplant unit]. Unpublished master's thesis, University of Montreal, Quebec, Canada. (Supervisor: Dr. Fabie Duhamel) [in French]

Robitaille, J. (2003). *Évaluation d'interventions systémiques auprès de couples dont un membre est atteint d'un problème cardiaque* [Co-constructive evaluation of family systems nursing in cardiology]. Unpublished master's thesis, University of Montreal, Quebec, Canada. (Supervisor: Dr. Fabie Duhamel) [in French]

Hong Kong

Ran, M., Xiang, M., Simpson, P., & Chan, C.L. (2005). *Family based mental health care in rural China.* Hong Kong: Hong Kong University Press.

Simpson, P.B. (2003). Family beliefs about diet and traditional Chinese medicine for Hong Kong women with breast cancer. *Oncology Nursing Society, 30*(5), 834-840.

Simpson, P. (2005). Hong Kong families and breast cancer: Beliefs and

Beliefs and Illness: A Model for Healing
adaptation strategies. *Psycho-Oncology, 14*(8), 671-683.

Japan

Araki, A., Ito, R., & Sato, N., & Ishigaki, K. (2009). *Special needs children in transition to home and independent living: Parents' beliefs.* Paper presented at the 9th International Family Nursing Conference, Reykjavik, Iceland.

Araki, A., Ito, R., Sato, N., & Ishigaki, K. (2009). *The beliefs of parents of children with special needs in transition to home and maintaining daily living.* Paper presented at the 9th International Family Nursing Conference, Reykjavik, Iceland.

Hohashi, N., Yamashita, T., Kobayashi, K., & Ishigaki, K. (2009). *Beliefs held by families of sick children at hospital discharge: A review of literature.* Paper presented at the 9th International Family Nursing Conference, Reykjavik, Iceland.

Ishigaki, K., & Tsujimura, M. (2009). *Beliefs held by families with older adults who need care upon hospital discharge in Japan (Second Report): From interviews with discharge planning staff.* Paper presented at the 9th International Family Nursing Conference, Reykjavik, Iceland.

Kamachi, C., & Kinoshita, M. (2000). Family members' beliefs about illness: Using Calgary Family Nursing Model. *St. Mary's Medical Journal, 25,* 121-122. [in Japanese]

Katakura, N., & Ishigaki, K. (2009). *Beliefs in the family that are considered to be unacceptable related to relatives with chronic psychiatric illnesses living in the community: A review of literature in Japan.* Paper presented at the 9th International Family Nursing Conference, Reykjavik, Iceland.

Kobayashi, N. (2006). *Group learning in family nursing: Introduction to Calgary Family Assessment Model/Calgary Family Intervention Model.* Tokyo, Japan: Ishiyaku Publishers. [in Japanese]

Kobayashi, N. (2009). *Family assessment workbook Part I: How to use genograms & ecomaps with the Calgary Family Nursing Models.* Tokyo, Japan: Ishiyaku Publishers. [in Japanese]. [Chapter 2: Calgary Family Nursing Models; Chapter 7: Prologue of advanced family nursing practice.].

Kobayashi, N., Bell, J. M., Wright, L.M., & Moules, N.J. (2005). *Understanding beliefs about aging, illness, and suffering among Japanese-Canadian elderly families.* Poster presented at the 7th International Family Nursing Conference. Victoria, British Columbia, Canada.

Kobayashi, N., Fukita, K., Takatsuka, S., & Nakamura, Y. (2009). *Using the intervention of "speaking the unspeakable": A case study using the Illness Beliefs Model.* Paper presented at the 9th International Family Nursing Conference, Reykjavik, Iceland.

Toima, M., Fujimoto, T., Yamaguchi, R., Shono, I., & Eguchi, C. (2006). Illness Beliefs: of patients' family who did not agree with discharge – Effectiveness of the therapeutic conversation. *Family Nursing, 4*(2), 116-126. [in Japanese]

Toima, M.,Yamaguchi, R., & Fujimoto, T. (2003). The effect of an intervention: Changing family members' constraining beliefs about illness into facilitative beliefs. *Japanese Journal of Research in Family Nursing, 9*(2), 126. [in Japanese]

Tsujimura,, M., Ishigaki, K., & Watanabe, M. (2009). *Beliefs held by families with older adults who need care upon hospital discharge in Japan (First Report): Review of the literature.* Paper presented at the 9th International Family Nursing Conference, Reykjavik, Iceland.

Watanabe, Y., & Endo, M. (2005). A father's suffering over his son's disability and the process and effect of their change: Approach to constraining beliefs. *Family Nursing, 3*(1), 139-146. [in Japanese]

Sweden

Benzein, E., Hagberg, M., & Saveman, B-I. (2008). Being appropriately unusual—A challenge for nurses in health promoting conversations with families. *Nursing Inquiry, 15*, 106-115.

Benzein, E., Johansson, P., Franzén, K., & Saveman B-I. (2008). Nurses attitudes towards families' importance in nursing care: A random sample survey. *Journal of Family Nursing, 14*, 162-180.

Benzein, E., Johansson, B., & Saveman, B-I. (2004). Families in home care: A resource or a burden? District nurses´ beliefs. *Journal of Clinical Nursing, 13*, 867-875.

Benzein, E., & Saveman, B-I. (2008). It´s like a purging bath. Health promoting conversations about hope and suffering with couples in palliative care: *International Journal of Palliative Nursing, 14*, 439-445.

Clausson, E., & Berg, A. (2008). Family intervention sessions: One useful way to improve schoolchildren's mental health. *Journal of Family Nursing,14*(3), 289-313.

James, I., Andershed, B., & Ternestedt, B.-M. (2007). A family's beliefs about cancer, dying, and death in the end of life. *Journal of Family Nursing, 13*(2), 226-252.

Saveman, B-I., Måhlén, C., & Benzein, E. (2005). Nursing students´ beliefs about families in nursing care. *Nurse Education Today, 25*, 480-486.

Söderström, I-M., Saveman, B-I., & Benzein, E. (2006). Interactions between family members and staff in intensive care units—An observational and interview study. *International Journal of Nursing Studies, 43*, 707-716.

Thailand

Areerungruang, W.(2008). *Effects of a family nursing intervention based on The Illness Belief Model on the health behaviors in coronary heart disease patients and their families.* Unpublished master's thesis, Burapha University, Chonburi, Thailand. (Supervisors: Dr. Chintana Wacharasin and Dr. Wannee Deoisres) [in Thai]

Chamnarnaksorn, W. (2008). *Effects of nursing intervention program based on The Illness Belief Model on the health behavior, suffering, and family support of osteoarthritis elderly patients and families.* Unpublished master's thesis, Burapha University, Chonburi, Thailand. (Supervisors: Dr. Chintana Wacharasin and Dr. N. Chaimongkol) [in Thai]

Channipar, P. (2008). *Effects of changing belief program on belief and intention of having cancer screening among women.* Unpublished master's thesis, Burapha University, Chonburi, Thailand. (Supervisors: Dr. Chintana Wacharasin and Dr. Wannee Deoisres) [in Thai

Kirdphon, N., (2005). *The effects of family relationship program on self-esteem and spiritual well-being of stroke patients.* Unpublished master's thesis, Burapha University, Chonburi, Thailand. (Supervisors: Dr. Chintana Wacharasin, Dr. Wannee Deoisres and Dr. N. Chaimongkol) [in Thai]

Kongkrajang, N. (2008). *The effect of family nursing intervention based on The Illness Belief Model on health behaviors of the diabetes mellitus patients and their families.* Unpublished master's thesis, Burapha University, Chonburi, Thailand. (Supervisors: Dr. Chintana Wacharasin and Dr. Wannee Deoisres) [in Thai]

Nanna, P., Wacharasin, C., & Deoisres, W. (2008). Effects of the Illness Belief Model program on suffering of hemodialysis patients and their families. *Journal of Faculty of Nursing, Burapha University, 16*(2), 24-38. [in Thai]

Tongdenok, A. (2008). *The effect of The Illness Belief Model nursing intervention program on the anxiety of pregnant women and their families.* Unpublished master's thesis, Burapha University. Chonburi, Thailand. (Supervisors: Dr. Wannee Deoisres and Dr. P. Suppasri) [in Thai]

Wacharasin, C., Homchampa, P., & Suwan, T. (2006). *Family care giving to the persons living with HIV/AIDS: Evaluation of problems, potential, needs, and family care-giving model in Rayong province.* Unpublished research report, Burapha University, Chonburi, Thailand. [in Thai]

Wacharasin, C., & Thienpichet, S. (2008). Family education, research, and practice: What is happening in Thailand? *Journal of Family Nursing, 14*(4), 429-435.

Wacharasin, C., & Wright, L.M. (submitted for publication). *Families suffering with HIV/AIDS: What family nursing interventions promote and pave the way for healing?*

United States of America

Astorga, P. (1998). *Children's beliefs about divorce and family relationships: A family case study using a story writing intervention.* Unpublished master's thesis, Brigham Young University, Provo, Utah. (Supervisor: Dr. Wendy Watson Nelson)

Binder, J.A. (2004). A case study of a married couple living with multiple sclerosis. *Rehabilitation Nursing, 29*(6): 183-186. (Advisor: Dr. Susan Heady)

Black, A.G. (1997). *Couples' relationship belief similarity and marital satisfaction.* Unpublished master's thesis, Brigham Young University, Provo, Utah. (Supervisor: Dr. Wendy Watson Nelson)

Cobb, N. (1997). *Development of a scale to measure constraining beliefs about mate selection.* Unpublished master's thesis, Brigham Young University, Provo, Utah. (Supervisor: Dr. Wendy Watson Nelson)

Cobb, N.P.G. (2001). *A grounded theory of change for married couples in chronic conflict from the couples' perspective.* Unpublished doctoral dissertation, Brigham Young University, Provo, Utah. (Supervisor: Dr. Wendy Watson Nelson)

Feetham, S. (1997) [Review of the book Beliefs: The heart of healing in families and illness]. *Journal of Family Nursing, 3*(2), 213-214.

Fife, S. (2003). *Uncovering the process of change in marital therapy: Therapists' perspectives.* Unpublished doctoral dissertation, Brigham Young University, Provo, Utah. (Supervisor: Dr. Wendy Watson Nelson)

Grant, J. (2007). *Death and families: Disruption and adaptation.* Unpublished master's synthesis project, Webster University, Kansas City, Missouri. (Advisor: Dr. Margo Thompson)

Harden, T. (2006). *Utilizing the Calgary Family Model with the Hispanic family in tuberculosis therapy.* Unpublished master's synthesis project, Webster University, Kansas City, Missouri. (Advisor: Dr. Mary Ann Drake)

Harrold, B.J. (2001). *Virtual affairs: A qualitative study of the meaning of computer - mediated extramarital relationships.* Unpublished doctoral dissertation, Brigham Young University, Provo, Utah. (Supervisor: Dr. Wendy Watson Nelson)

Hughes, P. (2006). *Case study: A family experiencing illness.* Unpublished master's synthesis project, Webster University, Kansas City, Missouri. (Advisor: Dr. Margo Thompson)

Kelly, A, (2003). *The effect of the autistic child on marital satisfaction.* Unpublished master's thesis, Brigham Young University, Provo, Utah. (Supervisor: Dr. Wendy Watson Nelson)

Manning, J. C. (2006). *A qualitative study of the supports women find most beneficial when dealing with a spouse's sexually addictive or compulsive sexual behavior.* Unpublished doctoral dissertation, Brigham Young University, Provo, Utah. (Supervisor: Dr. Wendy Watson Nelson)

Mazzola, J. (2006). *Gay and lesbian adoption: Creating social awareness.* Unpublished master's synthesis project, Webster University, Saint Louis, Missouri. (Advisor: Dr. Mary Ann Drake)

Mitchell, G. (2007). *Case study: End of life and family adaptation.* Unpublished master's synthesis project, Webster University, Kansas City, Missouri. (Advisor: Dr. Margo Thompson)

Phillips, C. (2007). *Case study: A family experiencing Alzheimer's disease.* Unpublished master's synthesis project, Webster University, Kansas City, Missouri. (Advisor: Dr. Margo Thompson)

Reitz, R. (2001). *"Curing" diabetes: Family therapy participant explanations of longitudinal biopsychosocial diabetes functioning.* Unpublished doctoral dissertation, Brigham Young University, Provo, Utah. (Supervisor: Dr. Wendy Watson Nelson)

Riley-Doucet, C. (2005). Beliefs about the controllability of pain: Congruence between older adults with cancer and their family caregivers. *Journal of Family Nursing, 11*(3), 225-241.

Robinson, W.D. (1999). *Co-creating family therapy interventions through the use of participatory action research for families experiencing the crucible of cancer.* Unpublished doctoral dissertation, Brigham Young University, Provo, Utah. (Supervisor: Dr. Wendy Watson Nelson)

Ross, K. (2008). *The appropriateness of using the Calgary Family Assessment and Intervention Models in Parish Nursing.* Unpublished master's synthesis project, Webster University, Saint Louis, Missouri. (Advisor: Dr. Mary Ann Drake)

Stephens, K. (2007). *End of life decisions: Using a family assessment model to facilitate the process.* Unpublished master's synthesis project, Webster University, Saint Louis, Missouri. (Advisor: Dr. Mary Ann Drake)

Tingle, A.M. (1996). *Attention Deficit Hyperactivity Disorder (ADHD) and family members' beliefs.* Unpublished master's thesis, Brigham Young University, Provo, Utah. (Supervisor: Dr. Wendy Watson Nelson)

Tingle, A.M. (1999). *Evaluation of a systemic belief treatment for Attention Deficit Hyperactivity Disorder (ADHD) families.* Unpublished doctoral dissertation, Brigham Young University, Provo, Utah. (Supervisor: Dr. Wendy Watson Nelson)

Resource Three

Instruments that Examine Illness Beliefs in Research and Clinical Practice

Bates, A.S., Fitzgerald, J.F., Wolinsky, F.D. (1994). Reliability and validity of an instrument to measure maternal health beliefs. *Medical Care, 32,* 832–846.

Broadbent, E., Petrie, K.J. Main, J., & Weinman, J. (2006). The Brief Illness Perception Questionnaire. *Journal of Psychosomatic Research, 60,* 631-637.

Furze, G., Bull, P., Lewin, R.J.P., & Thompson, D.R. (2003). Development of the York Angina Beliefs Questionnaire. *Journal of Health Psychology, 8*(3), 307-315.

Ginzburg, K., Arnow, B., Hart, S., Gardner, W., Koopman, C., Classen, C.C., Giese-Davis, J., & Spiegel, D. (2006). The Abuse-Related Beliefs Questionnaire for survivors of childhood sexual abuse. *Child Abuse and Neglect, 30(*8), 929-943.

Horne, R., Weinman, J., & Hankins, M. (1999). The Beliefs about Medicines Questionnaire: The development and evaluation of a new method for assessing the cognitive representation of medication. *Psychology and Health, 14*(1), 1-24.

Kazak, A.E., McClure, K.S., Alderfer, M.A., Hwang, W-T., Crump, T.A., Le, L.T., Deatrick, J., Simms, S., & Rourke, M.T. (2004). Cancer-related parental beliefs: The Family Illness Beliefs Inventory (FIBI). *Journal of Pediatric Psychology, 29*(7), 531-542.

Waddell, G., Newton, M., Henderson, I., Somerville, D., & Main, C.J. (1993). A Fear-Avoidance Beliefs Questionnaire (FABQ) and the role of fear-avoidance beliefs in chronic low back pain and disability. *Pain, 52*(2), 157-168.

Weinman, J., Petrie. K.J., & Moss-Morris, R., & Horne, R. (1996). The Illness Perception Questionnaire: A new method for assessing the cognitive representation of illness. *Psychology and Health, 11,* 431-435. (Website: http://www.uib.no/ipq/index.html)

CHAPTER NOTES

CHAPTER ONE—NOTES
From Illness Suffering to a Clinical Practice Model for Healing

Research project—*Exploring the Process of Therapeutic Change in Family Systems Nursing Practice* (Wright, Watson, & Bell, 1996) Funding from Alberta Foundation for Nursing Research.

Practice Units (established for education, research and/or service) where a Family Systems approach is used to guide practice with families experiencing illness
- Family Nursing Unit, University of Calgary, Canada (1982–2007)
- Family Therapy Program, Alberta Health Services, Calgary, Canada (1985–2010)
- Calgary Family Therapy Centre, Canada (1973–present) Website: www.familytherapy.org
- Denise Latourelle Family Nursing Unit, University of Montreal, Canada (1993–present)
- Chicago Center for Family Health, an affiliate of the University of Chicago, USA (1991- present) Website: www.ccfhchicago. org
- Institute for the Family, Family Therapy Services, Department of Psychiatry, University of Rochester, USA (1970–present) Website: http://www.urmc.rochester.edu/smd/psych/clin_ serv/amb_serv/fam_thrpy_serv.cfm
- Family Nursing Center, University of Wisconsin-Eau Claire, USA (1990–1998)
- Family Focused Nursing Unit, Kalmar University, Sweden (2004–present)
- Family Stress and Illness Program, Behavioral Health Center, The Children's Hospital of Philadelphia (2000–present)

This list is not exhaustive but provides a sampling of practice units that we are aware of throughout North America and Europe.

Journals that address a Family Systems perspective for practice and research
- *Journal of Family Nursing*
- *Families, Systems, & Health*
- *Family Process*
- *Journal of Marital and Family Therapy*
- *Journal of Family Psychology*
- *Family Relations*
- *Contemporary Family Therapy*
- *Psychotherapy Networke*r

Publications—Family Nursing Unit
- The legacy of family-focused clinical scholarship that began at the Family Nursing Unit continues to develop. Many of the publications of the faculty and graduate associated with the Family Nursing Unit (1982–2007) are available for public access at the Family Nursing Unit Collection, DSpace at the University of Calgary Library: https://dspace.ucalgary.ca/handle/1880/44060
- See also Part III, Resource One, in this book for a current list of these publications and productions.

Research project—Examining the Pedagogical Practices of Teaching Advanced Nursing Practice *[in Family Systems Nursing].* (Bell, Wright, Moules, & Paton, 2007; Moules, Bell, Paton, Wright, & Thirsk, 2007) Funding from Social Sciences and Humanities Research Council of Canada.

Dianne Tapp, **RN, PhD,** special case doctoral dissertation—*Exploring Therapeutic Conversations between Nurses and Families Experiencing*

Ischemic Heart Disease—Supervisor: Dr. Janice M. Bell (Tapp, 1997, 2000a, 2000b, 2001, 2004) Funding from Heart & Stroke Foundation. (Email: dtapp@ucalgary.ca)

CHAPTER TWO—NOTES
Understanding Beliefs

Dr. John Gottman—The Gottman Institute
For more information on John Gottman's work: www.gottman.com
Address: The Gottman Institute, P.O. Box 15644, Seattle, WA, USA 98115

Gottman's "Repair Checklist" is a valuable clinical tool when working with couples experiencing illness.

Gottman's 5:1 ratio: Gottman discovered that in "master" marriages the ratio of positive to negative emotion is at least five to one. Couples who were in satisfying marriages offered five positive conversations of affirmation and affection to their partner to every one negative conversation of accusation and recrimination, negative characterization, etc.

CHAPTER THREE—NOTES
Beliefs about Families

Carole Robinson RN, PhD, special case doctoral dissertation—*Women, Families, Chronic Illness and Nursing Interventions*—Supervisor: Dr. Lorraine M. Wright (Robinson, 1994, 1998; Robinson & Wright, 1995) Funding from National Health Research Development Program (Canada) and Canadian Nurses Foundation. (Email: carole.robinson@ubc.ca)

Family Genograph
The Family Genograph is an innovative assessment tool designed to health care providers care for families in all settings. Developed by **Dr. Fabie**

Duhamel and **Lyne Campagna** at the Faculty of Nursing, University of Montreal, the Family Genograph is a specialized stencil to facilitate the drawing of a genogram and ecomap. The pocket-sized stencil is combined with a memory aid to help nurses accurately diagram the structure of the family (genogram) and document the connections between the family members and other significant relationships and systems (ecomap). Five important questions are included as part of the Family Genograph to help the health care provider ask useful interventive questions as they effectively care for families.

English, French, and Spanish versions of the Family Genograph are available. Order from:

Faculté des Sciences Infirmières, c/o Madame Johanne Goulet, C.P. 6128, Succursale Centre-Ville, Montréal, Quebec, Canada H3C 3J7

Fax: (514) 343-2306

E-mail: johanne.goulet@umontreal.ca

Genogram Software

Information about the use of genograms and software to support the inclusion of genograms in clinical documentation and as a teaching resource is available from Genogram Analytics: www.genogramanalytics.com

Using the full standard symbol set in McGoldrick et al. 3rd edition, this software is easy to use, extremely flexible and works on both PCs and MACs.

Contact: Tom West, President, Genogram Analytics, Phone: (231) 861-0404 email: info@genogramanalytics.com

Seeing Strengths

Gilbert, D. (2006). *Stumbling on happiness*. New York: Vintage. This Harvard psychologist offers many fascinating research findings about perception. He argues that the eyes see what the brain wants them to see which perhaps explains why a clinician who is operating within the domain of objectivity-in-parentheses can see strengths and resiliency rather than only pathology.

CHAPTER FOUR—NOTES
Beliefs about Illness

Selected Films about Families and Illness Suffering

Movies can highlight family stories about the experience of illness, portray illness suffering, and show how family members and health care providers respond to illness in helpful and not so helpful ways. One of the assignments Dr. Lorraine Wright developed and we have used in a graduate interdisciplinary course called "Families and Illness" was to ask students to view a movie from a selected list and write about their reflections about it. Here are the trigger questions the student was asked to reflect on:

- How has the movie impacted/influenced you personally and professionally?
- What stood out for you as you watched this movie?
- Identify one belief of yours that was challenged by watching this movie.
- Identify one belief of yours that was strengthened or affirmed by watching this movie.
- What will you do differently in your clinical practice with families experiencing illness as a result of viewing this movie and your reflections about it?

Here's a list of our *Top Ten Favorite Movies* about illness suffering and families. The list includes movies that focus on mental illness and physical illness—both life-shortening and chronic illness. The short plot descriptions have been taken from www.imdb.com

The Diving Bell and the Butterfly (2007)—The true story of Elle editor Jean-Dominique Bauby who suffers a stroke and has to live with an almost totally paralyzed body; only his left eye isn't paralyzed.

Away From Her (2006)—A man coping with the institutionalization of his wife because of Alzheimer's disease faces an epiphany when she transfers her affections to another man…

A Beautiful Mind (2001)—After a brilliant but asocial mathematician accepts secret work in cryptography, his life takes a turn to the nightmarish; a story of schizophrenia.

The Savages (2007)—A sister and brother face the realities of familial responsibility as they begin to care for their ailing father.

Invasion of the Barbarians (English sub-titles) [Les invasions barbares] (2003, French)—During his final days, a dying man is reunited with old friends, former lovers, his ex-wife, and his estranged son.

Stepmom (1998)—Anna and Ben, the two children of Jackie and Luke, have to cope with the fact that their parents divorced and that there is a new woman...dealing with death and grief.

Iris (2001)—True story of the lifelong romance between novelist Iris Murdoch and her husband John Bayley, from their student days through her battle with Alzheimer's disease.

Philadelphia (1993)—When a man with AIDS is fired by a conservative law firm because of his condition, he hires a homophobic small-time lawyer as the only willing advocate for a wrongful dismissal suit.

Ordinary People (1980)—Beth, Calvin, and their son Conrad are living in the aftermath of the death of the other son. Conrad is overcome by grief...

My Left Foot (1989, Irish)—The story of Christy Brown, who was born with cerebral palsy. He learned to paint and write with his only controllable limb—his left foot.

Selected Books about Individual/Family Experiences of Illness
A. Biographies and Autobiographies

Albom, M. (1997). *Tuesdays with Morrie: An old man, a young man, and life's greatest lesson.* New York: Doubleday.

Broyard, D. (1992). *Intoxicated by my illness.* New York: Fawcett Columbine.

Cohen, R.M. (2004). *Blind-sided. Lifting a life above illness: A reluctant memoir.* New York: HarperCollins.

Cohen, R.M. (2008). *Strong at the broken places. Voices of illness, a chorus of hope.* New York: HarperLuxe.

Cousins, N. (1979). *Anatomy of an illness as perceived by the patient.* New York: Bantam Books.

Estess, J. (2004). *Tales from the bed. On living, dying, and having it all.* New York: Atria Books.

Fox, M.J. (2003). *Lucky man: A memoir.* New York: Hyperion.

Frank, A. (1991). *At the will of the body: Reflections on illness.* Boston: Houghton Mifflin.

Geist, M.E. (2008). *Measure of the heart: A father's Alzheimer's, a daughter's return.* Boston: Grand Central Publishing.

Sontag, S. (1977). *Illness as metaphor.* New York: Doubleday.

Taylor, J.B. (2006). *My stroke of insight. A brain scientist's personal journey.* New York: Viking.

Wilber, K. (1993). *Grace and grit: Spirituality and healing in the life and death of Trey Killam Wilber.* London: Shambhala.

Woodruff, L, & Woodruff, B. (2007). *In an instant. A family's journey of love and healing.* New York: Random House.

B. Fiction
Franzen, J. (2002). *The corrections.* Toronto, Ontario, Canada: Harper Collins.

Lamb, W. (1999). *I know this much is true*. Toronto, Ontario, Canada: Harper Collins.

Mistry, R. (2002). *Family matters*. Toronto, Ontario, Canada: McClelland & Stewart.

Picoult, J. (2005). *My sister's keeper*. New York: Washington Square Press.

Research project—*Conversations of Illness Suffering between Nurses and Families* (Wright, 2005; Wright, Bell, & Moules, 2004). Funding from Social Sciences and Humanities Research Council of Canada.

CHAPTER FIVE—NOTES
Beliefs about Therapeutic Change

Institute for the Study of Therapeutic Change (www.talkingcure.com) An international group of researchers and clinicians dedicated to studying what works in psychotherapy. Many helpful resources related to therapeutic alliance are available from the Institute as well as a two measurement tools for clinical practice designed to assess therapeutic alliance: Outcome Rating Scale (ORS) and Session Rating Scale (SRS). The Institute also maintains a computerized database where clients can input their scores from the therapeutic alliance scales and a response with feedback is offered to both the clinician and the client.

CHAPTER SIX—NOTES
Beliefs about Clinicians

Jill Bolte Taylor, a neuroscientist who experienced a stroke offers a vivid account of her illness experience in her book, *My stroke of insight. A brain scientist's personal journey* (2006, New York: Viking). She describes how, as a patient, she could quickly distinguish between those health care providers who offered her compassion and those health care providers who did not offer compassion.

CHAPTER SEVEN—NOTES
Creating a Context for Changing Beliefs

Research—*Exploring the Process of Therapeutic Failure* (Bell, 1999; Wright & Leahey, 2005) Internal Funding.

10,000 Hours of Practice

Research has found that superior performance in any activity requires 10,000 hours of deliberate practice reaching for objectives just beyond one's level of proficiency. This body of knowledge by K. Anders Ericsson is explored by Scott Miller, Mark Hubble, and Barry Duncan in Supershrinks (*Psychotherapy Networker*, 2007, 31(6), 26-35, 56) and by Malcolm Gladwell in *Outliers: The story of success* (2009, Little, Brown and Company).

CHAPTER EIGHT—NOTES
Distinguishing Illness Beliefs

Florence Nightingale Quote:

> No mockery in the world is so hollow as the advice showered upon the sick. It is of no use for the sick to say anything, for what the adviser wants is, not to know the truth about the state of the patient, but to turn whatever the sick may say to the support of his own argument, set forth, it must be repeated, without any inquiry whatever into the patient's real condition...How little the real sufferings of illness are known or understood (p. 57).

Nightingale, F. (1992). *Notes on Nursing*. Philadelphia: J.B. Lippincott. (Original work published 1859)

John Rolland – Family Systems Illness Model

Dr. John Rolland, Professor of Psychiatry, University of Chicago Pritzker School of Medicine, and Co-Director and Co-Founder of the Chicago Center for Family Health, is an influential leader in the field of family health and healing. Many of his ideas have been useful to our clinical practice and research, including:

Psychosocial typology and time phases of illness

- Rolland, J. S. (1994). *Families, illness, & disability: An integrative treatment model.* New York: Basic Books. (read: The psychosocial typology of illness and time phases of illness, pp. 19-42).

Relationship skews

- Rolland, J. S. (1994). In sickness and in health: The impact of illness on couples' relationships. *Journal of Marital & Family Therapy, 20*(4), 327-347.

Anticipatory loss

- Rolland, J.S. (2004). Helping families with anticipatory loss and terminal illness. In F. Walsh & M. McGoldrick (Eds.), *Living beyond loss* (2nd ed., pp. 213-237). New York: W.W. Norton.

Family Systems Illness Model

- Rolland, J. S. (2000). Chronic illness and the family life cycle. In B. Carter & M. McGoldrick (Eds.), *The expanded family life cycle: Individual, family, and social perspectives* (4th ed., pp. 492-511). Boston: Allyn and Bacon.

- Rolland, J. S. (2003). Mastering family challenges in serious illness and disability. In F. Walsh (Ed.), *Normal family processes* (3rd ed., pp. 460-489). New York: Guilford.

The Chicago Center for Family Health, based on a resilience approach, offers many learning opportunities for practicing professionals who wish to develop their knowledge and skills to assist families experiencing serious illness. The center also offers counseling services and community programs. A list of workshops and training opportunities is available on the website: www.ccfhchicago.org.

For a full description of the Center's specialized programs in Families, Illness, and Collaborative Health care see:
Rolland, J.S., & Walsh, F.W. (2005). Systemic training for health care professionals: The Chicago Center for Family Health approach. *Family Process, 44*(3), 283-301.

Deborah McLeod, RN, PhD, doctoral thesis—*Opening Space for the Spiritual: Therapeutic Conversations with Families Living with Serious Illness*—Supervisor: Dr. Lorraine M. Wright (McLeod, 2003; McLeod & Wright, 2001, 2008) Funding from Social Sciences and Humanities Research Council of Canada. (Email: deborahl.mcleod@cdha.nshealth.ca)

Walsh, F. (Ed.). (2009). *Spiritual resources in family therapy* (2ⁿᵈ ed.). New York: Guilford. (Previous edition: 1999). Exploring the role of spirituality in couple and family relationships, this text illustrates ways to tap spiritual resources for coping, healing, and resilience. Leading experts in family therapy and pastoral care discuss how faith beliefs and practices can foster personal and relational wellbeing, how religious conflicts or a spiritual void can contribute to distress, and what therapists can gain from reflecting on their own spiritual journeys.

CHAPTER NINE—NOTES
Challenging Constraining Beliefs

Lori Limacher, RN, PhD, doctoral thesis—*Commendations: The Healing Potential of One Family Systems Nursing* **Intervention**— Supervisor: Dr. Lorraine M. Wright (Limacher, 2003, 2008; Limacher & Wright, 2003, 2006) Funding from Killam Fellowship (Canada). (Email:

drlori@shaw.ca)

Nancy Moules, RN, PhD, special case doctoral thesis—*Nursing on Paper: The Art and Mystery of Therapeutic Letters in Clinical Work with Families Experiencing Illness*—Supervisor: Dr. Janice M. Bell (Bell, Moules, & Wright, 2009; Moules, 2000, 2002, 2003, 2009a, 2009b) Funding from Alberta Heritage Foundation for Medical Research. (Email: njmoules@ucalgary.ca)

Resource for Couples Experiencing Illness
• Collinge, W. (2008). *Partners in healing: Simple ways to offer support, comfort, and care to a loved one facing illness.* Boston: Trumpeter.

Lorraine M. Wright Family Nursing Scholarship
This endowed scholarship was created to honor Dr. Lorraine Wright's outstanding efforts to create and disseminate nursing knowledge about caring practices with families experiencing illness. Dr. Wright's clinical scholarship has changed the face of family nursing with important contributions to theory, practice, and research. Her work has been valued by an international community of nurses and by a variety of health professionals who encounter families in their clinical practice. The scholarship is awarded to students entering or enrolled in the Faculty of Nursing, University of Calgary in a program leading to either a Master of Nursing or a PhD with specialization in Family Systems Nursing. To make a donation, please contact: The University of Calgary Development Office, Phone: 403-220-5854; email: uofcgiving@ucalgary.ca

CHAPTER TEN—NOTES
Strengthening Facilitating Beliefs

Wright, L.M., & Leahey, M. (2009). *Nurses and families: A guide to family assessment and intervention* (5th ed.). Philadelphia: F.A. Davis. Chapter 10: "How to terminate with families" offers ideas how to conclude with families in a way that leaves families with hope and confidence in their new and rediscovered strengths, resources, and abilities to manage their health and relationships.

CHAPTER ELEVEN—NOTES
Grief and Families: Applying the Illness Beliefs Model to Bereavement

Research project—*Grief, Beliefs, and Clinical Practice* (Moules, Simonson, Prins, Angus, & Bell, 2004; Moules, Simonson, Fleiszer, Prins, & Glasgow, 2007). Funding from University Research Grants Committee.

Helpful publications/productions about grief:
- Iversen, S. (Producer). (2005). *Out of order: Dealing with the death of a child* [DVD]. Grief Support Program, Calgary Health Region. Available from: University of Calgary Press (http://www.ucalgary.ca/imagecentre/marketing/out_of_order.htm). First person accounts from parents who have experienced the death of a child.
- Neimeyer, R.A. (2005). Defining the new abnormal: Scientific and social construction of complicated grief. *Omega, 52*(1), 95-97.
- Rosenblatt, P.C. (2008). Recovery following bereavement : Metaphor, phenomenology, and culture. *Death Studies, 32,* 6-16.
- Walsh, F., & McGoldrick, M. (Eds.). (2004). *Living beyond loss: Death in the family.* New York: W.W. Norton.
- Walter, T. (2005). What is complicated grief? A social constuctionist perspective. *Omega, 52*(1), 71-79.

Lorraine Thirsk, RN, PhD, doctoral thesis - *Understanding the nature of nursing practices and interventions with grieving families* - Supervisor: Dr. Nancy J. Moules. Funding from Social Sciences and Humanities Research Council of Canada. (email: lmthirsk@ucalgary.ca)

ACKNOWLEDGEMENTS

We believe it takes a village to write a book! Some "villagers" have been more influential and prominent than others, but all were supportive and essential to the completion of this long overdue and awaited project.

We are especially grateful to:

- **Dr. Wendy L. Watson Nelson,** esteemed colleague and friend, who contributed immeasurably to our original ideas about this clinical approach and offered her creative ideas and masterful clinical examples in co-authoring our first book about beliefs and illness entitled *Beliefs: The heart of healing in families and illness* published in 1996 by Basic Books in New York. We thank you so very much, Wendy, and hope you will be pleased how our original ideas have evolved.

- **Dr. Nancy J. Moules,** Associate Professor, University of Calgary, admired colleague and friend, who worked with us for many years in the Family Nursing Unit, University of Calgary, as a graduate student and faculty colleague and enthusiastically embraced the *Illness Beliefs Model*. We so admire your brilliant contribution of clinical research that unpacked the intervention of "writing therapeutic letters" within the *Illness Beliefs Model* and your ongoing thoughtful contributions about families experiencing grief and loss. We are honored to have your beautiful chapter in our book on the application of the *Illness Beliefs Model* to grieving families.

- **Johanna M. Bates,** President and Founder of 4th Floor Press, Inc., Calgary, Canada, for her willingness to take on our book project, and along the way, despite our stalls and stops, never lost faith in us.

- **Anne Bougie,** Vice President of 4th Floor Press, Inc, and Literary Agent for Johanna M. Bates Literary Consultants, who single-handedly managed all aspects of our book project from contracts to content, from encouraging and extolling, to nudging and prodding. Our meetings with Anne always left us more informed and inspired. Her emails also made us more willing and wanting to press on with our project even when at times it had to be set aside. She would begin numerous emails with "Okay, Ladies, when can I expect another chapter?" Her review of each and every line of our book and her invaluable feedback and commendations has made our book much more readable, appealing, and human. Anne, we will be forever appreciative to you.

- **Wendy Lukasiewicz,** Editor, 4th Floor Press, Inc. who served as our very able and efficient copy editor who readied our manuscript for production.

We are also very grateful to our many dear academic friends, colleagues, and doctoral students for their encouragement to update our ideas about beliefs, illness, and suffering and describe our *Illness Beliefs Model* in more depth and with more precision. In particular, we appreciate the following colleagues who have followed and supported our work about beliefs and families and have either taught the ideas and/or utilized them in their research and clinical practice and/or have translated the original ideas into French, Swedish, and Japanese.

- **Brazil:** Dr. Margareth Angelo and Dr. Regina Szylit Bousso
- **Canada:** Dr. Fabie Duhamel, Dr. France Dupuis, Dr. Laurie Gottlieb, Dr. Maureen Leahey, Anne Marie Levac-Wolfert, Dr. Lori Houger Limacher, Dr. Deborah McLeod, Dr. Nancy J. Moules, Dr. Carole Robinson, Dr. Dianne Tapp, Lorraine Thirsk, and Christina West
- **Chile:** Dr. Humberto Maturana
- **Iceland:** Dr. Erla Svavarsdottir
- **Japan:** the late Dr. Cheiko Sugishita, Dr. Michiko Moriyama, Dr. Nami Kobayashi, and Hiroko Miyashita Ukisu
- **Portugal:** Dr. Maria do Ceu Barbieri, Ana Albuquerque Queiroz, and Luisa Santos

- **Sweden:** Dr. Birgitta Andershed, Dr. Eva Benzein, Dr. Eva Clausson , and Dr. Britt-Inger Saveman
- **Thailand:** Dr. Wannee Deoisres, Dr. Suntharawadee Theinpichet, and Dr. Chintana Wacharasin
- **United States:** Dr. Kathryn Anderson, Dr. Catherine Chesla, Dr. Mary Ann Drake, Dr. Suzanne Feetham, Dr. Catherine Gilliss, Dr. Susan Heady, Dr. Kathleen Knafl, and Dr. Wendy Watson Nelson

We also wish to acknowledge two previous Deans of the Faculty of Nursing, University of Calgary, who were particularly supportive to our clinical scholarship in the Family Nursing Unit: Dr. Janet Storch and the late Dr. Margaret Scott Wright.

To the many practicing nurses, graduate students, and faculty who have studied the *Illness Beliefs Model* through graduate courses or **Family Nursing Externships** with us, we are very appreciative and humbled by your openness to the ideas and how you helped to clarify our thinking and improve our clinical practice.

We are also very indebted to the numerous families with whom we have been privileged to work and who have graciously invited us into their illness experience so that we could learn, assist, grow, and expand our knowledge and clinical skills. They continue to challenge and refine our beliefs about the most useful ways to soften suffering and promote healing.

Finally, to each other, we are most grateful, appreciative, and fortunate. It is indeed a bonus and a blessing to make a friend out of a colleague. For over twenty years, we have been through many joys, sufferings, triumphs, and losses together and with each passing year, those memories and moments become more precious.

Lorraine M. Wright and Janice M. Bell
April 2009

Index

reflection, 226-227

Language, 53-54

Languaging, 34, 67, 77, 95, 107, 254

Larger systems, 5, 12, 24, 47, 171, 275

Listening, 33, 39, 74, 76, 99, 113

Love: x, 20, 36-37, 45, 74, 78-80, 89,
112-114, 133-134, 228, 249, 300-
301, 305-306, 311; definition of, 36

Macromoves of the Illness Beliefs
Model: challenging constraining
beliefs 10-11, 141, 312-313; creating
a context for changing beliefs,
141, 311; distinguishing illness
beliefs, 141, 311-312; strengthening
facilitating beliefs, 141, 314

Map for Healing, (Illness Beliefs
Model), ix

Maturana, Humberto R.: biology
of cognition, 27-30; constraining
beliefs, 55; definition of a reflection,
227; family structures, 46;
objectivity 27-29; objectivity-in-
parenthese, x, 27-29, 35-41

Medical family therapy, 6

Micromoves: challenging constraining
beliefs: asking interventive
questions, 226-227; offering
alternative beliefs, 226, 241-252;
offering commendations, 226,
263-267; offering externalizing
conversations, 226, 256-258;
speaking the unspeakable, 226,
235-241; using reflecting teams, 226,
267-269; using research findings,
226, 252-256; writing therapeutic
letters, 226, 258-263

Micromoves: creating a context
for changing beliefs: creating a
collaborative relationship, 144-
151; focusing the therapeutic
conversation, 144, 151-155;

removing obstacles to change, 144,
155-171

Micromoves: distinguishing illness
beliefs: beliefs about diagnosis, ix,
47, 66-67, 181, 190-193; beliefs
about etiology, 61, 69, 156, 181,
193-196; beliefs about healing and
treatment, 181, 187, 196-206; beliefs
about mastery, control, and influence,
181, 200-206, 257-258; beliefs about
prognosis, 181, 206-212; beliefs
about religion/spirituality, 181, 212-
216; beliefs about illness suffering,
181, 188-190; beliefs about the place
of illness, 181, 216-221

Micromoves: strengthening facilitating
beliefs: celebrating change, 280,
291-295; exploring change, 280,
283-285; exploring effects of change,
280, 287-290; inviting explanations
of change, 280, 290-291; inviting
observations of others about change,
280, 285-287, publishing change,
280, 295-299; seeing change,
280-283; targeting new facilitating
beliefs, 280, 290-291

Neutrality, 118

Noncompliance, 117

Objectivism, 30

Objectivity, 27-41, 54, 88, 117-119

Objectivity-in-parentheses, x, 27-29,
35-41, 48, 87-93, 108, 111, 129, 134

Objectivity-without-parentheses,
36,54, 88, 90, 117

Obstacles: removing, 144, 155-174

Offering alternative beliefs, 226, 241-
252

One question question, 11, 99-100,

AUTHOR CONTACT INFORMATION

Book website: www.illnessbeliefsmodel.com

Lorraine M. Wright, RN, PhD
Email: lmwright@ucalgary.ca
Website: www.lorrainewright.com

Janice M. Bell, RN, PhD
Email: jmbell@ucalgary.ca
Website: www.janicembell.com

Contact us for information about Externships*, lectures, workshops, keynote addresses, and/or consultations related to:

- Clinical practice models for family-focused health care (Illness Beliefs Model, Trinity Model, Calgary Family Assessment Model and/or Calgary Family Intervention Model)
- Illness suffering and family healing
- Spirituality and illness
- Family intervention research
- Curriculum innovation and program development for collaborative practice with families

*Externships: intensive learning opportunities are available over five days (Level I and Level II) to provide health care providers with knowledge and skills to care for families with compassion, competence and confidence. Please visit our websites for dates/location.